T0229104

Surgery of the Nose and Paranasal Sinuses: Principles and Concepts

Guest Editors

ORRETT E. OGLE, DDS

HARRY DYM, DDS

ORAL AND MAXILLOFACIAL SURGERY CLINICS OF NORTH AMERICA

www.oralmaxsurgery.theclinics.com

Consulting Editor
RICHARD H. HAUG, DDS

May 2012 • Volume 24 • Number 2

SAUNDERS an imprint of ELSEVIER, Inc.

W.B. SAUNDERS COMPANY
A Division of Elsevier Inc.

1600 John F. Kennedy Blvd. • Suite 1800 • Philadelphia, PA 19103-2899

www.oralmaxsurgery.theclinics.com

ORAL AND MAXILLOFACIAL SURGERY CLINICS OF NORTH AMERICA Volume 24, Number 2
May 2012 ISSN 1042-3699, ISBN-13: 978-1-4557-3903-5

Editor: John Vassallo; j.vassallo@elsevier.com
Developmental Editor: Teia Stone

Oral and Maxillofacial Surgery Clinics of North America (ISSN 1042-3699) is published quarterly by Elsevier Inc., 360 Park Avenue South, New York, NY 10010-1710. Months of issue are February, May, August, and November. Business and Editorial Offices: 1600 John F. Kennedy Blvd., Suite 1800, Philadelphia, PA 19103-2899. Periodicals postage paid at New York, NY and additional mailing offices. Subscription prices are $355.00 per year for US individuals, $522.00 per year for US institutions, $159.00 per year for US students and residents, $414.00 per year for Canadian individuals, $621.00 per year for Canadian institutions, $476.00 per year for international individuals, $621.00 per year for international institutions and $216.00 per year for Canadian and foreign students/residents. To receive student/resident rate, orders must be accompanied by name or affiliated institution, date of term, and the *signature* of program/residency coordinator on institution letterhead. Orders will be billed at individual rate until proof of status is received. Foreign air speed delivery is included in all *Clinics* subscription prices. All prices are subject to change without notice. **POSTMASTER:** Send address changes to *Oral and Maxillofacial Surgery Clinics of North America,* Elsevier Periodicals Customer Service, 11830 Westline Industrial Drive, St. Louis, MO 63146. Tel: 1-800-654-2452 (U.S. and Canada); 314-447-8871 (outside U.S. and Canada). Fax: 314-447-8029. E-mail: journalscustomerservice-usa@elsevier.com (for print support); journalsonlinesupport-usa@elsevier.com (for online support).

Reprints. For copies of 100 or more, of articles in this publication, please contact the Commercial Reprints Department, Elsevier Inc., 360 Park Avenue South, New York, NY 10010-1710. Tel.: 212-633-3812; Fax: 212-462-1935; Email: reprints@elsevier.com.

Oral and Maxillofacial Surgery Clinics of North America is covered in *MEDLINE/PubMed (Index Medicus)*, *Science Citation Index Expanded (SciSearch®)*, *Journal Citation Reports/Science Edition*, and *Current Contents®/Clinical Medicine.*

Printed and bound by CPI Group (UK) Ltd, Croydon, CR0 4YY

Transferred to Digital Print 2012

Contributors

CONSULTING EDITOR

RICHARD H. HAUG, DDS
Carolinas Center for Oral Health,
Charlotte, North Carolina

GUEST EDITORS

ORRETT E. OGLE, DDS
Director, Residency Training Program, Oral
and Maxillofacial Surgery, Woodhull Hospital,
Brooklyn; Associate Clinical Professor,
Department of Oral Surgery, School of Dental
Medicine, Columbia University, New York;
Chief, Program Director, Oral and Maxillofacial
Surgery, Department of Dentistry; Department
of Oral and Maxillofacial Surgery, Woodhull
Medical and Mental Health Center, Brooklyn,
New York

HARRY DYM, DDS
Chairman of Department of Dentistry/Oral and
Maxillofacial Surgery, The Brooklyn Hospital
Center, Brooklyn; Clinical Professor, Oral and
Maxillofacial Surgery, Columbia University,
College of Dental Medicine, New York;
Attending, Oral and Maxillofacial Surgery,
Woodhull Medical and Mental Health Center;
Attending, Oral and Maxillofacial Surgery,
New York Harbor Healthcare System, The
Brooklyn VA Campus, Brooklyn, New York

AUTHORS

ABIB AGBETOBA, MD
Resident, Department of Otolaryngology,
The Mount Sinai Medical Center, New York,
New York

SAMUEL BECKER, MD
Director of Rhinology, Becker Nose and Sinus
Center, LLC, Princeton, New Jersey

PHILLIP BROWN, MBBS
Senior Resident, Department of Surgery,
University Hospital of the West Indies,
Mona, Jamaica

EARL I. CLARKSON, DDS
Program Director, Department of Oral and
Maxillofacial Surgery, The Brooklyn Hospital
Center, Brooklyn, New York

LEWIS CLAYMAN, DMD, MD
Private Practice, Oral and Maxillofacial
Surgery, Pinole, California; Clinical Associate
Professor, Department of Otolaryngology–
Head and Neck Surgery, Wayne State
University, Detroit, Michigan

LADI DOONQUAH, MD, DDS
Consultant Maxillofacial Surgeon, Department
of Surgery, University Hospital of the West
Indies; Associate Lecturer, Faculty of
Medicine, University of the West Indies,
Mona, Jamaica

HARRY DYM, DDS
Chairman of Department of Dentistry/Oral and
Maxillofacial Surgery, The Brooklyn Hospital
Center, Brooklyn; Clinical Professor, Oral and
Maxillofacial Surgery, Columbia University,
College of Dental Medicine, New York;
Attending, Oral and Maxillofacial Surgery,
Woodhull Medical and Mental Health Center;
Attending, Oral and Maxillofacial Surgery,
New York Harbor Healthcare System, The
Brooklyn VA Campus, Brooklyn, New York

R. JOSHUA DYM, MD
Assistant Professor of Radiology, Division of
Emergency Radiology, Department of
Radiology, Montefiore Medical Center, Albert
Einstein College of Medicine, Bronx, New York

EZRA FRIEDMAN, DDS
Illustrator, Former Resident, General Practice, Woodhull Medical and Mental Health Center, Brooklyn, New York

SATISH GOVINDARAJ, MD
Assistant Professor, Department of Otolaryngology, The Mount Sinai Medical Center, New York, New York

LESLIE ROBIN HALPERN, MD, DDS, PhD, MPH
Surgical Fellow, Center for Cosmetic and Corrective Jaw Surgery, New York, New York

RICHARD H. HAUG, DDS
Carolinas Center for Oral Health, Charlotte, North Carolina

MARSHA JAMES, MBBS, DM(ORL)
Consultant Otolaryngologist, Kingston Public Hospital; Associate Lecturer, University of the West Indies, Kingston, Jamaica

JOSHUA E. LUBEK, DDS, MD, FACS
Assistant Professor and Fellowship Director, Maxillofacial Oncology/Microvascular Surgery, Department of Oral and Maxillofacial Surgery, University of Maryland, Baltimore, Maryland

DANIEL MASRI, MD
Clinical and Research Fellow, Division of Neuroradiology, Montefiore Medical Center, Albert Einstein College of Medicine, Bronx, New York

STANLEY MATTHEWS, DDS
Resident, Oral and Maxillofacial Surgery, Department of Dentistry, Woodhull Medical and Mental Health Center, Brooklyn, New York

JASON A. MOCHE, MD
Division of Otolaryngology, Department of Surgery, Harlem Hospital Center; Assistant Clinical Professor, Columbia University, New York, New York

WARREN MULLINGS, MBBS
Resident, Department of Surgery, University Hospital of the West Indies, Mona, Jamaica

MOHAMMED NADERSHAH, BDS
Fellow, Oral and Maxillofacial Oncology and Reconstruction, Department of Oral and Maxillofacial Surgery, Boston Medical Center, Boston University, Boston, Massachusetts

LEVON NIKOYAN, DDS
Resident, Oral and Maxillofacial Surgery, Department of Dentistry, Woodhull Medical and Mental Health Center, Brooklyn, New York

ORRETT E. OGLE, DDS
Director, Residency Training Program, Oral and Maxillofacial Surgery, Woodhull Hospital, Brooklyn; Associate Clinical Professor, Department of Oral Surgery, School of Dental Medicine, Columbia University, New York; Chief, Program Director, Oral and Maxillofacial Surgery, Department of Dentistry; Department of Oral and Maxillofacial Surgery, Woodhull Medical and Mental Health Center, Brooklyn, New York

ORVILLE PALMER, MD, MPH, FRCSC
Assistant Clinical Professor, Otolaryngology-Facial Plastics and Reconstruction, Harlem Hospital Center, Columbia University, New York, New York

JOSEPH E. PIERSE, DMD, MA
Second Year Oral and Maxillofacial Surgery Resident, Prosthodontist, Department of Dentistry/Oral and Maxillofacial Surgery, The Brooklyn Hospital Center, Brooklyn, New York

ANDREW SALAMA, MD, DDS, FACS
Assistant Professor, Oral and Maxillofacial Surgery, Department of Oral and Maxillofacial Surgery, Boston Medical Center, Boston University, Boston, Massachusetts

KEIVAN SHIFTEH, MD
Associate Professor of Radiology and Chief of Head and Neck Radiology, Division of Neuroradiology, Department of Radiology, Montefiore Medical Center, Albert Einstein College of Medicine, Bronx, New York

AVICHAI STERN, DDS
Attending, Department of Dentistry/Oral and Maxillofacial Surgery, The Brooklyn Hospital Center, Brooklyn, New York

JONATHAN M. TAGLIARENI, DDS
Department of Oral and Maxillofacial Surgery, The Brooklyn Hospital Center, Brooklyn, New York

ROBERT J. WEINSTOCK, DDS
Resident, Oral and Maxillofacial Surgery,
Woodhull Medical and Mental Health Center,
Brooklyn, New York

JOSHUA C. WOLF, DDS
Resident, Department of Oral and Maxillofacial
Surgery, The Brooklyn Hospital Center,
Brooklyn, New York

Contents

The oral cavity and its bony components (maxilla and mandible), along with the nose and its related sinuses, constitute most of the face. Because of their proximity, disease in one may affect the other, whereas trauma of the midface will involve bones common to the oral cavity, nose, and paranasal sinuses. The two serve important life-supporting functions, being the portals for nutrition and respiration. The paranasal sinuses are pneumatic cavities lined by mucous membrane and communicate directly with the nasal cavity. This article presents a brief but relevant view of the surgical anatomy of the nasal cavity and paranasal sinuses.

Optimal and accurate management of any patient depends on a detailed history and thorough physical examination. The information garnered dictates the definitive management of the patient. Adequate examination of the head and neck, particularly the upper aerodigestive tract, presents a unique challenge because much of the area to be examined is not easily accessible to direct visualization. However, advances in medical technology have prompted the evolution of the instrumentation and the techniques used to examine this anatomic region. This evolution allows for a more informative assessment of the patient and a more comfortable experience.

Evaluation of the paranasal sinuses is often performed in a purely clinical fashion, without the need for imaging. However, in certain instances imaging may be deemed valuable or even necessary in helping to solve a diagnostic dilemma, confirm a suspected diagnosis, evaluate the extent of a known condition, or assess for an underlying cause of the condition. Computed tomography (CT) and magnetic resonance imaging (MRI) can be useful in confirming a suspected diagnosis or providing additional information regarding causes or complications. CT and MRI play complementary roles in evaluating the rare tumors that may involve the paranasal sinuses.

The endogenous normal flora of the nose and paranasal sinuses works to create an environment of homeostasis within the region. This homeostasis can be interrupted by eliminating the anatomic barriers created by the skin, bone, and mucosa, such as after trauma and/or surgery; by altering the atmosphere of the surroundings, such as the creation of an anaerobic environment by obstruction of the sinus ostia or foramina; or by a change in the normal flora of the region. To fully understand the microbiological environment of this region, the normal flora of the nose and paranasal sinuses must be understood.

Oral and maxillofacial surgeons are occasionally called on to diagnose, treat, and rule out peritonsillar abscesses. In this article, the anatomy of the peritonsillar area, its contents, surgical approaches, and possible complications are discussed.

Inflammatory diseases of the upper and lower airways act not as individual entities but more as an integrated unit–the concept of the unified airway. This article focuses on the role of allergic rhinitis (AR) in the unified airway. An overview of AR and its association with upper and lower airway diseases is provided. AR is described in terms of its epidemiology, pathophysiology, and recent options for successful treatment. The recent use of immunotherapy and its future potential as a prophylactic method for the treatment of AR and concomitant diseases within the unified airway are emphasized.

Epistaxis is a common medical problem that rarely requires surgical intervention. However, when medical or surgical intervention is required, epistaxis can sometimes be difficult to control. Knowledge of nasopharyngeal anatomy is absolutely essential to the proper management of epistaxis. This article begins with a discussion of the essential anatomy of the region and the basic epidemiology of epistaxis, followed by a review of initial treatment as well as devices and procedures specifically designed for the control of epistaxis. Advances and new devices for the control of epistaxis are described.

The proper evaluation of the patient with nasal obstruction relies on a comprehensive history and physical examination. Once the site of obstruction is accurately identified, the patient may benefit from a trial of medical management. At times however, the definitive treatment of nasal obstruction relies on surgical management. Recognizing the nasal septum, nasal valve, and turbinates as possible sites of obstruction and addressing them accordingly can dramatically improve a patient's nasal breathing. Conservative resection of septal cartilage, submucous reduction of the inferior turbinate, and structural grafting of the nasal valve when appropriate will provide the optimal improvement in nasal airflow and allow for the most stable results.

The practicing oral and maxillofacial surgeon treating patients with oroantral communication (OAC)/oroantral fistulas should be familiar and competent with the various treatment options available. Multiple techniques are available from purely soft tissue flaps, which have proved to be successful over time, to a combination of hard tissue grafts (autologous, alloplastic, or allograft), which can prove to be useful with the increased demand for implant restorations. Although different procedures have proved to be successful, all are premised on the treatment of any underlying sinusitis, which is associated with a higher risk of recurrent OAC.

To thoroughly understand the biology of any lesion and render the appropriate management, clear and accurate definitions are paramount. For benign cysts and tumors of the oral maxillofacial region, an accurate depiction of these lesions needs to be elucidated to provide both the treating surgeon and the patient with a clear understanding of the course of treatment and the outcome.

The traditional treatment of frontal sinus fractures is undergoing a review by many clinicians. This review will undoubtedly contribute to the existing controversy surrounding the management of patients with this condition. This article seeks to further the review and suggest the authors' perspective on a more appropriate approach to the care of patients with frontal sinus injuries.

Mucosal preservation is of paramount importance in the diagnosis and surgical management of the sinonasal tract. The endoscope revolutionized the practice of endoscopic nasal surgery. As a result, external sinus surgery is performed less frequently today, and more emphasis is placed on functional endoscopy and preservation of normal anatomy. Endoscopic surgery of the nose and paranasal sinus has provided improved surgical outcomes and has shortened the length of stay in hospital. It has also become a valuable teaching tool.

Revision sinus surgery for inflammatory disease has been revolutionized by endoscopic sinus surgery. Clinical trials have shown statistically significant positive outcome data for patient symptoms and quality of life, as well as improvements in objective findings on postoperative nasal endoscopy and computed tomography imaging for patients undergoing revision sinus surgery. The keys to successful revision surgery are adjunctive medical management, aggressive postoperative debridement, mucosal preservation, and removal of osteitic bone. Both the physician and patient should also understand the underlying disease process and comorbid factors so that anticipated postoperative outcomes can be met with realistic expectations.

Oral and Maxillofacial Surgery Clinics of North America

THE CLINICS ARE NOW AVAILABLE ONLINE!
Access your subscription at:
www.theclinics.com

Preface

Surgery of the Nose and Paranasal Sinuses: Principles and Concepts

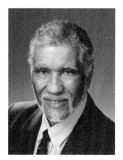 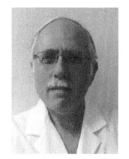

Orrett E. Ogle, DDS	Harry Dym, DDS

Guest Editors

The human head is without doubt the most complex anatomical portion of the human body. It is affected by a vast array of developmental conditions, malformations, and diseases. The number of medical practitioners (dentists, maxillofacial surgeons, craniofacial surgeons, neurosurgeons, otorhinolaryngologists, ophthalmologists, and plastic surgeons) that specialize in this area of the body attests to its complexity. Each specialized group has its unique compilation of facts in its own publications, with its own diagnostic criteria and surgical procedures. They practice independently, often with little knowledge of the other medical specialties, and information about other subspecialties can only be obtained by an extensive search of various sources.

The anatomic area treated by oral and maxillofacial surgeons is intimately related to the paranasal sinuses, and diseases that affect one area may extend to the other. In addition, the paranasal sinuses are involved in midface maxillofacial trauma as well as in orthognathic, craniofacial, and certain implant surgical procedures. Nasal anatomy and function are often altered by maxillary orthognathic surgery and function of the paranasal sinuses by trauma. For this reason, we believed that it would be a good idea for the oral and maxillofacial surgeon to become familiar with surgical procedures performed on the paranasal sinuses and indications for the procedures. This would allow us to educate our patients better on surgical options when such need arises. To cover the subject adequately, topics on surgical anatomy, radiology, physical exam, microbiology, pathology, and medical conditions such as rhinitis had to be included. We also took the editorial privilege of including closely related topics such as epistaxis

Oral Maxillofacial Surg Clin N Am 24 (2012) xiii–xiv
doi:10.1016/j.coms.2012.02.001
1042-3699/12/$ – see front matter © 2012 Elsevier Inc. All rights reserved.

oralmaxsurgery.theclinics.com

and frontal sinus fractures, in addition to not so closely related topics such as an update on cancer management, throat infection, and salivary gland surgery.

We have tried to combine experienced clinicians with younger writers to get a diversity of opinions. We believed that this would give exposure to younger clinicians as well as provide the reader with different thought processes and therapeutic approaches that may result in better patient care. We express our sincerest thanks and appreciation to all the writers who contributed to this issue, and we hope that their efforts will lead to a better understanding of this complex region.

Orrett E. Ogle, DDS
Oral and Maxillofacial Surgery
Department of Dentistry
Woodhull Medical and Mental Health Center
760 Broadway, Brooklyn, NY 11206, USA

Harry Dym, DDS
Department of Dentistry/Oral and
Maxillofacial Surgery
The Brooklyn Hospital
121 DeKalb Avenue, Box 187
Brooklyn, NY 11201, USA

E-mail addresses:
Orrett.Ogle@woodhullhc.nychhc.org (O.E. Ogle)
Hdymdds@yahoo.com (H. Dym)

Surgical Anatomy of the Nasal Cavity and Paranasal Sinuses

Orrett E. Ogle, DDS[a],*, Robert J. Weinstock, DDS[b],
Ezra Friedman, DDS[c]

KEYWORDS

- Paranasal sinuses • Nasal anatomy • Sinus anatomy
- Maxillary sinus • Ethmoid sinus • Frontal sinus
- Sphenoid sinus • Surgical anatomy

The oral cavity and its bony components (maxilla and mandible), along with the nose and its related sinuses, constitute most of the face. Because of their proximity, disease in one may affect the other, whereas trauma of the midface will involve bones common to the oral cavity, nose, and paranasal sinuses. The two serve important life-supporting functions, being the portals for nutrition and respiration. The nasal cavity receives air and conditions the air that is passed on to the other areas of the respiratory tract. The paranasal sinuses are pneumatic cavities lined by mucous membrane and communicate directly with the nasal cavity. The paranasal sinuses are the frontal sinus, ethmoid cells, maxillary sinus, and sphenoid sinus. This article presents a brief but relevant view of the surgical anatomy of the nasal cavity and paranasal sinuses that will be germane to the topics discussed in other articles elsewhere in this issue.

THE NASAL CAVITY

The nasal cavities are located in the middle of the face between the frontal sinus above, the oral cavity below, and the orbits and maxillary sinuses to the sides (**Figs. 1** and **2**). The nasal cavity is encased in a pyramidal-shaped osseo-cartilaginous framework and is divided into two compartments by the nasal septum. The osseous portion consists of two nasal bones that articulate with the nasal process of the frontal bone superiorly and fuses with the maxilla laterally. Their lower borders are beveled on their inner surfaces where they articulate with the upper lateral nasal cartilages. The upper lateral nasal cartilages project up below the nasal bones and are attached to them with dense connective tissue.

The cartilaginous portion of the framework consists of two components: the upper lateral and lower lateral nasal cartilages.

Upper Lateral Nasal Cartilages

The upper lateral nasal cartilage is roughly triangular-shaped. Its superior edge is thin and articulates with the nasal bones via dense connective tissue and fuses to the maxilla. The inferior border is also thin and inserts below the border of the lower lateral cartilage (this is not always a consistent relationship, however).[1] This inferior end is free and is the site of the intercartilaginous incision during rhinoplasty. The medial border is thick and continuous with the septal cartilage.

The authors have nothing to disclose.
[a] Oral and Maxillofacial Surgery, Department of Dentistry, Woodhull Medical and Mental Health Center, 760 Broadway, Brooklyn, NY 11206, USA
[b] Oral and Maxillofacial Surgery, Woodhull Medical and Mental Health Center, 760 Broadway, Room 2C-320, Brooklyn, NY 11206, USA
[c] General Practice, Woodhull Medical and Mental Health Center, 760 Broadway, Room 2C-320, Brooklyn, NY 11206, USA
* Corresponding author. Oral and Maxillofacial Surgery, Woodhull Medical and Mental Health Center, 760 Broadway, Room 2C-320, Brooklyn, NY 11206.
E-mail address: orrett.ogle@woodhullhc.nychhc.org

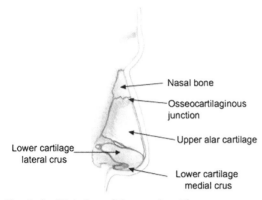

Fig. 1. Sagittal view of the nasal cartilages.

The upper lateral cartilage is fused to the dorsal septum in the midline, where the angle formed between them is normally 10° to 15°. The angle formed by the septum and upper lateral cartilage constitutes the internal valve. This angle between the septum and upper lateral cartilage is important during respiration, and obstruction of the angle by scar tissue or trauma will produce symptoms of nasal obstruction. The total composition of the internal nasal valve encompasses the area bounded by the angle of the upper lateral cartilage and septum, the nasal floor, and the superior portion of the inferior turbinate.

Lower Lateral Nasal Cartilages

Two lower lateral nasal cartilages, each having medial and lateral crus, form the shape of the nasal tip and maintain the patency of the nostrils. The upper border of the lateral crus is in contact with the upper lateral cartilage. Laterally, the extension is variable, but it is always connected to the maxilla with a thick fibrous membrane, with several lesser alar cartilages embedded in it. The lower border is free but does not reach the clinical border of the nose, which is formed by a double layer of skin. In the midline they are loosely connected to each other by the interdomal ligament. In this area, the structure is supported only by the septal cartilage,

subcutaneous tissue, and the thickness of the overlying skin. The external valve is a variable area dependent on the size, shape, and strength of the lower lateral cartilages.

The medial crus is the downward continuation of the lateral crus from the apex. It extends inferiorly to the region of the area of the anterior nasal spine of the maxilla, passing anterior to the free end of the nasal septum. It is more slender than the lateral crus, and these are loosely joined to each other and to the inferior border of the septal cartilage with connective tissue. The medial crus and lateral crus form the nostril, which is the opening into the nasal cavity itself.

The Nasal Cavity

The nasal cavity is divided by a vertical septum into two similarly paired cavities. Each half has a medial wall (the nasal septum) and a lateral wall that contains ridges called conchae or turbinates that participate in the drainage and ventilation of the paranasal sinuses. The roof of the nasal cavity consists of the crista galli, the cribriform plate, and the body of the sphenoid containing the sphenoid sinus. The cribriform plates contain nerves associated with the sense of smell passing through tiny openings in them. The bony floor is made up anteriorly of the palatine process of the maxilla and posteriorly by the horizontal process of the palatine bone.

Nasal septum

The nasal septum is a midline bony and cartilaginous structure that is composed of five parts **(Fig. 3)**:

- Perpendicular plate of ethmoid bone
- Vomer bone
- Crest of the maxillary bone
- Crest of the palatine bone
- Cartilage of the septum.

The vertical or perpendicular ethmoid plate forms the upper half of the bony nasal septum and is continuous superiorly with the cribriform

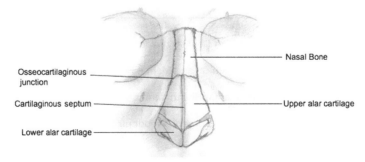

Fig. 2. Frontal view of nasal cartilages.

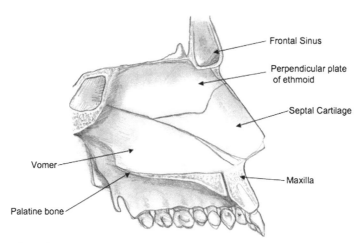

Frontal Sinus

Perpendicular plate of ethmoid

Septal Cartilage

Vomer

Maxilla

Palatine bone

Fig. 3. Sagittal view of nasal septum.

plate. It is generally deflected a little to one or the other side. It articulates with the frontal and nasal bones anterosuperiorly, the crest of the sphenoid bone posteriorly, the vomer posteroinferiorly, and with the septal cartilage anteroinferiorly. At its superior aspect, numerous grooves and canals lead from the medial foramina on the cribriform plate and carry filaments of the olfactory nerves.

The vomer is the posteroinferior portion of the septum. It articulates with the sphenoid, the ethmoid, the left and right palatine bones, and the left and right maxillary bones. It also articulates anteriorly with the septal cartilage of the nose. Separation of the cartilage from the vomer can occur in traumatic injuries.

The palatine process of maxillary and nasal crest of the palatine bone are midline bony projections that contribute small portions to the septum. Both the inferior borders of the vomer and the septal cartilage articulate with these structures. With nasal trauma, a common finding is dislocation of the septal cartilage off the maxillary crest.

The cartilage of the septum is somewhat quadrilateral in shape and provides dorsal support and helps to maintain the position of the columella and nasal tip. It is thicker at its margins than at its center. Its superoanterior margin is the thickest and is connected with the nasal bones, and is continuous with the medial margins of the upper lateral cartilages. Below, it is connected to the medial crura by fibrous tissue. Its posterior margin is connected with the perpendicular plate of the ethmoid, its posteroinferior margin with the vomer, and its base is along the palatine processes of the maxilla. The articulation of the septal cartilage inferiorly with the vomer and the maxilla may form horizontal "premaxillary wings," which make elevation of the mucoperichondrium difficult.[2] (These are sharp angulations seen in the nasal

septum occurring at the junction of the vomer below, with the septal cartilage and/or ethmoid bone above.)

The cartilage of the septum is firm but bendable and is covered by mucosa that has a substantial supply of blood vessels. This blood supply derives contribution from the anterior and posterior ethmoidal arteries, the sphenopalatine artery, the septal branch of the superior labial artery, and the greater and ascending palatine arteries. The vasculature of the septum runs between the perichondrium and the mucosa. Thus the subperichondrial space is the recommended avascular dissection plane when raising the mucoperichondrial flap during the first step in septoplasty. The anterior part of the septum, known as *Little's area*, is richly endowed with blood vessels and is the source of most nose bleeds. Little's area is an area of confluence of the labial, sphenopalatine, and ethmoidal arteries known as *Kiesselbach's plexus*.

The membranous septum (septum mobile nasi) is the narrow portion at the lower end of the nasal septum, lying between the semirigid columella and the more-rigid septal cartilage. It is the most flexible part of the septum and is formed by a union of the septum mucous membranes that envelop the septal cartilage. This united membrane then blends with the skin of the columella. This mucocutaneous junction is often the site of incisions for septal surgery.

Lateral wall
On examination of the nasal cavity, only a small section of the anatomy of the lateral nasal wall will be visible (**Fig. 4**). Its most prominent features are the turbinates, which project from the lateral wall. They are usually three or sometimes four in number. The superior turbinate is situated on the

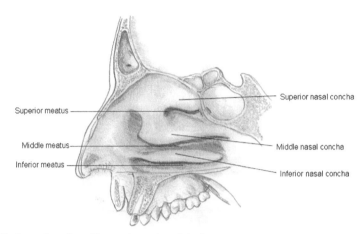

Fig. 4. Lateral wall of nasal cavity with nasal conchae intact.

upper part of the outer wall in the posterior one-third of the cavity, with its anterior and highest portion opposite the medial canthal tendon. The middle turbinate extends along the posterior two-thirds and the inferior turbinate bone extends along the entire length of the nasal floor (about 60 mm). The turbinates are vertical and slightly curved. The medial surface, which is directed toward the septum, is convex and the lateral surface is concave. The inferior turbinate is the largest and is an independent bone, whereas the middle and superior turbinates and a variable supreme turbinate are parts of the ethmoid bone. The middle and superior turbinates are incompletely separated from each other by fissures that start at the posterior border of the conchal plate of the ethmoid bone and extends anteriorly to end slightly behind the anterior end of these turbinates. At the superior attachment of the middle turbinate, a prominence known as the *agger nasi air cells* may be seen. These agger nasi cells are the most anterior ethmoidal air cells, and the mound is formed by mucous membrane that is covering the ethmoidal crest of the maxilla. They lay below the lacrimal sac from which they are separated by only a very thin layer of bone.

The passage in the nasal cavity formed by the projection of the turbinates are referred to as a *nasal meatus*, of which there are three. The inferior meatus is between the inferior turbinate, the floor of the nose, and the lateral nasal wall. It opens chiefly downward and backward so that more exhaled than inhaled air passes through it.[3] The nasal opening of the nasolacrimal duct opens in the anterior third of the inferior meatus. This opening is covered by a mucosal valve known as *Hasner's valve*. The course of the nasolacrimal duct from the lacrimal sac lie under the agger nasi cells.

The middle meatus lies between the inferior turbinate inferiorly, middle turbinate superiorly, and the lateral nasal wall. The middle meatus has a significant anatomic relationship with the paranasal sinuses and is the most complex of the meatuses. It is the major drainage area for the paranasal sinuses, which are divided into an anterior group and a posterior group. The anterior group of sinuses are frontal, maxillary, and anterior ethmoidal sinuses. These anterior sinuses drain into a curved fissure along the lateral wall of the middle meatus called the *hiatus semilunaris*, which acts as a pool for all the secretions from the anterior group of sinuses.

The features of the lateral wall of the meatus cannot be satisfactorily studied, however, unless the turbinates are removed (**Fig. 5**).

The hiatus semilunaris will be seen after removal of the middle and inferior turbinates. The hiatus semilunaris is bordered inferiorly by the thin sharp edge of the uncinate process of the ethmoid and superiorly by an elevation known as the *bulla ethmoidalis*. The ethmoid bulla is the largest and most constant air cell of the anterior ethmoid complex. The middle ethmoidal cells are contained within this bulla, and their opening is slightly superior and posterior to the bulla. Below the bulla ethmoidalis and hidden by the uncinate process of the ethmoid is the ostium for the maxillary sinus, which opens posteriorly and is the largest ostium within the semilunar hiatus. Following the curvature of the hiatus semilunaris anterosuperior leads to a communication with another curved passage called the *infundibulum*. The infundibulum then communicates in front with the anterior ethmoidal cells, and in approximately 77% of the population it is continued upward into the frontal sinus as the frontonasal duct. In 23% of individuals, the anterior end of the uncinate process fuses with the

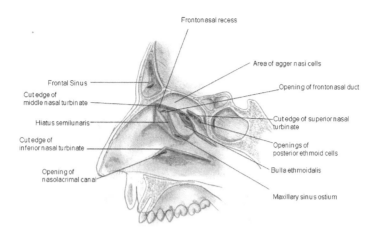

Fig. 5. Lateral wall of nasal cavity with nasal conchae removed.

front part of the bulla and the continuity is interrupted. In these people, the frontonasal duct drains directly into the anterior end of the meatus via a frontal sinus ostium.[4]

The uncinate process is a concaved wing-shaped projection of the ethmoid and forms the first lamella of the middle meatus. It attaches anteriorly to the posterior edge of the lacrimal bone and inferiorly to the superior edge of the inferior turbinate. The superior attachment is highly variable, because it may be attached to the lamina papyracea, the roof of the ethmoidal sinus, or to the middle turbinate. The configuration of the infundibulum and its relationship to the frontal recess depends largely on the superior attachment of the uncinate process.

The basal lamella of the middle turbinate separates the anterior and posterior ethmoid cells. The basal lamella as an important anatomic landmark to the posterior ethmoidal system, which has separate drainage systems from the anterior system. When disease is limited to the anterior compartment of the osteomeatal complex, the ethmoid cells can be opened and diseased tissue removed as far as the basal lamella. Leaving the basal lamella undisturbed will minimize the surgical risks.

Blood supply to the lateral nasal wall is from the sphenopalatine artery. The sphenopalatine artery is a branch of the maxillary artery that passes into the nasal cavity through the sphenopalatine foramen at the back part of the superior meatus. Here it gives off its posterior lateral nasal branches. It ends on the nasal septum as the posterior septal branches. In 72% of people, the feeding vessel to the superior turbinate is from the septal artery. The feeding vessel to the middle turbinate is from the proximal portion of the posterior lateral nasal artery just after exiting the

sphenopalatine foramen in 88% of people. In most people (98%), the inferior turbinate branch is the end artery of the posterior lateral nasal artery.[5]

The pattern of blood supply to the inferior turbinate is pretty consistent, with a single branch of the sphenopalatine artery entering its substance from above at the superior aspect of its lateral attachment at 1 to 1.5 cm from its posterior border. This large vessel crosses the middle meatus posteriorly and will be at risk of injury if surgery proceeds too far posteriorly. As the artery travels anteriorly within the turbinate, it remains close to the bone or travels most often within a bony canal. On its forward path it gives off several branches, forming an arterial arcade, which also remains close to or within the bone. Trimming of any part of the turbinate bone may be followed by brisk and prolonged bleeding. The artery travels mostly within a bony canal and will be splinted open by fibrous attachments to the bone, making it unable to contract. Because the artery at the posterior tip of the inferior turbinate is not in a bony canal, it provides a location to ligate the artery in the presence of persistent bleeding from the inferior turbinate. The diameter of the artery widens as it passes anteriorly, which may be from anastomosis with the facial artery via the pyriform aperture or with other intranasal vessels.[6]

ETHMOIDAL SINUS
Ethmoid Air Cell Development

The ethmoid sinus begins forming in the third to fourth month of fetal life as evaginations of the lateral nasal wall. At birth the anterior ethmoid cells are aerated, whereas the posterior ethmoid cells are fluid-filled. The posterior ethmoid air cells pneumatize with advancing age, and air replaces the fluid in these cells. The last air cells to finish forming are the anterior-most agger nasi and bulla cells. When pneumatization is complete, the average size of the anterior ethmoid cells are 20 to 24 mm × 20 to 24 mm × 10 to 12 mm and the average size of the posterior ethmoid cells are 20 to 21 mm × 20 to 22 mm × 10 to 12 mm.[7]

Ethmoid Bone

The ethmoid bone consists of five distinct components: cristae galli, cribriform plate, perpendicular plate, and paired ethmoidal labyrinths that contain the ethmoid air cells. The cristae galli marks the superior extent of the ethmoid bone as it rises into the anterior cranial fossa to provide attachment for the falx cerebri. The cristae galli ends inferiorly at the cribriform plate. The ethmoid bone continues inferior to the cribriform plate as the perpendicular plate of the ethmoid. The bilateral ethmoidal labyrinths come off the perpendicular plate at the level just inferior to the cribriform plate. The paired labyrinths continue inferiorly and terminate as the middle nasal concha. The perpendicular plate continues inferiorly, between the labyrinths, where it terminates at its articulations with the nasal septum anteriorly and the vomer posteriorly.

The cristae galli is a vertically oriented, triangular-shaped, superior-most extension of the ethmoid bone. The cristae galli provides attachment for the falx cerebri, which is the dural partition of the cerebral hemispheres at the level of the longitudinal fissure of the brain. The cristae galli ends inferiorly at the cribriform plate.

The cribriform plate is a thin horizontally oriented plate of bone that supports the olfactory bulb on its superior aspect. Vertical perforations throughout the cribriform plate allow for passage of olfactory

nerve terminals to reach the nose. The cribriform plate is 2 mm thick × 20 mm long × 5 mm wide.[8] Facial trauma may fracture this thin cribriform plate, resulting in a cerebrospinal fluid rhinorrhea. Anosmia can also result from traumatic damage to olfactory nerve terminals. The optic nerve also may potentially be damaged with overzealous exenteration of the posterior ethmoidal air cells. The ethmoid continues inferior to the cribriform plate as the perpendicular plate.

The perpendicular plate forms the superior portion of the nasal septum and gives off the ethmoid labyrinths bilaterally. The perpendicular plate articulates with the frontal bone anterosuperiorly, the nasal septal cartilage anteroinferiorly, and the vomer posteroinferiorly.

The ethmoid labyrinths project from the perpendicular plate at a point just inferior to the cribriform plate. Following their horizontal projection from the perpendicular plate, the labyrinths rise superiorly to a point one-eighth of an inch superolaterally to the cribriform plate.[9] The labyrinths are quadrangular-shaped structures situated between the orbit and olfactory portion of the nasal fossa. The labyrinths are formed by the laminae papyracea externally and the superior and middle turbinates internally; they are bordered anteriorly by the lacrimal and frontal bones and posteriorly by the body of the sphenoid.[10] The lamina papyracea forms part of the medial wall of the orbit and lateral nasal wall (**Fig. 6**).

Ethmoid Air Cells

Within the labyrinth lie the ethmoid air cells, which are lined by pseudostratified ciliated columnar epithelium. The ethmoid air cells are bordered medially by the nasal cavity, laterally by the lamina papyracea, and superiorly by the fovea ethmoidalis. The basal lamina of the middle turbinate divides

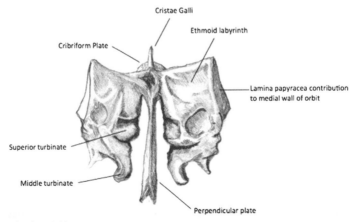

Cristae Galli

Ethmoid labyrinth

Cribriform Plate

Lamina papyracea contribution to medial wall of orbit

Superior turbinate

Middle turbinate

Perpendicular plate

Fig. 6. Frontal view of ethmoid bone.

the ethmoid cells into anterior and posterior divisions.[11] The anterior cells empty into the middle meatus and the posterior cells drain into the superior meatus.

Hajek[12] presented a simplified scheme to describe the location of the ethmoid air cells. Hajek's scheme depicted the air cells as existing in three sets of grooves, which form as valleys between four lamellar projections of bone. Anteriorly the unciform groove (hiatus semilunaris) is formed by the unciform process anteriorly and the ethmoid bulla posteriorly; the hiatus semilunaris is the site of orifices to the frontal sinus, maxillary sinus, and anterior ethmoidal cells. The second groove is the middle meatus, which lies between the ethmoid bulla anteriorly and the middle turbinate posteriorly; the ethmoid bulla located in this lamella is often involved in nasofrontal duct obstruction. The third groove is the superior meatus that is formed between the middle and superior turbinates (**Fig. 7**).[13]

The numbers of ethmoid cells vary by individual; however, seven smaller anterior cells and four larger posterior cells are typically present. The posterior air cells occasionally present as two very large air cells. The previous paragraph discussed the grooves in which the air cells are present. The uncinate groove is the most anterior and has three to four air cells at its superior border. At the middle meatus are one to two agger nasi cells, and posterior to the agger nasi is the ethmoid bulla that contains a superior and inferior cell.[9] The posterior ethmoid air cells drain via the superior meatus. The anterior ethmoid air cells drain via the middle meatus.

Blood Supply and Innervation

Blood supply to the ethmoid air cells is via the ethmoidal arteries that are branches from the ophthalmic artery. The anterior ethmoidal artery enters the anterior ethmoid foramen 24 mm posterior to the anterior lacrimal crest and supplies the anterior ethmoid air cells. The posterior ethmoidal artery enters the posterior ethmoid foramen 36 mm posterior to the anterior lacrimal crest[14] and supplies the posterior ethmoidal air cells. Venous drainage is via the named veins accompanying the arteries to the superior ophthalmic vein or pterygopalatine plexus. Lymphatic drainage from the anterior ethmoid cells is via the submandibular nodes, and the posterior ethmoid cells drain via the retropharyngeal nodes. Innervation is via anterior and posterior ethmoid nerves of the ophthalmic nerve (V_1) and the posterior nasal branch of the maxillary nerve (V_2) (**Fig. 8**).[7]

MAXILLARY SINUS
Development

The maxillary sinus begins developing in the third week of gestation. In the twelfth week of gestation, the maxillary sinus forms as an ectodermal invagination from the middle meatal groove and grows internally to a size that at birth is approximately 7 × 4 × 4 mm and has a volume of 6 to 8 mL. In utero the maxillary sinus is fluid-filled; however, after birth the maxillary sinus pneumatizes in concordance with biphasic rapid growth: during the first 3 years of life and then again from ages 7 to 12 years. By 12 years of age, the sinus is level with the floor of the nasal cavity[15]; however, as further pneumatization occurs into adulthood, with the eruption of the adult molars, the floor of the sinus descends to approximately 1 cm below the floor of the nasal cavity.[16]

Size and Location

The maxillary sinuses are paired paranasal sinuses that develop around the adult dentition to a volume of 15 mL, although the volume is smaller in

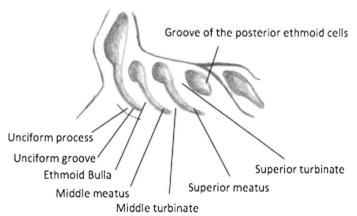

Groove of the posterior ethmoid cells

Unciform process

Unciform groove

Ethmoid Bulla

Middle meatus

Superior turbinate

Superior meatus

Middle turbinate

Fig. 7. Diagrammatic representation of ethmoid air cell anatomy.

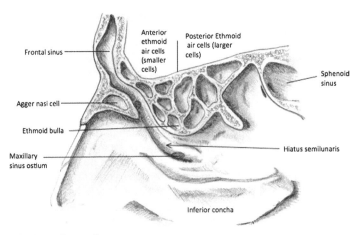

Fig. 8. Sagittal view of ethmoid air cells.

children and enlarges with sinus pneumatization that occurs with advancing age. The span of these sinuses is from the region of the third molar posteriorly to the premolar teeth anteriorly. The dimensions of the sinus vary and range from 25 to 35 mm mesiodistal width, 36 to 45 mm vertical height, and 38 to 45 mm deep anteroposteriorly.[17] Mesiodistal width differences are usually attributed to growth toward the zygomatic arch posteriorly rather than toward the canine teeth anteriorly.

The maxillary sinus is shaped like a quadrangular pyramid, with the base facing the lateral nasal wall and the apex oriented at the zygomatic arch. The roof of the sinus contributes to the floor of the orbit, the floor faces the alveolar process, and the sinus proceeds deep and adjacent to the palate. The Schneiderian membrane lines the maxillary sinus and is composed of pseudostratified ciliated columnar epithelium. The concentration of cilia increases with proximity to the sinus ostium. The thickness of this membrane is 0.8 mm. Compared with the nasal mucosa, the antral mucosa is thinner and less vascular.[18]

Pneumatization of the Sinus with Age

At birth, the maxillary sinus begins medial to the orbit and its dimensions are largest anteroposteriorly. At 2 years of age, the sinus continues inferiorly below the medial orbit and continues to pneumatize laterally. By 4 years of age, the sinus reaches the infraorbital canal and continues laterally. By 9 years of age, inferior growth reaches the region of the hard palate. Pneumatization continues as the permanent teeth erupt.[19]

VITAL STRUCTURES

The roof of the maxillary sinus contributes to the floor of the orbit. The roof contains the infraorbital

neurovascular bundle. The infraorbital foramen opens approximately 1 cm below the infraorbital rim.[20] The floor of the maxillary sinus abuts the alveolar process of the maxilla, frequently approximating the apices of the molar teeth, as is discussed in the next section. The inferior extent of the sinus floor is 1 cm inferior to the floor of the nasal cavity. The medial wall of the maxillary sinus houses the sinus ostium (os) at its superomedial aspect and the nasolacrimal duct, through which drainage of the lacrimal apparatus occurs. The maxillary os empties into the posterior aspect of the semilunar hiatus. The nasolacrimal duct runs 4 to 9 mm anterior to the os and empties at the anterior portion of the inferior meatus.[17]

Anatomic Relationship of Maxillary Sinus with Teeth

Sinus development follows a three-compartment model described by Underwood[21] in which these compartments, frequently separated by septae, are associated with three different dental milestones. The anterior compartment forms around the primary molars between 8 months and 2 years of age. The middle compartment forms around the adult first and second molars from 5 to 12 years of age. The posterior compartment forms around the third molars from 16 to 30 years of age.[21,22] The most inferior portion of the maxillary sinus is in the region of the first molar.[18] The distance from the sinus floor to the root tips of the teeth is longest for the first premolar and shortest for the second molar distobuccal root tip.[23] The roots of the maxillary first and second molars communicate with the floor of the maxillary sinus with an incidence of 40%.[24] The palatine roots of these teeth are 50% closer to the antral floor than to the palate, and in 20% of cases apical communication is present between the palatal roots of the maxillary first and second molars with the maxillary sinus (**Fig. 9, Table 1**).[25]

Clinical Significance of Septa

A *septum* is defined as a strut of bone that is at least 2.5 mm in height. Septae within the maxillary sinus are of two varieties. The first, discussed in the last section, are formed as part of the three-compartment model of sinus development and act as dividers of the anterior, middle, and posterior components. These septae are referred to as *primary septae* and are found between the roots of the second premolar and the first molar and the roots of the first and second molars, and distal to the roots of the third molar. Septae extrinsic to those of maxillary development are called *secondary septae* and occur as a result of pneumatization after dental extraction. The overall prevalence of septae present in any given maxillary sinus is 35%.[21] Septae in edentulous regions tend to be larger than those in partially edentulous regions that are larger still than dentate regions of the alveolus. The presence of septae is pertinent for sinus lift procedures, because they complicate the process of luxating the boney window to expose the sinus and increase the likelihood of sinus membrane perforation.

Ostium of Maxillary Sinus

The size and numbers of maxillary sinus ostia are variable. Simon[26] found that the sinus ostium existed as a canal greater than 3 mm in mesiodistal width from the infundibulum to the antral opening in 82.7% of individuals, in contrast to the 13.7% in whom the ostium existed as just an opening. The average length of the sinus ostium is 5.55 mm and is oriented inferolaterally from the infundibulum to the antrum to drain the maxillary sinus into the hiatus semilunaris. Approximately 16% of individuals have an accessory ostium (ie, an ostium

opening outside the infundibulum and semilunar hiatus). The accessory ostium typically exists only as an opening and not a canal, with an average length of 1.5 mm. The clinical significance of the ostium existing as a canal is an appreciation for how readily a canal obstruction can occur (**Fig. 10**).

The Superior Alveolar Nerves

Harrison[8] presented the anatomic location of the superior alveolar nerves described in this section. The superior alveolar nerves are in close apposition to the maxillary sinus and are therefore discussed. The anterior superior alveolar nerve (ASA) arises 15 mm behind the infraorbital foramen and runs inferiorly in the anterior wall of the maxilla. Occasionally the ASA forms an elevation at the anterior part of the sinus cavity approximately 6 mm inferior to the infraorbital foramen on its way to supply the lateral nasal wall and septum, and the anterior maxillary teeth. The middle superior alveolar nerve (MSA) often arises off the infraorbital nerve and courses along the posterolateral or anterior wall of the sinus to supply the premolar teeth. The posterior superior alveolar nerve (PSA) is a branch of the infraorbital nerve given off at the posterior end of the infraorbital canal. Two branches of this nerve are usually present: a smaller superior branch and the larger inferior branch. The superior branch of the PSA passes through the antrum and runs posteriorly along the maxillary tuberosity. The inferior branch supplies the molar teeth and joins the MSA and ASA to form the alveolar plexus. The significance of this presentation of the superior alveolar nerves is to present a safe area at the anterior region of the maxilla where bone can be safely removed (eg, Caldwell-Luc procedure), with minimal risk of damage to the superior alveolar nerves.

Blood Supply and Innervation

The maxillary sinus possesses rich anastomoses and receives its arterial supply from the infraorbital,

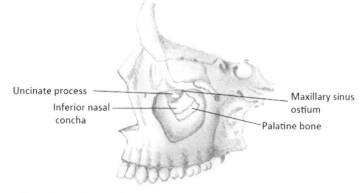

Uncinate process

Inferior nasal concha

Maxillary sinus ostium

Palatine bone

Fig. 9. Sagittal view of maxillary sinus anatomy.

Table 1
Distance from the roots of maxillary teeth to maxillary sinus floor

Root	Distance (mm)	SD
Buccal first premolar	6.18	1.60
Lingual first premolar	7.05	1.92
Second premolar	2.86	0.60
Mesiobuccal first molar	2.82	0.59
Palatal first molar	1.56	0.77
Distobuccal first molar	2.79	1.13
Mesiobuccal second molar	0.83	0.49
Palatal second molar	2.04	1.19
Distobuccal second molar	1.97	1.21

Data from Eberhardt JA, Torabinejad M, Christiansen EL. A computed tomographic study of the distances between the maxillary sinus floor and the apices of the maxillary posterior teeth. Oral Surg Oral Med Oral Pathol 1992;73(3): 345–6.

sphenopalatine, posterior lateral nasal, facial, pterygopalatine, greater palatine, and posterior superior alveolar arteries. Venous return from the maxillary sinus occurs anteriorly via the cavernous plexus that drains into the facial vein and posteriorly via the pterygoid plexus and to the internal jugular vein. Innervation of the maxillary sinus is via the anterior superior, middle superior, and posterior superior alveolar nerves. Lymphatic drainage occurs through the infraorbital foramen via the ostium to the submandibular lymphatic system.[16]

FRONTAL SINUS

The frontal sinuses are the most superior of the anterior sinuses. They are situated in the frontal bone between inner and outer plates. The inner plate, or posterior wall (separates the frontal sinus from the anterior cranial fossa), is much thinner than the outer wall and may be penetrated accidentally during surgery.[2] The septum between right and left is almost always asymmetrically placed and divides the frontal sinuses into two unequal sinuses. The larger sinus may pass across the midline and overlap the other. The sinuses often have incompletely separated recesses, which make the anatomy highly variable. Superficial surgical landmarks for the frontal sinus was described by Tubbs and colleagues[27] from adult cadaveric frontal sinus dissections. In their study of 70 adult cadavers, these investigators reported that the lateral wall of the frontal sinus never extended more than 5 mm lateral to a midpupillary line. At this same line and at a plane drawn through the supraorbital ridges, the roof of the frontal sinus was never higher than 12 mm, and in the midline, the roof of the frontal sinus never reached more than 4 cm above the nasion. The frontal sinus is separated from the orbit by a thin triangular plate.

Regarding the lateral extension of the frontal sinuses, the authors have observed several cases in which the lateral extension of the frontal sinuses extended more lateral than described by Tubbs and colleagues.[27] Further, Maves[28] states that the degree of pneumatization of the frontal sinuses varies and that it may extend laterally as far as the sphenoid wing.

The ostium of the frontal sinus lies in the posteromedial aspect of the sinus floor. The frontonasal duct opens into the anterior part of the middle meatus and the frontal recess, or directly into the anterior end of the infundibulum (**Fig. 11**).

This relationship to the infundibulum and middle meatus serves to protect the frontal sinus from the spread of disease in the osteomeatal complex. The agger nasi is intimately involved, in that the posterior wall of the agger nasi forms the anterior border of the frontal recess, which

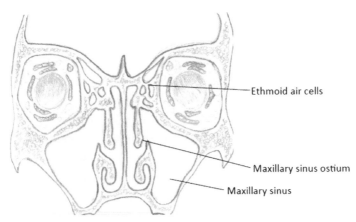

— Ethmoid air cells

— Maxillary sinus ostium

— Maxillary sinus

Fig. 10. Coronal view of osteomeatal complex.

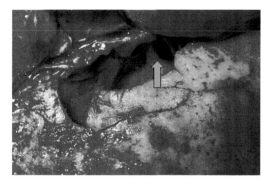

Fig. 11. Frontonasal duct in situ (*arrow*).

then passes posteromedially to the agger nasi and supraorbital cells. This recess is present in 77% of patients. In the other 23%, drainage occurs via a frontal sinus ostium.[4] There are also two patterns to the frontal sinus outflow tract: those that drain medial to the uncinate process and those that drain lateral to the uncinate process. Those that drain medially are more common and are significantly related to the presence of frontal sinusitis. The borders of the frontonasal duct are the 1) anterior border, which is the superior portion of the uncinate process; 2) posterior border, which is the superior portion of the bulla ethmoidalis; 3) medial border, which is formed by the conchal plate; and 4) lateral border, which is the suprainfundibular plate.[29] The nasofrontal duct can safely be widened through removing the upper portion of the ground lamella of the ethmoid bulla at the posterior boundary of the nasofrontal duct with cutting forceps.[29]

Blood Supply

The supraorbital and supratrochlear arteries, which branch off the ophthalmic artery, form the arterial supply of the frontal sinus. The superior ophthalmic vein provides venous drainage. Actual venous drainage for the inner table, however, is through the dura mater and the cranial periosteum for the outer table. These veins are in addition to the diploic veins and all venous structures that communicate in the venous plexuses of the inner table, periorbita, and cranial periosteum.

REFERENCES

1. Dion MC, Jafek BW, Tobin CE. The anatomy of the nose: external support. Arch Otolaryngol 1978; 104(3):145–50.
2. Janfaza P, Montgomery WW, Salman SD. Nasal cavities and paranasal sinuses. In: Janfaza P, Nadol JB, Galla RJ, et al, editors. Surgical anatomy of the head and neck. Philadelphia: Lipincott Williams and Wilkins; 2000. p. 266, 286.
3. Deaver JB. The nose. In: Deaver JB, editor. Surgical anatomy of the head and neck. Philadelphia: P. Blakiston's Son & Co; 1904. p. 284–98.
4. Metson R. Endoscopic treatment of frontal sinusitis. Laryngoscope 1992;102(6):712–6.
5. Lee HY, Kim HU, Kim SS. Surgical anatomy of the sphenopalatine artery in lateral nasal wall. Laryngoscope 2002;112(10):1813–8.
6. Padgham N, Vaughan-Jones R. Cadaver studies of the anatomy of arterial supply to the inferior turbinate. J R Soc Med 1991;84:729–30.
7. Snow JB Jr, Ballenger JJ. Section 26: Anatomy and Physiology of the Nose and Paranasal Sinuses. Ballenger's Otorhinolaryngology Head & Neck Surgery. 16th edition. Hamilton (ON): BC Decker Inc; 2003. p. 549–52.
8. Harrison DF. Surgical anatomy of maxillary and ethmoidal sinuses—a reappraisal. Laryngoscope 1971;81(10):1658–64.
9. Mosher HP. The applied anatomy and the intra-nasal surgery of the ethmoidal labyrinth. Laryngoscope 1913;23(9):881–907.
10. Gardner E, Gray DJ, O'Rahilly RO. Nose and paranasal sinuses. In: Anatomy: a regional study of human structure. 4th edition. Philadelphia (PA): WB Saunders Co; 1975. p. 732–41.
11. Stammberger HR, Kennedy DW. Paranasal sinuses: anatomic terminology and nomenclature. The Anatomic Terminology Group. Ann Otol Rhinol Laryngol Suppl 1995;167:7–16.
12. Hajek M. Pathologie und Therapie der entziindlichen Erkrankungen der Nebenhohlen der Nase. Leipzig (Germany): Deuticke; 1909.
13. Braun A. The diagnosis of suppurative disease of the nasal accessory sinuses. The medical record, Volume 78. Chicago (IL): William Wood & Company; 1910. p. 95–8.
14. Ellis E III, Zide MF. Section 3: Coronal approach. Surgical approaches to the facial skeleton. 2nd edition. Philadelphia (PA): Lippincott Williams & Wilkins; 2006. p. 85–7.
15. Lawson W, Patel ZM, Lin FY. The development and pathologic processes that influence maxillary sinus pneumatization. Anat Rec 2008;291(11):1554–63.
16. Smiler DG, Soltan M, Shostine MS, et al. Oral and maxillofacial surgery, vol 17, 2nd edition. St Louis (MO): Elsevier; 2009. p. 458–60.
17. Van den Bergh JP, ten Bruggenkate CM, Disch FJ, et al. Anatomical aspects of sinus floor elevations. Clin Oral Implants Res 2000;11(3):256–65.
18. Woo I, Le BT. Maxillary sinus floor elevation: review of anatomy and two techniques. Implant Dent 2004;13:28–32.
19. Scuderi AJ, Harnsberger HR, Boyer RS. Pneumatization of the paranasal sinuses: normal features of importance to the accurate interpretation of CT scans and MR images. AJR Am J Roentgenol 1993;160:1101–4.

20. Hitotsumatsu T, Matsushima T, Rhoton AL. Surgical anatomy of the midface and the midline skull base. Operat Tech Neurosurg 1999;2(4):160–80.

21. Underwood AS. An inquiry into the anatomy and pathology of the maxillary sinus. J Anat Physiol 1910;44(Pt 4):354–69.

22. Maestre-Ferrín L, Galán-Gil S, Rubio-Serrano M, et al. Maxillary sinus septa: a systematic review. Med Oral Patol Oral Cir Bucal 2010;15(2):e383–6.

23. Cenk K, Kivanc K, Selcen PY, et al. An assessment of the relationship between the maxillary sinus floor and the maxillary posterior teeth root tips using dental cone-beam computerized tomography. Eur J Dent 2010;4(4):462–7.

24. Wallace JA. Transantral endodontic surgery. Oral Surg Oral Med Oral Pathol 1996;82:80–3.

25. Waite DE. Maxillary sinus. Dent Clin North Am 1971; 15:349–68.

26. Simon E. Anatomy of the opening of the maxillary sinus. Arch. Otolaryng 1939;29:640–9.

27. Tubbs RS, Elton S, Salter G, et al. Superficial surgical landmarks for the frontal sinus. JNSPG Online 2002;96(2). Available at: http://thejns.org/doi/abs/10.3171/jns.2002.96.2.0320?journalCode=jns. Accessed October, 2011.

28. Maves MD. Surgical anatomy of the head and neck. In: Bailey BJ, Johnson JT, Newlands SD, editors. Head and Neck Surgery—Otolaryngology, vol 1. Philadelphia: Lippincott Williams & Wilkins; 2006. p. 8.

29. Kim KS, Kim HU, Chung IH, et al. Surgical anatomy of the nasofrontal duct: anatomical and computed tomographic analysis. Laryngoscope 2001;111(4):603–8.

Instrumentation and Techniques for Examination of the Ear, Nose, Throat, and Sinus

Marsha James, MBBS, DM(ORL)[a],*,
Orville Palmer, MD, MPH, FRCSC[b],*

KEYWORDS

• Patient history • Ear • Nose • Instrumentation

Optimal and accurate management of any patient depends on a detailed history and thorough physical examination. The information garnered dictates the definitive management of the patient. The importance of obtaining a detailed patient history cannot be overemphasized because it is the basis on which the examiner places all available information for the physical examination. Adequate examination of the head and neck, particularly the upper aerodigestive tract, presents a unique challenge because much of the area to be examined is not easily accessible to direct visualization. A comprehensive system, therefore, must be developed for both obtaining the history and the clinical examination to minimize the possibility of missing the underlying pathologic condition. The examiner must develop an approach to the examination of the head and neck that allows the patient to feel comfortable while the physician performs a complete and thorough evaluation. Hence a rapport must be established with the patient before proceeding with the examination in an orderly manner. The examiner should also be prepared by ensuring that all necessary instrumentation to facilitate the process is available and accessible. The physician should be familiar with the variety of instruments and techniques, as each patient may present a unique challenge. A knowledgable

and adaptable examiner builds confidence and comfort in the patient.

RELEVANT ANATOMY

Knowledge of surgical anatomy is essential for the accurate diagnosis and successful surgical management of all patients. A familiarity with the anatomy allows for a more comprehensive examination and an accurate diagnosis. The anatomy presented here is far from exhaustive, but highlights the areas accessible throughout examination.

Ear

The ear is divided into the external, middle, and inner ear. The external ear comprises the auricle and the external auditory canal, which terminates at the tympanic membrane. The middle ear or tympanic cavity is an irregular space in the temporal bone that houses the auditory ossicles (malleus, incus, and stapes) and communicates with the nasopharynx via the Eustachian tube. The inner ear lies medial to the middle ear, and contains the auditory and vestibular apparatus.[1]

The pinna has a cartilaginous skeleton that is thrown into folds and is covered by adherent skin. There is soft fibrofatty tissue but no cartilage in the lobule. The blood supply is derived mainly from the posterior auricular artery and the

[a] Kingston Public Hospital, University of the West Indies, North Street, Kingston, Jamaica
[b] Otolaryngology-Facial Plastics and Reconstruction, Harlem Hospital Center, Columbia University, 506 Lenox Avenue, New York, NY 10037, USA
* Corresponding authors.
E-mail addresses: njerijames@hotmail.com; odp3@columbia.edu

Oral Maxillofacial Surg Clin N Am 24 (2012) 167–174
doi:10.1016/j.coms.2012.01.002
1042-3699/12/$ – see front matter © 2012 Elsevier Inc. All rights reserved.

superficial temporal artery. The veins accompany the corresponding arteries. Lymphatic drainage is to the preauricular, mastoid, and superficial cervical lymph nodes. The sensory nerves are the great auricular and the auriculotemporal nerve.

The external auditory canal is a sinuous conduit, which is about 4 cm in length from the adult tragus. It has an outer third portion that is cartilaginous and contains a thin layer of subcutaneous tissue between the skin and cartilage. The inner portion is osseous and is formed primarily by the tympanic ring, and contains very scant soft tissue between the skin, periosteum, and bone. The average length of the adult external auditory canal is 2.5 cm. Because of the oblique position of the tympanic membrane, the posterosuperior part of the canal is about 6 mm shorter than the anteroinferior portion. Related to the meatus, in front of the osseous portion is the condyle of the mandible, with the mastoid air cells lying posteriorly. Branches of the posterior auricular, internal maxillary, and temporal vessels supply blood to the external auditory canal. Lymphatic drainage is similar to that of the pinna, and the sensory supply is provided by the auriculotemporal nerve and the auricular branch of the vagus nerve.[1,2]

The tympanic membrane is a thin fibrous membrane, which is oval in shape and has a depressed central part called the umbo, wherein the handle of the malleus attaches to the membrane. The lateral process of the malleus is located in the superior-anterior region, and is identified as a prominent bony point from which the anterior and posterior malleolar folds project. Superior to these folds is the lax pars flaccida, which lacks the radial and circular fibers present in the larger pars tensa and forms the remainder of the eardrum. The tympanic membrane is thickened at its circumference and is slotted into a groove, the tympanic sulcus. The blood supply is derived from the deep auricular and tympanic artery. The nerve supply is from the auriculotemporal and glossopharyngeal nerves.

The tympanic cavity is an air-filled space in the petrous bone, containing the bony ossicles (malleus, incus, and stapes). The tympanic membrane bulges into the cavity within millimeters of the promontory on the medial wall. Posterosuperior to the promontory is the oval window, closed by the stapes. The roof of the cavity is the tegmen tympani. The floor is a thin plate of bone separating the cavity from the jugular fossa and the carotid canal. The anterior wall is perforated by the opening of the bony portion of the eustachian tube. The posterior wall is deficient superiorly where the aditus leads into the antrum. Below the aditus, the fossa incudis and the pyramid are located. The chorda tympani emerges through a canal in the posterior wall that is located close to the posterior margin of the tympanic membrane.

The blood supply of the middle ear is derived from the tympanic branch of the maxillary, stylomastoid, and stapedial arteries. Venous drainage is toward the pterygoid plexus and superior petrosal sinus. The nerve supply is from the tympanic plexus with inputs from the glossopharyngeal nerve, facial nerve, and twigs from the sympathetic plexus.[1,2]

Nose and Paranasal Sinuses

External nose

The external nose has an anterior dorsum and 2 lateral projections. The apex is called the tip; the septum divides the nose into the anterior nares, is pyramidal in shape, and has a bony, cartilaginous, and membranous framework. The nasal bones articulate superiorly with the nasal part of the frontal bone and with each other laterally, and with the nasal process of the maxilla. Superiorly, the paired nasal bones are attached to the frontal bone and superolaterally, they are connected to the lacrimal bones. Inferolaterally, they are attached to the ascending processes of the maxilla. Posterosuperiorly, the bony nasal septum comprises the perpendicular plate of the ethmoid. The vomer lies posteroinferiorly, in part forming the choanal opening into the nasopharynx. The floor consists of the premaxilla and the palatine bones.

The chief arterial supply of the external nose is from the facial artery through the angular artery and superior labial arteries anteriorly, as well as branches of the anterior ethmoidal artery. The lymphatic drainage is to the submandibular lymph nodes. The nerve supply is provided by the external nasal nerve and branches of the infraorbital nerve.

The nasal septum consists of the nasal septal cartilage, the nasal crest of the maxilla, the nasal crest of the palatine bone, the vomer, and the perpendicular plate of the ethmoid bone. The lateral nasal wall is formed by the prominent nasal turbinates. The lateral nasal wall is formed by the superior, middle, and inferior turbinates as well as the corresponding meati. The ostiomeatal complex is an area of the anterior middle meatus, which is paramount in the understanding of sinonasal disease and endoscopic sinus surgery. The ostiomeatal complex refers collectively to several middle meatal structures, including the uncinate process, ethmoid infundibulum, hiatus semilunaris, and the ostia of the anterior ethmoid, maxillary, and frontal sinuses.[1,3,4]

The blood supply of the nasal cavity is primarily from the sphenopalatine branch of the maxillary artery, the anterior ethmoidal artery from the ophthalmic artery, the greater palatine artery, and the superior labial branch of the facial artery. The blood supply of the lateral nasal wall can be divided into quadrants. All of these vessels anastomose with each other on the anteroinferior nasal septum as the Kiesselbach plexus. Lymphatic drainage is to the retropharyngeal, submandibular, and deep cervical nodes. The nerve supply is provided by the branches of the ophthalmic and maxillary division of the trigeminal nerve and the olfactory nerves.

Paranasal sinuses

The paranasal sinuses consist of paired frontal, ethmoid, maxillary, and sphenoid sinuses. The maxillary sinus usually is the largest of the paranasal sinuses and is situated in the body of the maxilla. Its anterior wall is the facial surface of this bone, its posterior wall is the infratemporal surface, and its medial wall is that of the nasal cavity. The roof of the maxillary sinus is also the floor of the orbit, and it also may be affected by trauma to the orbit and by the extension of neoplastic or inflammatory processes. The ethmoid sinuses consist of a variable number of separate cavities that honeycomb the ethmoid bone between the upper part of the lateral nasal wall and the medial wall of the orbit. These cavities are separated into anterior and posterior ethmoidal cells by the basal lamella of the middle turbinate overlap, the bullar cells spreading backward, or the posterior cells spreading forward. The posterior ethmoid cells drain into the superior meatus. The sphenoid sinus usually opens into the sphenoethmoidal recess above and behind the superior nasal concha.

The blood supply to the ethmoid sinuses is provided by the sphenopalatine and ethmoidal arteries. The sphenoid sinus is supplied by the posterior ethmoidal vessels. The frontal sinus is supplied by the anterior ethmoid and supraorbital vessels. The facial, maxillary, infraorbital, and greater palatine vessels supply the maxillary sinuses. The nerve supply is provided by branches of the ophthalmic and maxillary divisions of the trigeminal nerves. Lymphatics drain to the submandibular and retropharyngeal nodes.[1,2]

Pharynx

The pharynx is a fibromuscular tube that extends from the skull base to the esophagus and communicates anteriorly with the nose, mouth, and larynx.

The nasal part of the pharynx, the nasopharynx, is continuous anteriorly through the posterior choanae with the nasal cavities. The floor is the upper surface of the soft palate. The roof, the mucosa of which is attached close to the base of the skull, slopes downward and backward to become continuous with its posterior wall. The eustachian tubes are prominent on the lateral aspect of the nasal pharynx. The fossa of Rosenmuller lies behind the posterior margin of the torus and the posterior wall.

The oropharynx is continuous anteriorly through the fauces, or oropharyngeal isthmus, with the oral cavity. The boundaries of the fauces are the posterior border of the soft palate above, the palatine arches laterally, and the dorsum of the tongue. The anterior wall of the oropharynx is the mobile posterior dorsum of the tongue. The posterior wall of the oropharynx is formed by all 3 constrictors. Within the lateral wall of the fauces lie the large palatine tonsils.

The laryngeal part of the pharynx, or hypopharynx, extends from just above the level of the hyoid bone superiorly to the lower border of the cricoid cartilage inferiorly, to become continuous with the esophagus. The anterior wall is formed laterally by mucosa on the medial surface of the thyroid cartilage, and centrally or medially by the larynx and its appendages. Above are the epiglottis and the aditus of the larynx. Below the aditus, the anterior wall of the pharynx is also the posterior wall of the larynx. Lateral to the epiglottis are the lateral glossoepiglottic folds that form the anterolateral boundary between the oral and the laryngeal parts of the pharynx. Below these folds, the hypopharynx extends forward around the sides of the larynx between this area and the thyroid cartilage. These bilateral extensions are the piriform sinuses.

The pharynx is supplied by branches of the external carotid (ascending pharyngeal) and subclavian (inferior thyroid) arteries. The motor and most of the sensory supply to the pharynx is via the pharyngeal plexus. Lymphatic drainage is to the deep cervical lymph nodes, especially the jugulodigastric nodes.

Larynx

The larynx extends from the epiglottis and the aryepiglottic folds to the cricoid cartilage, communicating with the laryngopharynx above through the laryngeal aditus and with the trachea below. The lateral walls have 2 infoldings of mucous membrane, the vestibular folds above and the true vocal folds below. The space between the 2 vestibular folds is called the rima vestibuli, and the space between the 2 vocal folds is called the rima glottis. The laryngeal ventricle lies between the rima vestibule and the rima glottis. The ventricle has a lateral extension, the saccule, between the vestibular fold and the thyroid cartilage.

The skeletal framework of the larynx consists of cartilages, joints, ligaments, and membranes. The 3 single cartilages are the shield-shaped thyroid cartilage, epiglottis, and cricoid cartilage. There are 3 paired cartilages, the largest of which are the arytenoids. The paired arytenoid cartilages provide an attachment for the vocal ligament and movement of the vocal folds. The cartilages are connected by the cricothyroid and cricoarytenoid joints. Overlying the structure of this skeletal framework are the infrahyoid muscles, which include the paired sternohyoid, sternothyroid, omohyoid, and thyrohyoid muscles. The ligaments and membranes are classified as intrinsic (quadrangular and conus elasticus) and extrinsic (thyrohyoid and cricotracheal membranes, and hyoepiglottic and thyroepiglottic ligaments). The intrinsic muscles of the larynx alter the shape and size of the inlet, and move the vocal cords. The movement of the true vocal cords is produced by the posterior and lateral cricoarytenoids, thyroarytenoids, vocalis, transverse arytenoids, and the cricothyroids.

The blood supply is divided at the level of the vocal folds. Above the vocal folds the superior laryngeal vessels supply the larynx, while the lower half is supplied by the inferior laryngeal vessels. The intrinsic muscles of the larynx are innervated by the recurrent laryngeal nerve. The exception is the cricothyroid muscle, which is innervated by the external laryngeal nerve. The recurrent laryngeal nerve on the left originates over the aortic arch and ascends in the neck to innervate the larynx. On the right, the nerve goes around the subclavian artery. The lymphatic drainage is to the deep cervical nodes and the prelaryngeal and pretracheal nodes.

Neck

The neck can be divided into 6 levels for the classification of the neck masses and adenopathy. Level I is defined by the body of the mandible, anterior belly of the contralateral digastric muscle, and the stylohyoid muscle. The anterior belly of digastric muscle divides it into level IA, containing the submental nodes, and level IB, consisting of the submandibular nodes. These 2 levels are separated by the anterior belly of the digastric muscle. The jugulodigastric lymph nodes from the skull base to the inferior border of the hyoid bone are located in level II, whereas the middle and lower third represent levels III and IV, respectively. The spinal accessory nerve divides these

levels into sublevels A and B. Level III extends from the inferior border of the hyoid bone to the inferior border of the cricoid cartilage, and level IV extends from the inferior border of the cricoid to the superior border of the clavicle. Level V includes the spinal accessory and supraclavicular nodes, and extends from the lateral border of the sternocleidomastoid muscle to the anterior border of the trapezius.

The visceral structures of the neck include the thyroid and parathyroid glands, a portion of the pharynx, the larynx, the trachea, the esophagus, and sometimes portions of the thymus. The thyroid gland lies below and on the side of the thyroid cartilage, covered anteriorly by the infrahyoid muscles. A pyramidal lobe of the thyroid may extend superiorly from the isthmus that connects the 2 lobes of the thyroid gland. On the posterior surface of the thyroid gland lie the paired parathyroid glands.[1,2]

INSTRUMENTATION

The instrumentation for ear, nose, and throat examination has evolved alongside the advances in medical technology. Before the invention of the electric light by Thomas Edison in 1879, examination was performed only by daylight or with a candle. The traditional concave mirror with the central perforation was introduced as a handheld device in 1841, and the headband was added in 1845. Head mirrors and lamps have now been replaced by powered headlights, and otoscopes now have built-in light sources. The introduction of the Hopkins rod and fiberoptic light sources in 1954 revolutionized the examination of previously inaccessible regions of the nose, pharynx, and larynx.[5]

Before beginning the examination, all necessary instrumentation should be carefully laid out in an orderly manner and should be readily accessible. The instrumentation should include, but not be limited to, the following (**Fig. 1**):

> Headlight
> Nasal speculum
> Rigid nasal endoscope 0° and 30° (optional 70°, 90°, 110°)
> Flexible nasoendoscope
> Light source and fiber-optic cable
> Tongue depressor
> Laryngeal mirrors
> Aural speculum
> Otoscope with pneumatic attachment
> Tuning forks
> Crocodile forceps
> Suction tips

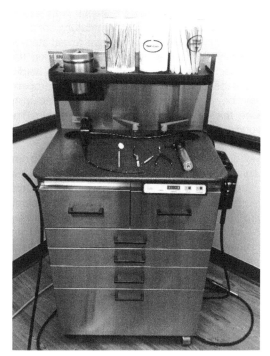

Fig. 1. Typical ear, nose, and throat instrumentation.

Cotton-tip applicators
Antifog solution
Topical anesthesia
Gauze
Gloves.

THE EXAMINATION

Throughout the examination, the patient should be informed of each step and what is to be expected. Consent should be obtained before embarking on this process. This engaging manner puts the patient at ease and allows for a more comfortable examination. The patient should sit upright and should not slouch in the chair. Constant repositioning of the head is necessary to obtain adequate visualization of the various anatomic regions. The examiner should be positioned across from the patient, preferably seated on an adjustable wheeled chair. The examination proceeds with inspection and palpation, as well as percussion and auscultation whenever applicable. After the general examination the ear is examined initially, followed by the nose and paranasal sinuses. The mouth, pharynx, and larynx are then examined and, for completeness, the neck and cranial nerves are also examined.

General Appearance

The general appearance of the patient provides important clues to the pathologic processes that may be existent. Changes in appearance, such as weight loss, anorexia, and fatigue, could indicate malignancy. The face should be analyzed for facial asymmetry by positioning the head squarely in front of the examiner. Facial asymmetry may indicate bony disorders, such as fibrous dysplasia, soft tissue involvement from trauma, or tumor infiltration. Facial nerve palsy also presents as facial asymmetry. The appearance of the skin is inspected for color, mass lesions or ulcerations, abrasions, and ecchymoses. The facial skeleton then should be carefully palpated for bony deformities while taking note of any areas of tenderness, which holds especially true for patients with recent facial trauma. The periorbital rims may be irregular because of fractures involving the zygomatic arches or orbital floor.

Ear

The ear is examined with reflected light from a head mirror or a headlight, and may be complemented with an otoscope. The patient should be seated sideways while the examiner sits opposite to the ear to be examined and reflects light on to it. The patient should be asked about areas of tenderness before the examination is begun. The pinna and preauricular and postauricular regions are examined for any surgical scars, sinuses, or masses. The sun-exposed pinna is a common site for basal cell carcinoma. The pinna should be drawn upward, outward, and backward in adults, whereas in infants the pinna is pulled downward and backward to straighten the external auditory canal, which improves the visualization of the auditory canal and tympanic membrane and facilitates insertion of the aural speculum. The size of the auditory canal and the presence of discharge, polyps, exostoses, or foreign bodies should be noted. An appropriate-sized aural speculum should be carefully inserted after the examination of the pinna and the external auditory canal. Cerumen impaction may be removed by several techniques, such as careful curetting, gentle suctioning, or irrigation with warm water. The external canal may be filled with wax, which obscures the view of the external auditory canal and the tympanic membrane. The tympanic membrane is then examined, paying attention to the position of the lateral process and handle of the malleus, transparency of the membrane, and the presence of the light reflex. The presence of any perforations, or middle ear masses or fluid should be noted. An otitis media with effusion may appear as a clear fluid, and hemotympanum may be present if there has been a recent head trauma. A pulsatile mass in the hypotympanum is suggestive of a glomus tumor. A magnified view of the tympanic membrane can be obtained with an otoscope. The presence and intensity of the light source of the otoscope is checked before use. An appropriate-sized speculum is chosen and attached to the end of the otoscope. The otoscope is held in the hand of the same side as the ear about to be examined. The otoscope is held in a pen/pencil or hammer grip. The former is preferred, as it allows for more control of the patient's head and is especially useful for restless children. An insufflator can be attached to a port in the otoscope and thus used for pneumatic otoscopy. Pneumatic otoscopy should be used to assess the mobility of the tympanic membrane. Immobility may be due to fluid, a perforation, or tympanosclerosis.

Hearing tests, including free-field speech testing and tuning-fork tests, complete the ear examination. Free-field testing is performed by asking the patient to repeat spoken words with a whispered voice, conversation voice, and shouted voice, at 60 cm from the ear. The nontest ear can be masked by gently massaging the tragus or by using a Barany noise box. Tuning forks, preferably 512 Hz, are used to perform the Rinne and Weber hearing tests, which are useful in differentiating between conductive and sensorineural hearing loss.[6] In the Rinne test, the tuning fork is struck against the heel of the shoe or the physician's elbow; the vibrating fork is first held lateral to the pinna and then held firmly on the mastoid process. The patient is asked which sound is louder. The process is then repeated for the other ear. A positive result in the Rinne test infers that air conduction is louder than bone conduction. The Weber test is performed by placing the vibrating tuning fork on the middle of the forehead or the bridge of the nose, and the patient is then asked whether the sound is heard loudest in the midline or preferentially to one side. A conductive hearing loss or contralateral sensorineural hearing loss is marked by lateralization to one side.

Nose and Paranasal Sinuses

The examiner should be seated with knees together to the right of the patient and not astride the patient. The examination begins with inspection of the external nose and paranasal sinuses after clear explanation to the patient. The convexity or concavity of the nasal dorsum, the width or the projection of the tip, the deviation of the nose, and the shape of the columella should be closely examined. Possible findings include deformity of the nasal dorsum, surgical scars, and cutaneous abnormalities. The paranasal sinuses may be palpated directly to elicit any tenderness. Palpation of the sinuses, particularly the frontal

and maxillary ones, can be useful, with severe tenderness indicating an inflammatory condition of the sinuses. Palpation may also reveal step-off deformity in facial trauma. Transillumination has low specificity and sensitivity, but may be helpful in the absence of nasal endoscopy. This property may be due to anatomic variations including bone thickness, which makes it unreliable. The technique involves direct placement of a strong light in the sublabial region (for maxillary sinus) and supraorbital rim (frontal sinus) while comparing both sides, which is preferably done in a darkened room to optimize the effects. Decreased light transmission when compared with the normal side suggests significant fluid collection or marked mucosal edema.

Anterior rhinoscopy, using a headlamp and nasal speculum, allows assessment of the nasal septum and inferior turbinates. The patient is asked to tilt the head backward for better visualization, and the nasal speculum is inserted with the blades closed. A standard nasal speculum is then introduced carefully into the vestibule, avoiding the sensitive mucosa of the nasal septum by directing the instrument toward the lateral wall of the nose while observing the nasal mucosa for color, vascularity, and crusting. The position of the septum is also noted for deviation or dislocation, as well as septal spurs, hematoma, or perforation. The inferior turbinate and middle turbinate can also be seen clearly when this method is used. The mucosa of the inferior turbinate may range from the boggy, edematous, pale mucosa seen in those with allergic rhinitis to the erythematous, edematous mucosa seen in those with sinusitis. Patency of the airway is assessed by asking the patient to occlude one nostril and then breathe through the opposite nostril, observing the fogginess of a mirror or the surface of a metal tongue depressor held below the nasal cavities while the patient exhales.

The posterior nasal space can be assessed by using a postnasal space or dental mirror and a headlight. The patient is asked to open the mouth, and a tongue depressor is used to depress the tongue to facilitate passage of the mirror. The mirror, previously coated with antifog to prevent misting, is introduced face up and directed posterior to the soft palate. The posterior choanae and eustachian tube cushions are also inspected. This procedure is limited by poor visualization and the patient's gag reflex, which is overcome by the use of a flexible nasoendoscope.

Nasal Endoscopy

The advent of the Hopkins rod in the 1950s revolutionized the visualization of the nasal and sinus cavities. Diagnostic nasal endoscopy allows the characterization of intranasal anatomy and the identification of pathologic conditions not usually visible with traditional examination techniques.[7] Anterior rhinoscopy offers limited information about the middle meatal cleft and no visualization of the maxillary sinus orifice, whereas nasal endoscopy precisely assesses this area for the evidence of sinonasal or for anatomic defects that affect ventilation and mucociliary clearance.

After anterior rhinoscopy, the nasal cavities are sprayed with a topical decongestant and local anesthetic. A 4% cocaine solution or 2% lidocaine solution is often used if there are no contraindications. It is helpful to view the nasal anatomy in both the native state and the state after decongestant use, so that the effect of the decongestant may be seen.

The patient is positioned in the sitting or supine position while the examiner is seated to the right of the patient. A 0° telescopic endoscope is most often used.

The endoscope is held by the shaft using the thumb and the first 2 fingers and is then passed carefully along the floor of the nose to visualize the anatomy, state of the nasal mucosa, and presence of polyps. The inferior meatus and sometimes the nasolacrimal duct can be seen with this view. The endoscope is then advanced into the nasopharynx. The orifices of the eustachian tube are easily identified, and the fossa of Rosenmuller should be examined for any fullness or masses. Secretions from the ostiomeatal complex may also be seen in this region. The final passage of the endoscope is between the middle and inferior turbinates. Advancing the scope allows the visualization of the middle meatus, fontanelles, and any accessory maxillary sinus ostia. Rotation of the scope superiorly provides a view of the superior turbinate and the ostia of the sphenoidal sinus. The eustachian tube cushion and orifice are inspected as well as the fossa of Rosenmuller. The midline is observed for lymphoid tissue, masses, or ulceration. A flexible nasoendoscope may also be used because this allows the visualization of the entire nasopharynx via one nostril rather than through both sides, as is done with the rigid endoscope.

Another method for viewing the nasopharynx involves the use of a 90° rigid telescope that is introduced through the mouth with the beveled edge pointed upward. The entire nasopharynx can be seen once the endoscope is passed beyond the soft palate.

The inspection of the larynx and hypopharynx may be done with a headlight and laryngeal mirrors, and is referred to as indirect laryngoscopy. The procedure should be attempted without local anesthesia initially. If this is not well tolerated, topical 2% or 4% lidocaine spray may be used to anesthetize the soft palate. The patient should then be instructed to breathe normally through the mouth while the mirror is slowly directed up to the soft palate. The mirror is used to inspect the tongue, vallecula, and the epiglottis. The mirror is redirected to visualize the piriform fossa, aryepiglottic folds, arytenoids, ventricular folds, and the true vocal cords. Abnormalities arising in this area include neoplastic and inflammatory lesions. The movements of the vocal cords are assessed by asking the patient to phonate a high-pitched "eee" followed by a deep breath, and to repeat the exercise. Any abnormal movements or fixation should be noted. The patient should be reminded to avoid food and drink for the next hour because of the impaired gag reflex and to avoid aspiration or burning of the throat by hot beverage.

Some patients are unable to tolerate indirect laryngoscopy because of an overactive gag reflex. Flexible nasopharyngoscopy can be offered to these patients. In this case, local anesthetic and decongestants are applied to facilitate comfortable and easy passage of the flexible nasoendoscope. While waiting for the local anesthetic to take effect, the procedure should be explained to the patient, and he or she should be warned about avoiding hot food or beverages for the next 30 minutes or until the anesthetic has worn off. The scope is then prepared by applying antifog solution to increase visibility. In some centers, a protective sheath may be applied. After achieving the best possible focus, a small amount of water-soluble lubricant is applied to facilitate the passage of the nasoendoscope. The instrument is then passed along the floor of the nose into the nasopharynx; the tip should be directed downward until the epiglottis comes into view. The base of tongue, vallecula, and epiglottis can be inspected initially, and the view is changed to observe the laryngeal inlet. The true vocal cords are then inspected for appearance and movement, and the subglottis is also examined. The piriform fossae are also examined for pooling of saliva or any abnormal lesions.

Rigid endoscopy using 70°, 90°, or 110° endoscopes provides a good view, especially in patients with trismus. The procedure is similar to that of the mirror examination but allows for photographic documentation.

Neck/Lymph Node

Inspection of the neck is conducted with the examiner facing the patient. The whole neck should be exposed up to and including the clavicles. The presence of any obvious scars, skin lesions, or masses should be noted. The patient may then be asked to swallow, which emphasizes a thyroid swelling. Palpation of the neck should be done with the physician standing behind the patient, and performed in a systematic manner while checking for size and consistency of the cervical nodes. The examiner stands behind the seated patient and begins the bimanual palpation of the cervical nodes at the parotid, preauricular, retroauricular, and mastoid regions. The examination continues from the mastoid bone down to the line of the trapezius into the posterior triangle and then toward the supraclavicular fossa. On reaching the suprasternal notch, palpation continues superiorly along the anterior border of the sterno-cleidomastoid muscle. The patient's neck should be flexed to the examining side to allow for adequate displacement of the sternocleidomas-toid muscle and, thus, deep palpation. Alternate sides are flexed to avoid simultaneous com-pression of the carotid arteries. The submental and submandibular nodes are then palpated to complete the cervical node assessment. The thyroid gland is also palpated at this time. The neck can then be auscultated for carotid or thyroid bruits.

Cranial Nerves

Assessment of the cranial nerves complements the examination of the nose and paranasal sinuses. Tumors of the maxillary sinus may result in dysfunction of cranial nerves III, IV, V, and VI, resulting in ophthalmoplegia. The optic nerve may become involved in extensive tumors. Naso-pharyngeal tumors may extend intracranially to affect the lower 4 cranial nerves as well as the abducens nerve. The facial nerve may be affected by ear infections or Bell palsy.

SUMMARY

The examination of the ear, nose, throat, and sinuses continues to present a challenge to medical personnel because of the intricate anatomy. However, advances in medical tech-nology have prompted the evolution of the instru-mentation and techniques used to examine this anatomic region. This evolution allows for a more informative assessment of and more comfortable experience for the patient. A detailed examination provides vital information for the definitive man-agement and subsequent outcome.

REFERENCES

1. McMinn RM. Last's anatomy regional and applied. 9th edition. Edinburgh (UK): Churchill Livingstone; 1994.
2. Williams PL, Warwick R, Dyson M, editors. Gray's anatomy. 37th edition. Edinburgh (UK): Churchill Livingstone; 1989.
3. Stammberger H. Functional endoscopic sinus surgery. Philadelphia: BC Decker; 1991.
4. Constantinides M, Doud Galli SK, Miller PJ. A simple and reliable method of patient evaluation in the surgical treatment of nasal obstruction. Ear Nose Throat J 2002;81:734–7.
5. Stammberger H. The evolution of functional endo-scopic sinus surgery. Ear Nose Throat J 1994;73(7): 451, 454–5.
6. Douglas G, Nicol F, Robertson C, editors. Macleod's clinical examination. Edinburgh (UK): Churchill Livingstone; 2005.
7. Kennedy DW. Functional endoscopic sinus surgery: technique. Arch Otolaryngol 1985;111:643–9.

Imaging of the Paranasal Sinuses

R. Joshua Dym, MD[a],*, Daniel Masri, MD[b],
Keivan Shifteh, MD[b]

KEYWORDS

- Paranasal sinuses • Imaging • Radiology
- Computed tomography • Magnetic resonance imaging

Evaluation of the paranasal sinuses is often performed in a purely clinical fashion, without the need for imaging. However, in certain instances imaging may be deemed valuable or even necessary in helping to solve a diagnostic dilemma, confirm a suspected diagnosis, evaluate the extent of a known condition, or assess for an underlying cause of the condition. Although evaluation of the effects of trauma is beyond the scope of this article, imaging of the facial bones, including the paranasal sinuses, is certainly essential in this setting to evaluate for fractures and associated injuries.

METHODS

In the past, plain radiographs were considered a useful imaging examination of the paranasal sinuses. With the advent of more advanced imaging such as computed tomography (CT), the use of plain radiographs has mostly fallen by the wayside because of its relatively low sensitivity and specificity for most conditions.[1] Although plain radiography is still used at times in the setting of trauma or to assess for sinus opacification (or air-fluid levels) in the setting of suspected sinusitis, it is now generally accepted that CT is the imaging examination of choice for these indications.[1–4] Iodinated intravenous contrast may be used to improve CT evaluation in certain situations, but it is not routinely administered for initial examinations.

CT with use of a bone algorithm reconstruction has the advantage of providing excellent anatomic depiction of the paranasal sinuses, including the fine details of the outflow tracts. Standard CT with soft tissue windows best displays the internal contents of the sinuses and can depict complications of various sinus conditions. Furthermore, with newer multidetector CT scanning, examination time is brief and easily tolerated while providing images of very high resolution. Coronal images are useful to the surgeon, as they correlate well with their endoscopic perspective. With the isotropic imaging provided by 64-slice CT, reconstructions can easily be created in any plane, with equally high resolution as standard axial plane images.[5] Moreover, this allows for the creation of 3-dimensional reconstructions that may aid in surgical planning. Sinus surgery can also be greatly facilitated by preoperative imaging, often performed with a stereotactic headset on the patient, which enables precise intraoperative imaging-guided navigation.[6]

One disadvantage of CT relative to plain radiography is the increased radiation exposure, which has received much attention within the medical community and lay press in recent years. Regarding imaging of the sinuses, the primary concern is the increased risk of cataracts resulting from the effects of radiation on the radiosensitive lenses. However, studies have shown that even after multiple CT examinations, the radiation dose

The authors have nothing to disclose.
[a] Division of Emergency Radiology, Department of Radiology, Albert Einstein College of Medicine, Montefiore Medical Center, 111 East 210th Street, Bronx, NY 10467, USA
[b] Division of Neuroradiology, Department of Radiology, Albert Einstein College of Medicine, Montefiore Medical Center, 111 East 210th Street, Bronx, NY 10467, USA
* Corresponding author.
E-mail address: joshdym@yahoo.com

Oral Maxillofacial Surg Clin N Am 24 (2012) 175–189
doi:10.1016/j.coms.2012.01.004
1042-3699/12/$ – see front matter © 2012 Elsevier Inc. All rights reserved.

oralmaxsurgery.theclinics.com

to the lens is still well below known thresholds of clinical damage.[7] Nevertheless, for certain indications such as evaluation for sinusitis, particularly in younger patients, a low-dose CT protocol is usually sufficient and therefore warranted.[8]

With its superior tissue contrast discrimination, magnetic resonance imaging (MRI) plays an important role in the evaluation of intracranial and intraorbital complications of sinusitis, and is also used in conjunction with CT to evaluate neoplasms of the paranasal sinuses.[9,10] However, with the exception of those uncommon situations, MRI of the paranasal sinuses is not routinely performed because of its higher cost and inferior depiction of fine bony detail in comparison with CT.[1,11] Nevertheless, when MRI is used for other (usually brain-related) indications, the paranasal sinuses are included in the examination and may yield findings. As such, a cursory knowledge of the MRI appearances of sinus disease is useful.

Positron emission tomography (PET), performed in tandem with CT or MRI, may be of value in the initial workup of certain malignancies involving the sinuses, and is also an excellent tool in the assessment of response to therapy and in screening for recurrence.[12] Nuclear imaging may also be used in the evaluation of a suspected cerebrospinal fluid (CSF) leak (see later discussion).[13]

ANATOMY

As the paranasal sinuses are essentially pockets of air enclosed by bone, CT, which provides the best definition of bony structures as well as the highest resolution, is considered the examination of choice in evaluating paranasal sinus anatomy (**Fig. 1**). The paranasal sinuses are composed of paired frontal, ethmoid, sphenoid, and maxillary sinuses. Unlike the other sinuses, which are generally composed of a single compartment, the ethmoid sinuses are actually a conglomerate of numerous air cells. Furthermore, they are best thought of as 2 separate zones, with the anterior/middle and posterior ethmoid air cells generally draining via separate outflow tracts. The ethmoid and maxillary sinuses are present at birth, whereas the frontal and sphenoid sinuses develop during early childhood.[9]

Outflow Tracts

Mucociliary clearance of the paranasal sinuses into the nasal cavity occurs via several different pathways. Maxillary sinus secretions drain through a superomedially located ostium and enter the infundibulum, which is a path located lateral to a bony extension called the uncinate process (see **Fig. 1A**). Mucus then traverses the infundibulum to reach the hiatus semilunaris, which is just superior to the uncinate process and inferior to the largest ethmoid air cell, the ethmoid (or ethmoidal) bulla. At this point, the secretions drain posteromedially via the middle meatus into the nasal cavity. The combination of the aforementioned anatomic structures and pathways comprise the ostiomeatal complex. Approximately 30% of persons also have

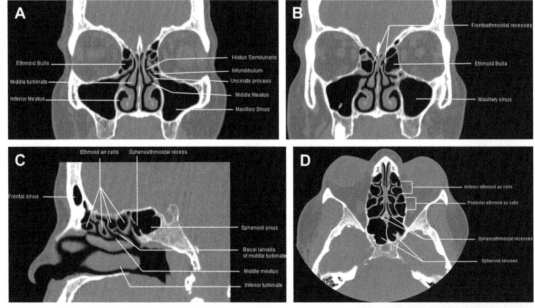

Fig. 1. (*A–D*) Coronal, sagittal, and axial CT images with bone windows demonstrate the anatomy of the paranasal sinuses, including outflow tracts.

an accessory maxillary sinus ostium, which provides an alternative pathway for drainage of mucus directly into the nasal cavity.[9]

The middle meatus is also a final common drainage pathway for the frontal and anterior/middle ethmoid air cells, which drain via the frontal (or frontoethmoidal) recess (see **Fig. 1**B). Secretions of the posterior ethmoid air cells and sphenoid sinus flow into the sphenoethmoidal recess to drain via the superior meatus (see **Fig. 1**C and D).[14]

Anatomic Variants

Paranasal sinus anatomic variations are extremely common, particularly involving the ethmoid air cells. In some instances, these variations may contribute to paranasal sinus outflow tract obstruction and may therefore be an important target of sinus surgery for chronic sinusitis. Furthermore, to avoid damaging adjacent structures it is important that before performing sinus surgery, the surgeon should be aware of certain anatomic variations, including those described here.[14,15]

Agger nasi cells

Present in most individuals, agger nasi cells are the anteriormost ethmoid air cells, just inferior to the frontal sinus (**Fig. 2**). In some cases, large agger nasi cells may contribute to blockage of the frontoethmoidal recess.[16]

Enlarged ethmoid bulla

The ethmoid (or ethmoidal) bulla is located superior and posterior to the infundibulum and hiatus semilunaris (see **Fig. 1**A). A congenitally large ethmoid bulla can therefore encroach on these structures and result in obstruction of the ostiomeatal complex.[9]

Haller cell

A Haller (infraorbital) cell is a commonly seen variant caused by inferolateral extension of ethmoid air cells below the orbital floor (**Fig. 3**). When enlarged, these Haller cells may result in narrowing of the infundibulum and/or ostium of the maxillary sinus.[9]

Concha bullosa

Pneumatization of the middle turbinate is termed a concha bullosa (**Fig. 4**). When enlarged, a concha bullosa may rarely result in sinusitis by obstructing the ostiomeatal complex, especially when present in conjunction with another anatomic variant contributing to the obstruction.[14]

Onodi cell

A posterior ethmoid air cell extending into the sphenoid bone is known as an Onodi (sphenoethmoid) cell (**Fig. 5**). Knowledge of this variation is important before undertaking endoscopic sinus surgery, because of its close relation to the optic nerve and internal carotid artery, and the necessity to avoid passing through this cell and damaging one of these structures.[8]

INFLAMMATORY SINUS DISEASE

Inflammatory disease of the paranasal sinuses is a ubiquitous condition that results in tens of millions of health care visits in the United States each year, with annual health care expenditures estimated at more than \$5.8 billion.[17] Most cases of acute sinusitis follow viral upper respiratory infections.[9] Aside from typical upper respiratory

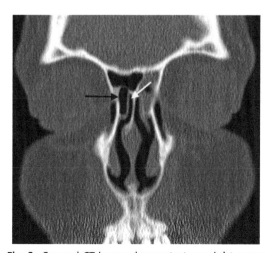

Fig. 2. Coronal CT image demonstrates a right agger nasi cell (*black arrow*) resulting in narrowing of the right frontoethmoidal recess (*white arrow*). Left frontal sinus disease is incidentally noted.

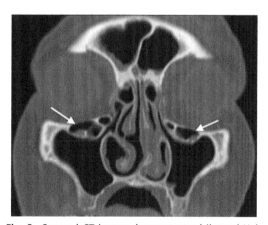

Fig. 3. Coronal CT image demonstrates bilateral Haller cells (*arrows*) narrowing the maxillary ostia. Also noted is mucosal thickening involving the frontal sinuses and left nasal cavity.

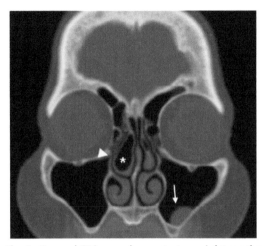

Fig. 4. Coronal CT image demonstrates a right concha bullosa (*asterisk*) narrowing the right maxillary ostium /infundibulum (*arrowhead*). Incidentally noted is a left maxillary sinus retention cyst or polyp (*arrow*).

symptoms, headache and/or facial pain often raises suspicion for sinusitis. Although this is a diagnosis that may be made clinically, in uncertain cases imaging is often performed for clarification, usually in the form of an unenhanced head CT. One situation that would certainly warrant imaging evaluation is generalized headache or orbital pain in the setting of sinusitis, as this may reflect intracranial or intraorbital extension of infection, respectively. MRI is considered the gold standard for detection and evaluation of these dangerous complications.[1,9]

Acute Sinusitis

Sinus mucosal inflammation results in submucosal edema, which is readily seen on CT or MRI as

mucosal thickening (see **Fig. 3**). Contrast-enhanced examinations will more clearly show enhancing mucosa with underlying edema, which will be low density on CT and high in signal intensity on T2-weighted MRI. However, mucosal thickening is an extremely common incidental finding, which is not necessarily related to an acute infection. Mucosal swelling may result in ostial obstruction with retention of secretions, providing a favorable environment for growth of pathogens. The resulting sinus opacification is more suggestive of sinusitis (**Fig. 6**). On the basis of pure imaging, however, sinus opacification does not establish acuity of the sinusitis; in fact, sinus opacification is often chronic and may be asymptomatic.[1,18] In addition, the finding of sinus opacification in children is of limited significance, as it may be a consequence of redundant mucosa and congestion caused by crying.[18]

One useful sign of acute bacterial sinusitis that is often relied on is an air-fluid level, which is usually a result of ostial obstruction preventing fluid drainage (**Fig. 7**). However, this finding is not very sensitive, as it is only believed to be present in 25% to 50% of cases of acute sinusitis.[18,19] Furthermore, there are a few other causes of air-fluid levels, first among them being sinonasal lavage, which is often performed by those with chronic sinus disease. This practice may result in residual saline within the sinuses for 2 to 4 days; acute sinusitis should not be diagnosed unless air-fluid levels remain for at least 7 days after lavage.[18] Air-fluid levels are also commonly seen in the setting of nasogastric tubes and/or prolonged supine positioning, which prevents normal sinus drainage. After a few days, diffuse sinus opacification may also develop; these findings all usually resolve following extubation and as soon

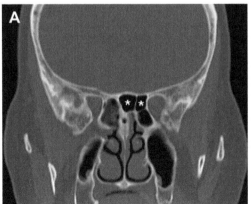

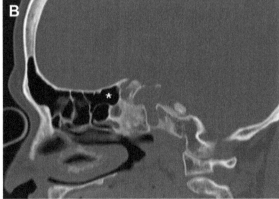

Fig. 5. (*A, B*) Coronal and sagittal CT images demonstrate posterior ethmoid air cells that extend into the sphenoid bone superior to the sinus; these are known as Onodi cells (*asterisks*); they are in close proximity to the optic nerve.

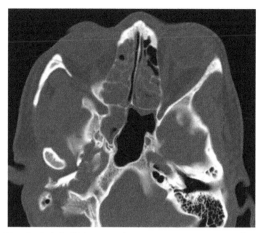

Fig. 6. Axial CT image demonstrates near complete opacification of the right sphenoid and bilateral ethmoid sinuses, as well as left sphenoid sinus mucosal thickening. This patient presented with complaints of headache for 1 week and fever.

as the patient can vary head position. Air-fluid levels caused by intrasinus blood may also be seen after trauma or in patients with bleeding disorders. This situation does not usually present a diagnostic dilemma; nevertheless, the high density on CT (or high signal intensity on T1-weighted MRI) usually helps confirm that the fluid is blood.[18] The presence of blood within the sinuses after trauma should prompt a more vigilant search for an associated fracture (**Fig. 8**).

There are various patterns of sinusitis. Diffuse sinusitis or pansinusitis is usually secondary to

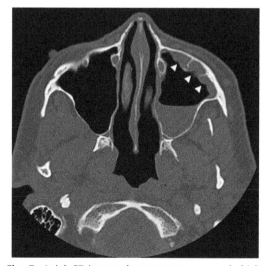

Fig. 7. Axial CT image demonstrates mucosal thickening of the anterior wall of the left maxillary sinus (*arrowheads*) with an associated air-fluid level, indicating acute sinusitis.

allergies. By contrast, asymmetric sinusitis involving only certain sinuses is usually a sign of bacterial sinusitis resulting from ostial obstruction.[18]

Knowledge of the anatomy of the paranasal sinus drainage pathways is critical to the understanding of the different patterns of sinusitis. Sonkens and colleagues[20] described 5 patterns of paranasal sinus obstructive disease. Disease involving the infundibulum of the maxillary ostiomeatal complex will result in obstruction of only the maxillary sinus, known as the infundibular pattern of obstruction. However, a more distal obstruction at the level of the hiatus semilunaris/middle meatus will also result in obstruction of the ipsilateral frontal sinus as well as the anterior and middle ethmoid air cells, known as the ostiomeatal unit pattern. In the sphenoethmoidal recess pattern, the sphenoid sinus and ipsilateral posterior ethmoid air cells are affected by obstruction at the level of the sphenoethmoidal recess. The latter 2 patterns comprise the sinonasal polyposis pattern, in which multiple nasal and sinus polyps produce a combination of the first 3 patterns, and the sporadic pattern, in which retention cysts, mucoceles, and/or postsurgical changes produce a pattern unrelated to a specific drainage pathway. The type of surgery required to resolve the obstruction and alleviate the symptoms is dictated by the specific pattern and the cause of the obstruction.[5,14]

Fungal Sinusitis

Fungal sinusitis may occur in several forms, ranging from benign and asymptomatic to extremely aggressive and life-threatening. Various fungi have been implicated in these varying forms of infection, but *Aspergillus* is the most common overall. Fungal sinusitis, including invasive and allergic types, should be considered in patients with chronic inflammation that has been unresponsive to antibiotics.[5]

Invasive fungal sinusitis

Invasive fungal sinusitis is generally attributable to *Aspergillus* or *Mucor* species, and usually occurs in immunosuppressed patients; this is especially true for the highly aggressive and often lethal fulminant form of fungal sinusitis.[9] Air-fluid levels are uncommon in fungal sinusitis. The maxillary or ethmoid sinuses are usually involved, with thickening, erosion, or remodeling of adjacent bone often seen, especially in the chronic invasive form (**Fig. 9**).[18] Fungal sinusitis often demonstrates high density on CT and low signal intensity on both T1- and T2-weighted MRI. Punctate calcifications in the center of the sinus are also strongly

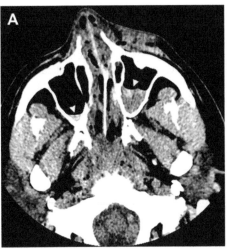
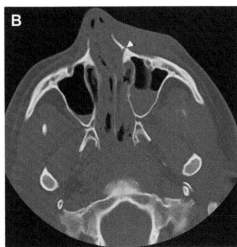

Fig. 8. (*A*) Axial CT image (in soft tissue windows) demonstrates premalar swelling/hematoma and high-density material layering in both maxillary sinuses (*arrowheads*) in a patient who experienced facial trauma. (*B*) When viewed in bone windows, the same axial CT image demonstrates fractures of the left lamina papyracea (*black arrowhead*) and frontal process of the maxilla (*white arrowhead*). The dense maxillary sinus fluid in *A* represents blood.

suggestive of fungal infection.[9] Soft tissue infiltration adjacent to the sinuses can occur and may also raise the possibility of invasive fungal sinusitis. Furthermore, fungal sinusitis tends to invade the orbit, cavernous sinus, and intracranial cavity, often spreading along vessels. MRI is of great value in detecting such invasion, especially in patients with the fulminant form of fungal infection.[2,5]

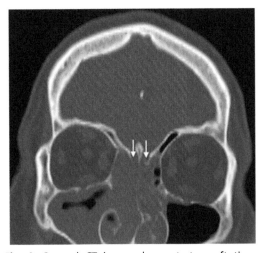

Fig. 9. Coronal CT image demonstrates soft tissue density material filling the nasal cavities and paranasal sinuses with dehiscence of the cribriform plates bilaterally (*arrows*), consistent with an aggressive process. This patient was diagnosed with invasive fungal sinusitis.

Noninvasive fungal sinus disease

Nonaggressive fungal colonization of the sinuses, usually with *Aspergillus*, may occur in immunocompetent patients. CT may demonstrate dense polypoid fungal balls, termed mycetomas or aspergillomas, often with dense foci at their center. The fungal ball may cause bony expansion, but only rarely does it produce erosion.[21] Allergic fungal sinusitis is another relatively benign entity resulting from a hypersensitivity reaction to fungi within the sinuses, usually in patients with a history of allergic sinusitis or asthma.[5] It is characterized by opacified sinuses containing material of low signal intensity on both T1- and T2-weighted MRI and increased density on CT (**Fig. 10**). Expansion of sinus walls, bony erosion, or remodeling and thinning are common features.[9]

Chronic Sinusitis

Chronic sinusitis is characterized clinically by repeated or persistent episodes of acute or subacute sinusitis. Up to one-third of patients with acute sinusitis may develop some evidence of chronic sinusitis.[18] Aside from mucosal thickening, retention cysts, and polyps (see later discussion) related to chronically inflamed mucosa, as well as other radiographic signs of acute sinus disease that may be present, chronic sinusitis is characterized by thickened, sclerotic bone surrounding the chronically infected sinus (**Fig. 11**). Although sinonasal secretions in acute sinusitis usually demonstrate low signal intensity on T1-weighted MRI and high signal intensity on

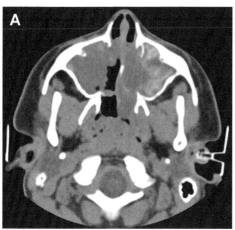
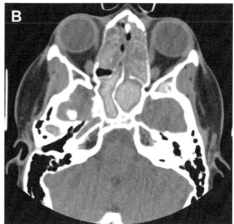

Fig. 10. (*A, B*) Axial CT images demonstrate high-density material along the wall of the left maxillary sinus, filling the ethmoid and sphenoid sinuses in this patient with allergic fungal sinusitis.

T2-weighted MRI, the higher protein concentration of the retained desiccated secretions often present in chronic sinusitis may result in different patterns of MRI signal intensity. Nevertheless, the peripheral enhancement pattern should still allow differentiation from neoplasm filling the sinus, which would be expected to have central enhancement. With chronic obstruction, the secretions within the involved sinus may also continue to accumulate with development of a mucocele (see later discussion).[18]

COMPLICATIONS OF SINUSITIS

There are several common complications of inflammatory sinus disease; these may persist even after resolution of acute inflammation and

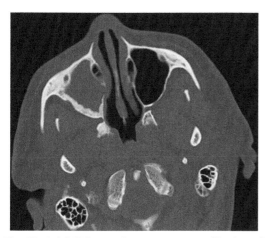

Fig. 11. Axial CT image demonstrates opacification of the right maxillary sinus with sclerosis and thickening of its wall, typical of chronic sinusitis. The left maxillary sinus has normal wall thickness.

are commonly detected incidentally. There are also several less common complications of sinusitis, some of which may cause significant morbidity.

Mucocele

A mucocele is a complication of sinusitis whereby a sinus, most commonly a frontal sinus, becomes obstructed and chronically filled with secretions, with complete opacification of the sinus. Over time, this condition results in bony remodeling and expansion of the sinus, with bony thinning and/or dehiscence. These bony changes are best seen on CT (**Fig. 12**A).[18] Although initially low density on CT, the secretions in the setting of a mucocele desiccate over time and become increasingly dense. The MRI appearance of a mucocele is variable, with signal characteristics also dependent on the chronicity of the condition (see **Fig. 12**B). However, one important differentiating imaging feature from a solid mass is that a mucocele may only demonstrate rim enhancement after contrast administration; any internal enhancement should lead to consideration of other lesions, such as polyps, inverted papillomas, or malignancies.[22] Mucoceles that become infected are termed mucopyoceles, which are more likely to demonstrate rim enhancement but may also develop more invasive features.[23] Mucoceles may present with signs and symptoms resulting from the mass effect of the lesion, typically proptosis caused by pressure on orbital contents (see **Fig. 12**).[18]

Retention Cyst

Unlike a mucocele, which is caused by obstruction of a sinus outflow tract, a retention cyst is the result of obstruction of a single submucosal

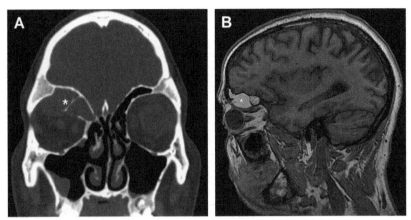

Fig. 12. (*A*) Coronal CT image demonstrates complete opacification and expansion of the right frontal sinus (*asterisk*), typical of a mucocele, with dehiscence of the inferior wall of the frontal sinus and mass effect on the orbital contents. The globe is displaced anterior to the plane of this image. (*B*) Sagittal MR image in the same patient again demonstrates a frontal sinus mucocele (*asterisk*) with mass effect on the globe. The secretions within the sinus demonstrate high signal intensity on this T1-weighted image, typical of desiccated secretions with high protein concentration.

mucinous gland within a sinus. These cysts have a characteristic convex appearance arising from the wall of a sinus, most commonly a maxillary sinus (see **Fig. 4**). When in a dependent location, their convex border should prevent confusion with a fluid level related to sinusitis. Serous retention cysts can also form, resulting from an accumulation of serous fluid in the submucosal space.[18] Retention cysts are commonly seen in studies performed for indications other than sinus disease and are frequently not associated with clinical symptoms.[10]

Polyps

Polyps may be related to allergic sinusitis or may be a result of hyperplasia caused by chronic inflammation.[9] The CT appearance of small polyps is usually indistinguishable from a retention cyst;

however, the distinction is inconsequential because intervention or follow-up is generally unnecessary for either of these benign diagnoses.[18] When a large polyp arising within the maxillary sinus extends through the maxillary sinus ostium into the posterior nasal cavity, it is termed an antrochoanal polyp (**Fig. 13**). The significance of this imaging diagnosis relates to surgical planning. Knowledge of the polyp's origin within the maxillary sinus should prevent incomplete resection whereby only the nasal portion of an antrochoanal polyp is removed; this would likely lead to recurrence.[10]

Sinonasal Polyposis

Sinonasal polyposis is a chronic inflammatory condition that may be associated with allergies, asthma, cystic fibrosis, and aspirin intolerance.

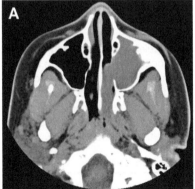
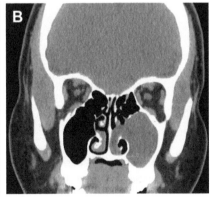

Fig. 13. (*A, B*) Axial and coronal CT images (in soft tissue windows) demonstrate an antrochoanal polyp filling the left maxillary sinus and extending through the accessory maxillary ostium into the nasal cavity.

As already described, sinonasal polyposis is the pattern of inflammatory paranasal sinus disease whereby numerous nasal and sinus polyps obstruct sinus outflow tracts.[20] In some cases the individual polyps cannot be discerned, because of the complete opacification of the sinuses and nasal cavity; however, their presence may be inferred by the secondary bone thinning and remodeling with expansion of outflow tracts (**Fig. 14**).[24] The CT and MRI appearance of multiple confluent polyps may overlap with that of certain malignancies; however, the typical peripheral enhancement pattern of polyps can often help in making this important distinction.[9] This condition may be treated surgically or with steroids, but recurrence is frequent.[15,24]

Extrasinus Extension of Infection

Acute sinusitis can occasionally spread to areas adjacent to the paranasal sinuses, with potentially serious effects. The most common example of this is intraorbital extension of ethmoid sinusitis, facilitated by the thin lamina papyracea and valveless ethmoidal veins (**Fig. 15**).[18] This condition results in the development of a subperiosteal abscess of the medial orbital wall, with displacement of the medial rectus muscle and orbital fat, often with associated preseptal or postseptal cellulitis.[25]

Less commonly, sinusitis may spread intracranially and result in meningitis or an epidural, subdural, or cerebral abscess (**Fig. 16**). Intracranial spread is most common with frontal sinusitis and is less commonly seen with ethmoid or sphenoid sinusitis, which may in part be due to the presence of a rich venous plexus between the frontal sinus mucosa and the meninges.[18] Although abscesses will usually be seen on unenhanced examinations, contrast is necessary to demonstrate the meningeal enhancement of meningitis.[9] Although CT is often performed first, contrast-enhanced MRI has greater sensitivity for intracranial or intraorbital extension of infection, and also better defines the full extent of disease.[2,26]

Frontal sinusitis may also spread externally to result in a subgaleal abscess overlying the frontal bone, known as a Pott puffy tumor (see **Fig. 16**). This tumor is often associated with osteomyelitis of the frontal bone, especially in the setting of chronic sinusitis.[18,27]

Silent Sinus Syndrome

Chronic maxillary sinusitis with ostial obstruction may lead to persistent negative pressure, resulting in retraction of sinus walls and orbital floor with a reduction of sinus volume, known as silent sinus syndrome (**Fig. 17**).[9] Although it may initially be asymptomatic, this condition is characterized by the eventual development of enophthalmos and facial asymmetry.[28] A congenitally hypoplastic maxillary sinus may have a similar radiographic appearance.[9]

BENIGN NEOPLASMS

In addition to the described inflammatory lesions resulting from sinusitis, there are several types of benign neoplasms that may arise within the paranasal sinuses. Similar to the aforementioned lesions, these may be clinically silent or may produce symptoms that lead to their detection.

Inverted Papilloma

There are several varieties of sinonasal papillomas, of which the most common is the inverted papilloma.[9] These benign neoplasms generally

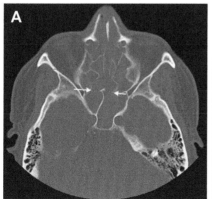
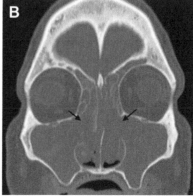

Fig. 14. (*A, B*) Axial and coronal CT images demonstrate soft tissue filling the paranasal sinuses and nasal cavities, with expansion of bilateral sphenoethmoidal recesses (*white arrows*) and bilateral ostiomeatal units (*black arrows*) in this patient with sinonasal polyposis.

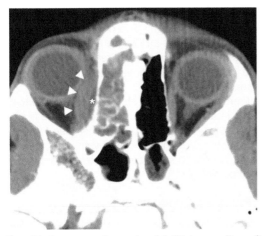

Fig. 15. Contrast-enhanced axial CT image (in soft tissue windows) demonstrates right ethmoid sinus inflammatory disease with an associated right lamina papyracea subperiosteal abscess (*asterisk*), which displaces the medial rectus muscle laterally (*arrowheads*).

arise from the lateral nasal wall and extend into the maxillary and/or ethmoid sinuses (**Fig. 18**). This lesion often presents a diagnostic dilemma because it has a similar radiographic appearance to malignancy, especially when it causes bone destruction.[5] Inverted papillomas commonly contain calcifications, which are believed to actually represent residual bone fragments.[29] On MRI, a striated cerebriform pattern on T2-weighted and contrast-enhanced T1-weighted images is supportive but not diagnostic.[30] In addition to being difficult to distinguish from malignancy, inverted papillomas coexist with squamous cell carcinoma in approximately 15% of cases. As such, it is generally resected with wide margins; nevertheless, recurrence is frequent.[5,9]

Osteoma

An osteoma is a benign growth of mature bone arising from within a bone. Osteomas are commonly seen in the membranous bones of the skull and face, frequently involving the frontal or ethmoid sinuses (**Fig. 19**).[29] These lesions may obstruct the frontal sinus, often producing intermittent headaches and/or sinusitis, and occasionally resulting in a mucocele. Occasionally they may extend into the orbit and cause a mass effect on intraorbital contents. Rarely an osteoma may breach the posterior wall of the frontal sinus and result in pneumocephalus. In most cases, however, osteomas are completely asymptomatic and clinically irrelevant. Osteomas are easily detected on CT as dense bony masses protruding into or from the sinus. However, they are usually invisible on MRI because of the lack of signal from dense compact bone.[9] Multiple osteomas may also be seen as a manifestation of Gardner syndrome, a rare autosomal dominant polyposis syndrome.[29] There are also several other benign osseous tumors, including osteochondromas and exostoses, which may have a similar imaging appearance.

Fibrous Dysplasia

Fibrous dysplasia is an idiopathic condition whereby medullary bone is replaced with abnormal fibro-osseous tissue (**Fig. 20**). Patients with the polyostotic form of this condition commonly have craniofacial involvement, including involvement of the paranasal sinuses, which can lead to obstruction of outflow tracts and may occasionally result in a mucocele.[29] Fibrous dysplasia anywhere in the skeleton has a classic ground-glass appearance on radiographs or CT, which may vary slightly depending on the amount

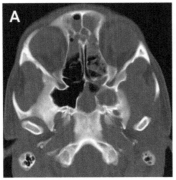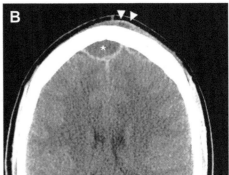

Fig. 16. (*A*) Axial CT image (in bone windows) demonstrates inflammatory disease involving the frontal, ethmoid, and left sphenoid sinuses. (*B*) Axial CT image from the same examination (in brain windows) at a slightly higher level than in *A* demonstrates that the frontal sinusitis has resulted in an epidural abscess (*asterisk*) as well as an overlying frontal bone subgaleal abscess (*arrowheads*), otherwise known as a Pott puffy tumor.

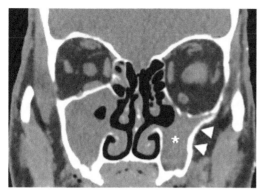

Fig. 17. Coronal CT image (in soft tissue windows) demonstrates an opacified left maxillary sinus (*asterisk*) with inferior retraction of the roof of the sinus (orbital floor) and medial retraction of the lateral sinus wall (*arrowheads*), typical of silent sinus syndrome.

of fibrous tissue present; the appearance may also overlap with ossifying fibroma, another benign fibro-osseous lesion. Fibrous dysplasia generally expands the medullary space, with a thin rim of surrounding cortex often remaining intact.[29]

Odontogenic Lesions

Although not directly arising from the sinuses, there are several types of developmental and odontogenic cysts and tumors that may secondarily involve the sinuses, including radicular and dentigerous cysts (**Fig. 21**), odontogenic keratocyst, and ameloblastoma.[29]

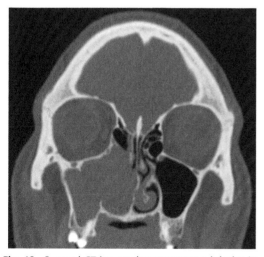

Fig. 18. Coronal CT image demonstrates a lobular inverted papilloma arising from the right nasal cavity, which has extended through and enlarged the middle meatus and infundibulum and has filled the maxillary sinus.

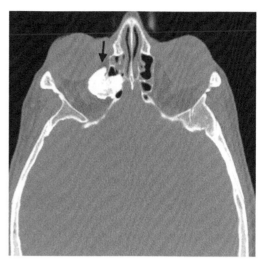

Fig. 19. Axial CT image demonstrates a large ossific mass (*arrow*) arising from the right ethmoid sinus and extending into the orbit, with mass effect on the intraorbital contents. This appearance is typical of an ethmoid osteoma.

MALIGNANT NEOPLASMS

Although uncommon, malignancies involving the paranasal sinuses are significant because they generally have poor outcomes, often the result of a delayed diagnosis made partly because such neoplasms may remain clinically silent until an advanced stage. In addition, coexisting inflammatory sinusitis resulting from neoplastic sinus obstruction may confound the clinical presentation. Furthermore, the complex location of these tumors and cosmetic considerations often limit aggressive surgical resection.[29] CT and MRI play complementary roles in the evaluation of sinonasal malignancies, with CT providing information regarding bony destruction and MRI providing superior soft tissue contrast and better definition of tumor invasion of the epidural space, meninges, orbit, or skull base. MRI is also superior in distinguishing tumor from the commonly coexisting sinus inflammatory disease.[9]

Squamous Cell Carcinoma

Squamous cell carcinoma usually presents as a large mass, with solid enhancement on CT and MRI helping to differentiate it from inflammatory disease or a mucocele.[9] Furthermore, as with most sinonasal tumors, squamous cell carcinoma demonstrates intermediate to slightly low signal intensity on T2-weighted MRI, which aids in the distinction of tumor from adjacent inflammatory tissue.[29] As already mentioned, contrast-enhanced MRI is also important in the assessment of epidural or meningeal invasion.

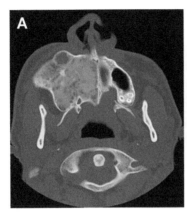
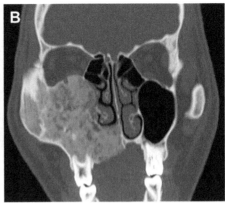

Fig. 20. (*A, B*) Axial and coronal CT images demonstrate bony expansion of the right maxilla with a ground-glass appearance typical of fibrous dysplasia. The right maxillary sinus is obliterated.

Once the presence of malignancy is established using CT and/or MRI, squamous cell carcinoma is the most likely diagnosis, as it comprises approximately 80% of all paranasal sinus malignancies. Although there is significant overlap with the imaging appearance of several other types of neoplasm, one characteristic feature of squamous cell carcinomas is their aggressive bone destruction (**Fig. 22**). However, it should be noted that such bony destruction may also be seen less commonly with certain types of sarcoma, lymphoma, and metastatic disease. By contrast, benign conditions such as mucoceles, polyps, and inverted papillomas will generally remodel bone rather than destroy it.[29] In addition, benign lesions can often be differentiated by their rounded, polypoid appearance.[9]

Sinonasal Undifferentiated Carcinoma

Sinonasal undifferentiated carcinoma is a very aggressive malignancy that has the appearance of an advanced squamous cell carcinoma. It favors the ethmoid sinuses and is often necrotic, with heterogeneous enhancement.[31]

Minor Salivary Gland Tumors

Approximately 10% of all sinonasal tumors are of glandular origin, with most arising in minor salivary glands.[29] This category includes adenoid cystic carcinoma, benign or malignant pleomorphic adenoma, mucoepidermoid carcinoma, adenocarcinoma not otherwise specified, and a few

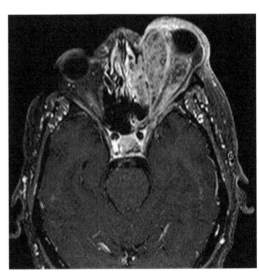

Fig. 22. Axial contrast-enhanced T1-weighted MR image (with fat suppression) demonstrates an enhancing squamous cell carcinoma arising from the left ethmoid sinus and extending through the lamina papyracea into the left orbit, causing significant proptosis.

Fig. 21. Coronal CT image demonstrates a cyst surrounding the crown of an unerupted tooth (*arrow*), typical of a dentigerous cyst.

rare others. As opposed to most sinonasal malignancies, minor salivary gland tumors may sometimes demonstrate high signal intensity on T2-weighted MRI, depending on their histology and the presence of cysts or necrosis.[9] This appearance helps in the differentiation from squamous cell carcinoma but may hinder its delineation from associated inflammatory disease, although contrast administration may help in this regard. MRI with contrast is particularly important in the evaluation of adenoid cystic carcinoma, as it tends to have perineural spread.[9]

Other malignancies in the sinonasal adenocarcinoma family include sinonasal neuroendocrine carcinoma and the so-called intestinal-type adenocarcinoma, both of which are essentially indistinguishable from squamous cell carcinoma on imaging (**Fig. 23**).[29]

Melanoma

Although it is more commonly seen in the nasal cavity, melanoma may also occur in the paranasal sinuses. One distinguishing feature of some melanomas is high signal intensity on T1-weighted MRI, due to the presence of melanin and/or hemorrhage.[32] Also, the presence of multiple lesions related to melanosis is suggestive of melanoma.[9]

Lymphoma

There are several forms of sinonasal lymphoma. T-cell lymphoma is more common and usually occurs in the nose or ethmoid sinuses; B-cell lymphoma favors the maxillary sinuses. T-cell/natural killer cell nasal lymphoma is in the spectrum of posttransplant lymphoproliferative disease and is usually more aggressive.[9] Sinonasal lymphomas appear as bulky, enhancing soft tissue masses on CT and MRI. Bone remodeling is common, although aggressive bone invasion may be present, especially with the natural killer cell phenotype.[29] Sinonasal lymphoma is also often associated with cervical lymphadenopathy.[9]

Metastases

Metastases of other primary malignancies may also rarely involve the paranasal sinuses. Of the remote malignancies, renal cell carcinoma is the most common. Multiple myeloma may also involve the walls of the paranasal sinuses. Of the local malignancies, nasopharyngeal carcinoma has a high rate of spread to the sinuses.[9] In addition, chondrosarcoma or osteosarcoma arising in the facial bones may invade the sinuses.[29]

POSTSURGICAL IMAGING

CT or MRI performed after endoscopic sinus surgery will demonstrate postsurgical changes with evidence of bone resection and widening of outflow tracts, including the ostiomeatal complexes. Sinus opacification commonly persists after surgery, even when symptoms have improved (**Fig. 24**). Mucosal thickening seen on postoperative imaging may represent fibrosis or

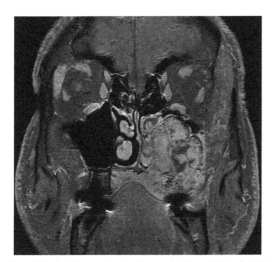

Fig. 23. Axial contrast-enhanced T1-weighted MR image (with fat suppression) demonstrates a destructive enhancing mass filling the left maxillary sinus and invading the nasal cavity in this patient with adenocarcinoma. The solid enhancement pattern aids in distinction of this neoplasm from inflammatory disease.

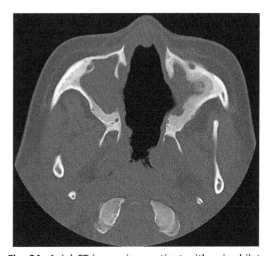

Fig. 24. Axial CT image in a patient with prior bilateral uncinectomies and ethmoidectomies demonstrates persistent or recurrent bilateral maxillary sinus inflammatory disease. There is also sclerosis involving the lateral walls of the maxillary sinuses bilaterally, consistent with chronic sinusitis.

inflammation; both may enhance and appear identical.[9,15]

In the acute setting of suspected postoperative complications, CT is usually the first imaging examination, and can assess for inadvertent resection of adjacent structures or the presence of an orbital hematoma compressing the optic nerve or its blood supply.[9,15] In obliterative frontal sinus surgery, fat may be used to plug the sinuses; incomplete obliteration may lead to mucoceles or recurrent sinusitis. Following such surgery, the postoperative frontal sinuses can be evaluated using MRI with fat suppression. With the progression of fibrosis, the signal intensity from fat will decrease.[9]

One serious complication of endoscopic sinus surgery is trauma to the cribriform plate resulting in a meningocele or encephalocele. An encephalocele is best diagnosed with MRI and must always be distinguished from sinus inflammation, scar tissue, or a mass, especially when biopsy of a sinus mass is being contemplated in a patient with a history of prior sinus surgery. Even without an encephalocele, damage to the cribriform plate and dura may result in a CSF leak, which may also lead to meningitis, epidural abscess, or pneumocephalus.[9] Aside from direct CT visualization of a bony defect, one method to assess for a CSF leak is to perform a CT cisternogram following intrathecal contrast instillation; the CT may demonstrate contrast localization at the site of the leak. MRI cisternography can also be used.[15]

A nuclear medicine examination, which has high sensitivity in the detection of a slow CSF leak, can also be used. Pledgets are placed in each nostril before intrathecal injection of indium-111–labeled diethylenetriamine pentaacetic acid. In addition to imaging of the head at half-hour intervals following lumbar puncture, the radioactivity of the pledgets is measured at 4 and 24 hours after placement and is compared with concurrently drawn blood samples.[13] Although this technique will detect any active leak of CSF during the 24-hour period and may also provide a general notion as to the side and location of the leak, it certainly does not afford the precise anatomic definition of CT or MRI techniques; these newer methods are therefore gradually replacing nuclear imaging, especially in cases of known CSF leaks.[9,15]

SUMMARY

Although imaging of the paranasal sinuses is unnecessary in most cases of inflammatory sinus disease, CT and MRI may often be useful or even vital in confirming a suspected diagnosis or providing additional information regarding causes or complications. CT provides exquisite anatomic detail and is a formidable aid in planning for endoscopic sinus surgery. Knowledge of the anatomy of the paranasal sinus outflow tracts and anatomic variants is essential for interpretation. CT and MRI play complementary roles in evaluating the rare benign and malignant tumors that may involve the paranasal sinuses.

REFERENCES

1. Yousem DM. Imaging of sinonasal inflammatory disease. Radiology 1993;188:303–14.
2. American College of Radiology. ACR Appropriateness Criteria®: sinonasal disease. Available at: http://www.acr.org/SecondaryMainMenuCategories/quality_safety/app_criteria/pdf/ExpertPanelonNeurologicImaging/SinonasalDisease.aspx. Accessed August 15, 2011.
3. Aalokken TM, Hagtvedt T, Dalen I, et al. Conventional sinus radiography compared with CT in the diagnosis of acute sinusitis. Dentomaxillofac Radiol 2003;32(1):60–2.
4. Yealy DM, Hogan DE. Imaging after head trauma: who needs what? Emerg Med Clin North Am 1991;9:707–17.
5. Momeni AK, Roberts CC, Chew FS. Imaging of chronic and exotic sinonasal disease: review. AJR Am J Roentgenol 2007;189(6):S35–45.
6. Anon JB, Klimak L. Stereotactic surgery. In: Levine HW, Clemente MP, editors. Sinus surgery: endoscopic and microscopic approaches. New York: Thieme; 2005. p. 219–30.
7. Bassim MK, Ebert CS, Sit RC, et al. Radiation dose to the eyes and parotids during CT of the sinuses. Otolaryngol Head Neck Surg 2005;133:531–3.
8. Zinreich SJ, Gotwald TF. Radiographic anatomy of the sinuses. In: Kennedy DW, Bolger WE, Zinreich SJ, editors. Diseases of the sinuses: diagnosis and management. Hamilton (Ontario): BC Decker; 2001. p. 13–28.
9. Grossman R, Yousem D. Sinonasal disease. In: Neuroradiology, the requisites. 2nd edition. Philadelphia: Mosby; 2003. p. 611–40.
10. Barakos JA. Head and neck imaging. In: Brant WE, Helms CA, editors. Fundamentals of diagnostic radiology. 3rd edition. Philadelphia: Lippincott Williams & Wilkins; 2007. p. 241–70.
11. Hahnel S, Ertl-Wagner B, Tasman AJ, et al. Relative value of MR imaging as compared with CT in the diagnosis of inflammatory paranasal sinus disease. Radiology 1999;210:171–6.
12. Czernin J, Dahlbom M, Ratib O, et al. Cancers of the head and neck. In: Atlas of PET/CT imaging in oncology. New York: Springer; 2004. p. 117–29.
13. Mettler FA, Guiberteau MJ. Cerebrovascular system. In: Essentials of nuclear medicine imaging. 5th

edition. Philadelphia: Saunders Elsevier; 2006. p. 53–73.

14. Zinreich SJ, Albayram S, Benson ML, et al. The ostiomeatal complex and functional endoscopic surgery. In: Som PM, Cutin HD, editors. Head and neck imaging. 4th edition. St Louis (MO): Mosby; 2003. p. 149–73.

15. Hudgins PA, Kingdom TT. Postoperative complications of functional endoscopic sinus surgery. In: Som PM, Cutin HD, editors. Head and neck imaging. 4th edition. St Louis (MO): Mosby; 2003. p. 175–92.

16. Gotwald TF, Zinreich SJ, Corl F, et al. Three-dimensional volumetric display of the nasal ostiomeatal channels and paranasal sinuses. AJR Am J Roentgenol 2001;176:241–5.

17. Ray NF, Baraniuk JN, Thamer M, et al. Healthcare expenditures for sinusitis in 1996: contributions of asthma, rhinitis, and other airway disorders. J Allergy Clin Immunol 1999;103(3):408–14.

18. Som PM, Brandwein MS. Inflammatory diseases. In: Som PM, Cutin HD, editors. Head and neck imaging. 4th edition. St Louis (MO): Mosby; 2003. p. 193–259.

19. Kuhn JP. Imaging of the paranasal sinuses: current status. J Allergy Clin Immunol 1986;77:6–9.

20. Sonkens JW, Harnsberger HR, Blanch GM, et al. The impact of screening sinus CT on the planning of functional endoscopic sinus surgery. Otolaryngol Head Neck Surg 1991;105:802–13.

21. Aygun NF, Yousem DM. Imaging of the nasal cavities, paranasal sinuses, nasopharynx, orbits, infratemporal fossa, pterygomaxillary fissure and base of skull. In: Snow JB, Wackym PA, editors. Ballenger's otorhinolaryngology: head and neck surgery. 17th edition. Hamilton (Ontario): BC Decker Inc; 2009. p. 501–18.

22. Lanzieri CF, Shah M, Krauss D, et al. Use of gadolinium-enhanced MR imaging for differentiating mucoceles from neoplasms in the paranasal sinuses. Radiology 1991;178:425–8.

23. Ada S, Yalamanchili M, Kambhampati G. Frontal sinus mucopyocele. Arch Intern Med 2002;162: 2487–8.

24. Drutman J, Babbel RW, Harnsberger HR, et al. Sinonasal polyposis. Semin Ultrasound CT MR 1991;12: 561–74.

25. Grossman R, Yousem D. Orbit. In: Neuroradiology, the requisites. 2nd edition. Philadelphia: Mosby; 2003. p. 469–516.

26. Younis RT, Anand VK, Davidson B. The role of computed tomography and magnetic resonance imaging in patients with sinusitis with complications. Laryngoscope 2002;112(2):224–9.

27. Kombogiorgas D, Solanki GA. The Pott puffy tumor revisited: neurosurgical implications of this unforgotten entity. Case report and review of the literature. J Neurosurg 2006;105(Suppl 2):143–9.

28. Illner A, Davidson HC, Harnsberger HR, et al. The silent sinus syndrome: clinical and radiographic findings. AJR Am J Roentgenol 2002;178(2):503–6.

29. Som PM, Brandwein MS. Tumors and tumor-like conditions. In: Som PM, Cutin HD, editors. Head and neck imaging. 4th edition. St Louis (MO): Mosby; 2003. p. 261–373.

30. Jeon TY, Kim HJ, Chung SK, et al. Sinonasal inverted papilloma: value of convoluted cerebriform pattern on MR imaging. AJNR Am J Neuroradiol 2008;29(8):1556–60.

31. Phillips CD, Futterer SF, Lipper MH, et al. Sinonasal undifferentiated carcinoma: CT and MR imaging of an uncommon neoplasm of the nasal cavity. Radiology 1997;202:477–80.

32. Yousem DM, Li C, Montone KT, et al. Primary malignant melanoma of the sinonasal cavity: MR evaluation. Radiographics 1996;16:1101–10.

Microorganisms of the Nose and Paranasal Sinuses

Richard H. Haug, DDS

KEYWORDS

- Microorganism • Nose • Paranasal • Sinus

From a teleologic standpoint, the human nose and paranasal sinuses developed from prehistoric ancestors with specific functions as the final outcome. The pneumatization of the craniofacial region by the nose and paranasal sinuses resulted in a lighter weight of the skull, allowing humans to begin standing upright, a departure from 4-legged mammalian relatives. The resonance provided by this pneumatization permitted the development of speech beyond simple barking and grunting to eventually more culturally unique capabilities such as chanting and ultimately singing. Although the vibrissae of the nose create physical barriers to foreign bodies ranging from insects to particulate matter, the moist mucosal lining of the nose and paranasal sinuses traps finer substances and microbes by mucostatic tension. The constant fasciculation by the villi of the pseudostratified columnar epithelial lining helps to eliminate these potentially disease-threatening foreign bodies and microbes. The moisture of this mucosa humidifies and warms the air before it enters the lungs. The endogenous normal flora of the nose and paranasal sinuses works to create an environment of homeostasis within the region. This homeostasis can be interrupted by eliminating the anatomic barriers created by the skin, bone, and mucosa, such as after trauma and/or surgery; by altering the atmosphere of the surroundings, such as the creation of an anaerobic environment by obstruction of the sinus ostia or foramina; or by a change in the normal flora of the region. To fully understand the microbiological environment of this region, it is first important to understand the normal flora of the nose and paranasal sinuses.

NORMAL MICROFLORA OF THE NOSE AND PARANASAL SINUSES

Nomenclature

Consistent nomenclature is the key to communication of the various microbes of the body from one health care professional to another. Taxonomy is the branch of biology that deals with classification, and the taxonomic classification system from the general to the most specific is kingdom, phylum, class, order, family, genus, and species.[1,2] To create consistency and uniformity during this review of microbes of the nose and paranasal sinuses, the descriptions of the Protista (bacteria, fungi, protozoa, and so forth), when speaking in general terms, will include only the genus. As an example, the genus *Staphylococcus* contains many different species. When speaking in more specific terms, both the genus and species are included. Using the same example, the genus and species might be *Staphylococcus aureus* or *Staphylococcus epidermidis*. Although the viruses also follow the same classification scheme, they are more frequently referred to by more common names. For instance, the common name for one of the viruses of the herpes genera is herpes simplex virus type 1.

Factors Affecting Microbial Flora

Most areas of the human body harbor an indigenous microbial flora that is specific to both that anatomic area and the individual human being.[1,3–5] As mentioned earlier, this specific ecosystem helps to play a role in protecting the individual from invasion by pathogenic organisms. There

Carolinas Center for Oral Health, 1601 Abbey Place, Charlotte, NC 28209, USA
E-mail address: Richard.Haug@carolinashealthcare.org

Oral Maxillofacial Surg Clin N Am 24 (2012) 191–196
doi:10.1016/j.coms.2012.01.001
1042-3699/12/$ – see front matter © 2012 Elsevier Inc. All rights reserved.

are numerous factors that may alter the type, frequency, and distribution of normally occurring microbes of the body. These factors include such entities as the individual host's immune system, the relative humidity of the specific anatomic region, the presence or lack of oxygen, local surface characteristics, the available nutrition, any interaction between the microbes present, and so forth.[1,3,4] Although there is generally a normal resident flora for any particular anatomic region, a transient flora may also be found to colonize for periods ranging from hours to weeks without being retained permanently. The author's discussions are limited to indigenous flora (not transient) and, for brevity, have been listed in box form.

Nasal and Paranasal Sinus Microflora

Unlike the skin and mouth, the nasal passages and paranasal sinuses are sterile at birth. Yet, within days, the infant acquires a flora, mostly associated with the mother, the nursing staff, and the specific hospital that the newborn resides in.[6–10] As the human breathes air and its contents, it pass through the nose. There the air is filtered, and most of the microorganisms are trapped by vibrissae and mucous secretions and are routinely swallowed. These mucous secretions contain enzymes and immunoglobulins that further kill or inhibit the growth of microorganisms. Yet, with time and altered host resistance, the adult human acquires an indigenous microflora and occasionally is subjected to colonization (**Box 1**).[6–11] *S aureus* and *Haemophilus influenzae* are the most common inhabitants of the nose and paranasal sinuses, although many others may inhabit this region (see **Box 1**).

NASAL AND PARANASAL SINUS INFECTIONS
Acute Maxillary and Ethmoid Sinusitis

Sinusitis is a disease that results from an infection of 1 or more of the paranasal sinuses.[13,14] Acute sinusitis is generally categorized by its etiology, as nosocomial or community acquired, or as viral, bacterial, or fungal.[13,14] Combinations of these etiologies are possible. Perhaps the most common cause for acute maxillary sinusitis is an infection secondary to a rhinovirus. The ability to accurately culture viruses is a relatively recent development, and thus changes and/or trends in viral pathogenicity have not yet been established.

The etiology of acute community-acquired bacterial sinusitis (ACABS) has been well substantiated for the past 6 to 7 decades (**Box 2**).[8,12–17] *S pneumoniae* and *H influenzae* account for most occurrences of this form of sinusitis. Yet other

---

> **Box 1**
> **Some of the most common indigenous and colonizing nasal and paranasal sinus flora**
>
> *Aerobic and facultative isolates*
>
> *Corynebacterium diphtheria*
>
> *Corynebacterium* species
>
> *H influenzae*
>
> *Haemophilus parainfluenza*
>
> *Neisseria* species
>
> *Staphylococcus* species
>
> *Streptococcus pneumoniae*
>
> *Moraxella* species
>
> *Micrococcus* species
>
> *Neisseria meningitidis*
>
> *S aureus*
>
> *S epidermidis*
>
> *Streptococcus viridans*
>
> *Anaerobic isolates*
>
> *Propionibacterium acnes*
>
> *Data from Refs.*[6–9,12]

Streptococcus species, *S aureus*, *Moraxella catarrhalis*, α-hemolytic *Streptococci*, and anaerobic bacteria have also been associated with this form of sinus infection. Complicating the diagnosis and treatment of this problem has been the observation that both viruses and bacteria may be identified as simultaneously causing an ACABS. When cultures fail to yield bacteria for an ACABS, which occurs approximately 40% of the time, a viral etiology should be suspected. Even fungi may be responsible for an ACABS but are more associated with nosocomial sinusitis and sinus disease developing in compromised hosts such as diabetic patients. *S aureus*, *Pseudomonas aeruginosa*, *Serratia marcescens*, *Klebsiella pneumoniae*, *Enterobacter* species, *Proteus mirabilis*, *and Legionella pneumophila* are also associated with nosocomial sinusitis and the compromised host.[13]

The relative distribution of microorganisms responsible for ACABS has not changed in either appearance or prevalence over the past 6 decades.[12,13,17] What has changed is their antimicrobial susceptibility. Penicillin-resistant *S aureus* has emerged as a difficult microbe to manage, along with β-lactam–resistant strains of *H influenza* and *M catarrhalis*. Worse yet has been the emergence of multiple strains of resistant *S pneumoniae*.

The emergence of these forms of resistant microbes is based on the acquisition of antibiotic

Chronic Maxillary Sinusitis

The specific etiology and pathogenicity of chronic sinusitis disease (CSD) remains unanswered, although its successful treatment modalities continue to evade the clinician.[16,17,37] Although some cases of CSD exist as separate and distinct entities, it has been assumed that most of these infections arise from treatment failures of ACABS. *S pneumoniae, H influenzae*, and other streptococcal species have been isolated from patients who have CSD (**Box 3**).[8,9,15–17] Of particular interest is that β-lactamase–producing strains of *S pneumoniae, H influenzae*, and *M catarrhalis* have been isolated in ACABS aspirates.[37,38] It would therefore seem likely that CSD is merely the continued manifestation of an ACABS caused by ineffective management.

Infectious Rhinitis

Infective rhinitis has been classified as acute, self-limiting, or chronic and is the major component of what many consider the common cold.[39] Viruses are the most frequent cause of infectious rhinitis, and rhinoviruses are the most frequent causative agent among viruses (**Box 4**).[7,9,10,39] Bacteria are an infrequent cause of isolated nasal infections but are common as causes of combination nasal/paranasal sinus infections.[39] Granulomatous nasal infections such as rhinoscleroma, tuberculosis, syphilis, aspergillosis, and mucormycosis are rare and caused by numerous microorganisms, including fungi, protozoa, and mycobacterium.[7,9,10,39]

The herpes simplex virus is a common cause of nasal/perinasal infection. This virus is usually introduced into the body through mucosal exposure. Although the initial infection may be subclinical, recurrences are common. More than 90% of

resistance mechanisms, either through mutation or by transfer of genetic information from other bacteria.[19–21] Thus, there has been an increase in the antibiotic resistance of important pathogenic genera. The most dramatic example in the development of resistance during the past 4 decades in terms of cost, both economic and human, has been the evolution of methicillin-resistant *S aureus* (MRSA). It is estimated that methicillin resistance in certain strains of *Staphylococcus* species has arisen from 2.4% in the 1970s to 29% by the end of the twentieth century and that the costs of hospitalization for these types of nosocomial infections could approach $3 billion annually in the United States alone.[13,22–36] Yet, it must be remembered that money is not the real issue and that the ultimate cost for humans is death. Post-surgical patients who develop nosocomial infections such as MRSA are twice as likely to die as those who do not.[32,33]

Box 4
Some common microorganisms responsible for rhinitis

Aerobic and facultative isolates
Klebsiella rhinoscleromatis

Mycobacteria
Mycobacterium tuberculosis

Spirochetes
Treponema pallidum

Fungi
Absidia species
Aspergillosis flavus
Aspergillosis fumigatus
Bipolaris species
Cladosporium species
Curvularia species
Exophiala species
Exserohilum species
Histoplasma capsulatum
Mucor species
Rhinosporidium seeberi
Rhizopus species
Wangiella species

Protozoa
Leishmaniasis

Viruses
Adenovirus
Enterovirus
Influenza virus
Parainfluenza virus
Respiratory syncytial virus
Rhinovirus

Data from Refs.[7,9,10,39]

Frontal and Sphenoid Sinusitis

The microbial flora of infected frontal and sphenoid sinuses is separate and distinct from that of maxillary and ethmoid sinuses. Acute sphenoid and frontal sinusitis is uncommon, difficult to diagnose, carries with it a significant degree of morbidity, and yet accounts for less than 5% of paranasal sinus infections.[18,40,41] Headache is the most common consistent finding and may be accentuated with activity or may become debilitating in the degree of pain associated with it. Several organisms have been identified with this disease (**Box 5**).[15,18,40,41] *S aureus*, *S pneumoniae*, *H influenza*, and other streptococcal species are the most frequent pathogens.[18,40,41] Although changes in the microbiology of the diseased frontal and sphenoid sinuses have not been identified by scientifically scrutinized investigations, changes in the clinical management point toward the use of antibiotics that address β-lactamase–producing strains of organisms. Especially problematic are β-lactamase–producing *Staphylococci*, *Streptococci*, and *H influenza*.

Box 5
Some common microorganisms responsible for sphenoid and frontal sinusitis

Aerobic and facultative isolates
β-hemolytic *Streptococci*
Citrobacter
Coliform bacilli
Enterococci
Escherichia coli
H influenzae
K pneumoniae
Pneumococci
Proteus
P aeruginosa
Serratia
S aureus
S epidermidis
S pneumoniae
S viridans

Anaerobic isolates
Anaerobic streptococci

Fungi
Aspergillus

Data from Refs.[15,18,40,41]

adults have antibodies to herpes simplex virus. The prevalence of this microorganism increases with decreasing socioeconomic status. It is more prevalent in African Americans than other Americans and more prevalent in Western Europe than the United States. Although relief and complacency was initially perceived in medical and lay populations after the discovery of acyclovir, consternation has again arisen with the isolation of acyclovir-resistant strains of herpes simplex virus with increasing frequency.

THE FUTURE

Although the taxonomic system described in the introduction and used throughout the article remains in clinical use, the development of a taxonomic system based on DNA and RNA has become of increasing importance in the potential for identifying and/or classifying microbes.[42–44] All living organisms of closely related individuals share some basis of gene sequence similarity. The use of sequence diversity in protein-coding genes shows that there are sequence clusters that correspond to unique ecological populations. With this in mind, it is possible to identify related and, conversely, unrelated individuals. The use of polymerase chain reaction allows the use of a single or very few strands of a DNA sequence and then amplification of these strands thousands or millions of times over, for the sequence to be more readily identified. This technology permits the identification and classification of living organisms and, for the sake of this discussion, the identification of microbes in a more precise and specific manner. Although an exciting concept and useful in benchtop research and forensics, this technology has not yet replaced the current system of nomenclature.

THE PRESENT

S pneumoniae, H influenza, and S aureus are the most common inhabitants of the healthy nose and paranasal sinuses. When homeostasis is interrupted by elective surgery, trauma, or a change in the environment (altered humidity or oxygen content), the normal flora will change. Although acute sinusitis is most frequently attributed to *S pneumoniae* and *H influenza*, acute rhinitis is most commonly associated with viral infection. From a microbial standpoint, chronic sinus infections seem to be mere failures of the treatment of acute sinus infections. Of increasing concern is the emergence of microbes that are resistant to common antimicrobial agents. Whether by direct mutation or transfer of genetic material from other microbes, these bacteria have become a challenge in antimicrobial management. At present, antibiotics that contain a β-lactamase inhibitor are preferred.

REFERENCES

1. Gallis HA. Normal flora and opportunistic infections. In: Joklik WK, Willett HP, Amos DB, et al, editors. Zinsser microbiology. 19th edition. Norwalk (CT): Appleton and Lange; 1988. p. 337–42.

2. Koneman EW, Allen SD, Dowell VR, et al, editors. Color atlas and textbook of diagnostic microbiology. 3rd edition. Philadelphia: Lippincott; 1988. p. xvii–xviii.

3. Schuster GS. Microbiology of the orofacial region. In: Topazian RG, Goldberg MH, Hupp JR, editors. Oral and maxillofacial infections. 4th edition. Philadelphia: WB Saunders Co; 2002. p. 30–42.

4. Shuster GS. Oral flora and pathogenic organisms. Infect Dis Clin North Am 1999;13:757–74.

5. Tramont EC, Hoover DL. Innate (general or nonspecific) host defense mechanisms. In: Mandell GL, Bennett JE, Dolin R, editors. Principles and practice of infectious disease. 5th edition. Philadelphia: Churchill Livingstone; 2000. p. 31–8.

6. Bamberger DM. Antimicrobial treatment of sinusitis. Semin Respir Infect 1991;6:77–84.

7. Larsen HS. Host-parasite interaction. In: Mahon CR, Manuselis G, editors. Textbook of diagnostic microbiology. 2nd edition. Philadelphia: WB Saunders; 2000. p. 213–6.

8. McCarter YS. Laboratory microbiological diagnostic techniques. In: Topazian RG, Goldberg MH, Hupp JR, editors. Oral and maxillofacial infections. 4th edition. Philadelphia: WB Saunders Co; 2002. p. 43–61.

9. Weiser JN, Kim JO. The respiratory tract microflora and disease. In: Tannock GW, editor. Medical importance of the normal microflora. Boston: Kluwer Academic Publishers; 1999. p. 47–73.

10. Volk WA, Gebhart BM, Hammarskjold M, et al, editors. Essentials of medical microbiology. 5th edition. Philadelphia: Lippincott-Raven Publishers; 1996. p. 315–32.

11. Lemonick MD. The killers all around us. Time Magazine. September 12, 1994;144:62.

12. Winther B, Vickery CL, Gross CW, et al. Microbiology of the maxillary sinus in adults with chronic sinus disease. Am J Med Sci 1998;316:13–20.

13. Gwaltney JM. Sinusitis. In: Mandell GL, Bennett JE, Dolin R, editors. Principles and practice of infectious disease. 5th edition. Philadelphia: Churchill Livingstone; 2000. p. 676–86.

14. Hamory BH, Sande MA, Sydor, et al. Etiology and antimicrobial therapy of acute maxillary sinusitis. J Infect Dis 1979;139:197–202.

15. Sandler NA, Johns FR, Braun TW. Advances in the management of acute and chronic sinusitis. J Oral Maxillofac Surg 1996;54:1005–13.

16. Snydor A, Gwaltney J, Cacchetto DM, et al. Comparative evaluation of cefuroxime axetil and cefaclor for treatment of acute bacterial maxillary sinusitis. Arch Otolaryngol Head Neck Surg 1989;115:1430–3.

17. Wald ER, Reilly JS, Casselbrant M, et al. Treatment of acute maxillary sinusitis in childhood: a comparative study of amoxicillin and cefaclor. J Pediatr 1984; 104:297–302.

18. Middleton WG, Briant TDR, Fenton RS. Frontal sinusitis—a 10 year experience. J Otolaryngol 1985;14:197–200.

19. Wald E. Microbiology of acute and chronic sinusitis. In: Lusk RP, editor. Pediatric sinusitis. New York: Raven Press; 1992. p. 43–7.

20. Neu HC. The crisis in antibiotic resistance. Science 1992;257:1064–73.

21. Satcher D. Emerging infections: getting ahead of the curve. Emerg Infect Dis 1995;1:1–6.

22. American Society of Health-System Pharmacists. ASHP therapeutics guidelines on antimicrobial prophylaxis in surgery. Am J Health Syst Pharm 1999;56:1839–58.

23. Barett F, McGehee R, Finland M. Methicillin-resistant *Staphylococcus aureus* at Boston City Hospital. N Engl J Med 1998;279:441–8.

24. Corey L. Herpes simplex virus. In: Mandell GL, Bennett JE, Dolin R, editors. Principles and practice of infectious disease. 5th edition. Philadelphia: Churchill Livingstone; 2000. p. 1564–80.

25. Crossley K, Loesch D, Landesman B, et al. An outbreak of infections caused by strains of *Staphylococcus aureus* resistant to methicillin and aminoglycosides, I: clinical studies. J Infect Dis 1979;139:273–9.

26. Fukatsu K, Saito H, Matsuda T, et al. Influences of type and duration of antimicrobial prophylaxis on an outbreak of methicillin-resistant *Staphylococcus aureus* and on the incidence of wound infection. Arch Surg 1997;132:1320–5.

27. Goldstein E, Citron D, Feingold S. Dog bite wounds and infection: a prospective clinical study. Ann Emerg Med 1980;9:508–12.

28. Bolger WE, Kennedy DW. Changing concepts in chronic sinusitis. Hosp Pract (Off Ed) 1992;27:20–8.

29. Dacre J, Emmerson A, Jenner E. Gentamicin-methicillin-resistant *Staphylococcus aureus*: epidemiology of an outbreak. J Hosp Infect 1986;7:130–6.

30. Stoll D, Dutkiewicz J, Boineau F, et al. Bacteriology of the nose and sinuses. Rev Laryngol Otol Rhinol 1996;117:179–82.

31. Chin CW, Yeak CL, Wang DY. The microbiology and the efficacy of antibiotic-based medical treatment of chronic rhinosinusitis in Singapore. Rhinology 2010; 48:433–7.

32. Kirkland KB, Briggs JP, Trivette SL, et al. The impact of surgical-site infections in the 1990's: attributable mortality, excess length of hospitalization, and extra costs. Infect Control Hosp Epidemiol 1999;20: 725–30.

33. Klimek J, Marsik F, Bartlett R, et al. Clinical, epidemiologic and bacteriologic observations of an outbreak of methicillin-resistant *Staphylococcus aureus* at a large community hospital. Am J Med 1976;61:340–5.

34. Almadori G, Bastiani L, Bistoni F, et al. Microbial flora of the nose and paranasal sinuses in chronic maxillary sinusitis. Rhinology 1986;24:257–64.

35. Panlilio AL, Culver DH, Gaynes RP, et al. Methicillin-resistant *Staphylococcus aureus* in US hospitals, 1975-1991. Infect Control Hosp Epidemiol 1992;13: 582–6.

36. Pavillard R, Harvey K, Douglas D, et al. Epidemic of hospital-acquired infection due to methicillin-resistant *Staphylococcus aureus* in Victorian hospitals. Med J Aust 1982;1:451–4.

37. Bikle DD. Effects of alcohol abuse on bone. Compr Ther 1988;14:16–20.

38. Brennen SR, Rhodes KH, Peterson HA. Infection after farm related injuries in children and adolescents. Am J Dis Child 1990;144:710–3.

39. Kopke RD, Jackson RL. Rhinitis. In: Bailey BJ, editor. Head and neck surgery—otolaryngology. Philadelphia: JB Lippincott; 1993. p. 269–89.

40. Kibblewhite DJ, Cleland J, Mintz DR. Acute sphenoid sinusitis: management strategies. J Otolaryngol 1988; 17:159–63.

41. Lew D, Southwick FS, Montgomery WW, et al. Sphenoid sinusitis: a review of 30 cases. N Engl J Med 1983;309:1149–54.

42. Zimmerley T, Sadowsky MJ. Use of repetitive DNA sequences and the PCR to differentiate Escherichia coli isolates from human and animal sources. Appl Environ Microbiol 2000;66:2572–7.

43. Palys T, Nakamura LK, Cohan FM. Discovery and classification of ecological diversity in the bacterial world: the role of DNA sequence data. Int J Syst Evol Microbiol 2010;60:2697–704.

44. Abe T, Sugawara H, Kinouchi M, et al. Novel phylogenetic studies of genomic sequence fragments derived from uncultured microbe mixtures in environmental and clinical samples. DNA Res 2005;12: 281–90.

Tonsillitis, Peritonsillar and Lateral Pharyngeal Abscesses

Jonathan M. Tagliareni, DDS*, Earl I. Clarkson, DDS

KEYWORDS

- Tonsillitis • Peritonsillar abscesses
- Lateral pharyngeal abscesses

PERITONSILLAR ANATOMY

The Waldeyer tonsillar ring forms a ring of lymphoid or adenoid tissue around the upper end of the pharynx. This ring consists of the lingual tonsils anteriorly, the palatine tonsils laterally, and the pharyngeal tonsils or adenoids posterosuperiorly. The structures of the Waldeyer ring have similar histology and similar functions.

Palatine Tonsil

The palatine tonsil represents the largest accumulation of lymphoid tissue in the Waldeyer ring and, in contrast to the lingual and pharyngeal tonsils, constitutes a compact body with a definite thin capsule on its deep surface.[1] The tonsillar capsule is a specialized portion of the pharyngobasilar fascia that covers the surface of the tonsil and extends into it to form septa that conduct the nerves and vessels.[1] The capsule is united by loose connective tissue to the pharyngeal muscles. The tonsillar fossa is composed of 3 muscles: the palatoglossus muscle, which forms the anterior pillar; the palatopharyngeal muscle, which is the posterior pillar; and the superior constrictor muscle of the pharynx, which forms the larger part of the tonsillar bed. The muscular wall is thin, and immediately against it on the outer wall of the pharynx is the glossopharyngeal nerve. The glossopharyngeal nerve can be injured if the tonsillar bed is violated, and not uncommonly the

nerve is temporarily affected by edema after tonsillectomy, which produces both a transitory loss of taste over the posterior third of the tongue and referred otalgia.[2] The arterial blood supply of the tonsil consists of the tonsillar branch of the dorsal lingual artery anteriorly, the ascending palatine artery posteriorly, and the tonsillar branch of the facial artery, which enters the lower aspect of the tonsillar bed. The ascending pharyngeal artery enters posteriorly, and the lesser palatine artery enters on the anterior surface of the upper pole. The tonsillar branch of the facial artery is the largest. Venous blood drains through a peritonsillar plexus. The plexus drains into the lingual and pharyngeal veins, draining into the internal jugular vein. The nerve supply of the tonsillar region is through the tonsillar branches of the glossopharyngeal nerve through the descending branches of the lesser palatine nerves, which travel through the pterygopalatine ganglion.[1]

Adenoids

Surrounding the oropharyngeal isthmus, the adenoid or pharyngeal tonsils form the central part of the ring of lymphoid tissue. Composed of lymphoid tissue, the apex of the adenoid points toward the nasal septum and its base toward the roof and posterior wall of the nasopharynx. The adenoid is covered by a pseudostratified ciliated columnar epithelium that is plicated to form numerous surface folds.[2] It develops as a midline

Department of Oral and Maxillofacial Surgery, The Brooklyn Hospital Center, 121 Dekalb Avenue, Brooklyn, NY 11201, USA
* Corresponding author.
E-mail address: jtagliarenidds@gmail.com

Oral Maxillofacial Surg Clin N Am 24 (2012) 197–204
doi:10.1016/j.coms.2012.01.014

oralmaxsurgery.theclinics.com

structure by the fusion of 2 lateral primordia that become visible during early fetal life, and is fully developed by the seventh month of gestation, and continues to grow until the fifth year of life, often causing some airway obstruction.[3] The adenoid gradually atrophies, the nasopharynx grows, and the airway improves.[4] The blood supply and drainage are from the ascending pharyngeal artery, the ascending palatine artery, the pharyngeal branch of the maxillary artery, the artery of the pterygoid canal, and contributing branches from the tonsillar branch of the facial artery.[3] Venous drainage is through the pharyngeal plexus, which communicates with the pterygoid plexus and then drains into the internal jugular and facial veins. The nerve supply is from the pharyngeal plexus. The efferent lymphatic drainage of the adenoids is to the lymph nodes in the retropharyngeal and pharyngomaxillary space (**Fig. 1**).[3]

IMMUNOLOGY OF THE ADENOIDS AND TONSILS

B cells account for 50% to 65% of all tonsillar lymphocytes.[5] T cells account for 40% of adenoid and tonsillar lymphocytes, with 3% mature plasma cells. Conversely, 70% of the lymphocytes in peripheral blood are T cells. The immunoreactive lymphoid cells of the adenoids and tonsils are found in 4 distinct areas: the reticular cell epithelium, the extrafollicular area, the mantle zone of the lymphoid follicle, and the germinal center of the lymphoid follicle.[5]

Both the adenoids and tonsils are favorably located to mediate immunologic protection of the upper aerodigestive tract, because they are exposed to airborne antigens. Both organs, specifically the tonsils, are particularly designed for direct transport of foreign material from the exterior to the lymphoid cells.[5] This characteristic is in contrast to lymph nodes, which depend on antigenic delivery through afferent lymphatics. The tonsillar crypts are covered by stratified squamous epithelium. There are 10 to 30 of these crypts in the tonsils, and they are ideally suited to trapping foreign material and transporting it to the lymphoid follicles.[5] Intratonsillar defense mechanisms eliminate weak antigenic signals. When additional higher antigenic concentrations are presented, dose proliferation of antigen-sensitive B cells occurs in the germinal centers. Low antigen doses affect the differentiation of lymphocytes to plasma cells, whereas high antigen doses produce B-cell proliferation. The generation of B cells in the germinal centers of the tonsils was considered by Siegel[6] to be one of the most essential tonsillar functions. T-cell functions, such as interferon-γ production and, presumably,

production of other important lymphokines, have been shown to be present in the tonsils and adenoids.[5]

The tonsils are immunologically most active between ages 4 and 10 years. Involution of the tonsils begins after puberty, resulting in a decrease of the B-cell population and a relative increase in the ratio of T to B cells.[7] Although the overall immunoglobulin-producing function is affected, considerable B-cell activity is still seen in clinically healthy tonsils even at age 80 years.[8] The situation is different in disease-associated changes, such as when recurrent tonsillitis and adenoid hyperplasia are observed. Inflammation of the reticular crypt epithelium results in shedding of immunologically active cells and decreasing antigen transport function with subsequent replacement by stratified squamous epithelium.[9] These changes lead to reduced activation of the local B-cell system, decreased antibody production, and an overall reduction in density of the B-cell and germinal centers in extrafollicular areas.[9]

INFECTIONS OF THE WALDEYER RING

Many organisms including aerobic and anaerobic bacteria, viruses, yeasts, and parasites can induce inflammation of the Waldeyer ring. Most of the infectious organisms are part of the normal oral pharyngeal flora, and others are external pathogens. Colonized by many organisms, most infections of the Waldeyer ring are polymicrobial. These organisms work synergistically and can be found in mixed aerobic and anaerobic infections.[10] Mixed infections have the ability to protect an organism susceptible to that agent by the production of an antibiotic-degrading enzyme that is secreted into the tissues. Because of its polymicrobial nature, it is often difficult to interpret data derived from clinical samples obtained from mucosal surfaces and to differentiate between organisms that are colonized and those that are invaders.[11]

Viruses

The common cold is the most frequent cause of tonsillar infection. Numerous offending viral pathogens have been implicated in causing pharyngitis, including rhinovirus, influenza virus, parainfluenza virus, adenovirus, Coxsackie virus, echovirus, reovirus, and respiratory syncytial virus. Viral pharyngitis is usually mild in manifestations, with patients complaining of a sore throat and dysphagia. Most patients have a fever, with erythema of the pharyngeal mucosa. The tonsils may be enlarged, but frequently there is no associated exudate. Herpangina caused by Coxsackie virus

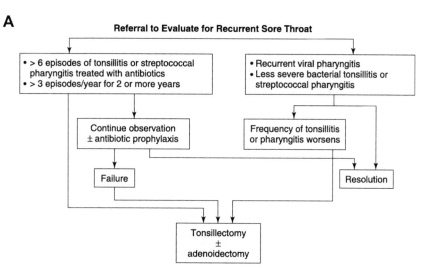

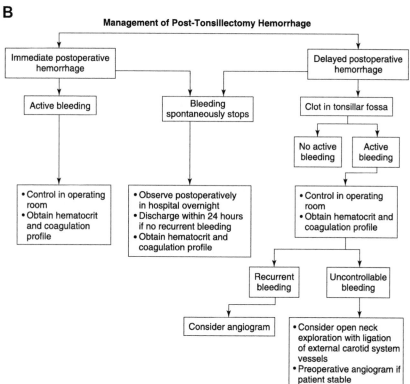

Fig. 1. Management algorithms for pediatric pharyngitis and adenotonsillar disease. (*A*) Algorithm for evaluation of a patient referred for recurrent sore throat. (*B*) Algorithm for management of posttonsillectomy hemorrhage. (*C*) Algorithm for evaluation of a patient referred for adenotonsillar hypertrophy. (*From* Flint PW, Haughey BH, Lund VJ, et al. Cummings otolaryngology: head and neck surgery. 5th edition. St Louis (MO): Mosby; 2010. p. 2783; with permission.)

is characterized by small vesicles with erythematous bases that become ulcers and are spread over the anterior tonsillar pillar, palate, and posterior pharynx (**Fig. 2**).[11]

Epstein-Barr Virus

Epstein-Barr virus (EBV) can induce the mononucleosis syndrome, which consists of general malaise, high fever, and large, swollen, gray tonsils.

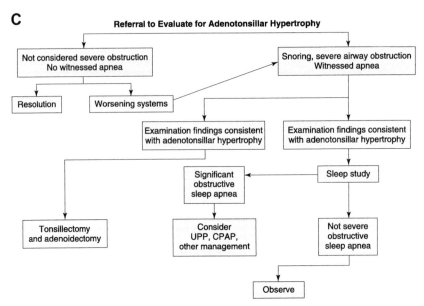

Fig. 1. (*continued*)

A differential blood count showing 50% lymphocytosis with 10% atypical lymphocytes is characteristic of EBV infection. Serologic studies include monospot and other serum heterophil antibody titer measurements. Results of these tests may be negative initially, and repeat testing in 1 to 2 weeks is warranted if clinical suspicion of EBV infection is strong. The heterophil antibody titers are detected by the Paul-Bunnell-Davidsohn or ox-cell hemolysis test. If the heterophil antibody agglutination test result is negative, the disease may still be present. Only 60% of patients with infectious mononucleosis have a positive result within the first 2 weeks after onset of the illness; 90% have a positive result 1 month after onset.[12] EBV-specific serologic assays have become the method of choice for confirmation of acute or convalescent EBV infection. Management of this condition is symptomatic. Upper airway obstruction from severely enlarged tonsils can be life-threatening and should be managed immediately with the insertion of a nasopharyngeal airway and short-term high-dose steroid therapy. If the obstruction is severe a tonsillectomy or tracheotomy may be indicated.

Streptococcal Tonsillitis-Pharyngitis

Group A streptococcus is the most common bacterial cause of acute pharyngitis.[12] Acute streptococcal tonsillitis is a disease of childhood, with a peak incidence at about 5 to 6 years of age, but can occur in children younger than 3 years and in adults older than 50 years.[13] Outbreaks may arise

in epidemic forms in institutional settings such as recruit camps and daycare facilities. Acute tonsillitis manifests as a dry throat, malaise, fever, fullness of the throat, odynophagia, dysphagia, otalgia, headache, limb and back pain, cervical adenopathy, and shivering. Examination reveals a dry tongue, erythematous, enlarged tonsils, and yellowish white spots on the tonsils. In severe cases, a tonsillar or pharyngeal membrane or purulent exudate may exist along with jugulodigastric lymph node enlargement (**Fig. 3**).[13]

The diagnosis of acute tonsillitis is made mainly on clinical grounds. The clinical manifestations of streptococcal and nonstreptococcal pharyngitis overlap frequently, making it difficult to diagnosis with certainty. For this reason, most authorities

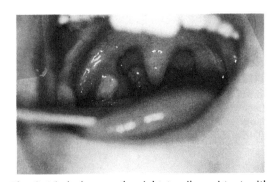

Fig. 2. Viral ulcer on the right tonsil consistent with Coxsackie virus infection. (*From* Flint PW, Haughey BH, Lund VJ, et al. Cummings otolaryngology: head and neck surgery. 5th edition. St Louis (MO): Mosby; 2010. p. 2786; with permission.)

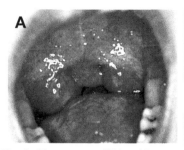 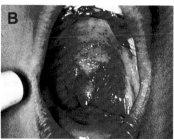 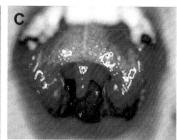

Fig. 3. Pharyngotonsillitis. This common syndrome has several causative pathogens and a wide spectrum of severity. (A) The diffuse tonsillar and pharyngeal erythema seen here is a nonspecific finding that can be produced by a variety of pathogens. (B) This intense erythema, seen in association with acute tonsillar enlargement and palatal petechiae, is highly suggestive of group A β-streptococcal infection, although other pathogens can produce these findings. (C) This picture of exudative tonsillitis is most commonly seen with either group A streptococcal or EBV infection. (*From* Yellon RF, McBride TP, Davis HW. Otolaryngology. In: Zitelli BJ, Davis HW, editors. Atlas of pediatric physical diagnosis. 4th edition. Philadelphia: Mosby; 2002. p. 852; with permission.)

recommend that the diagnosis of group A β-hemolytic streptococcal (GABHS) pharyngitis be verified or ruled out by microbiologic tests in patients who seem likely, from clinical and epidemiologic considerations, to have this illness.[14] The throat culture is the diagnostic tool most frequently used. The throat culture is a useful and simple test, but sampling must be skillfully performed by swabbing the posterior pharynx and tonsillar areas.[13] A delay in obtaining results has been a major problem in the use of throat cultures. Delays ranging from 18 to 48 hours are not uncommon, inadvertently delaying the start of management. If group A streptococcal pharyngitis is treated early in the clinical course, the period of communicability is reduced.[15] The streptococcal group A carbohydrate may be detected within minutes. Although the rapid detection tests are highly specific, they are not as sensitive as routine throat culture.[16,17] A negative rapid detection test result may prompt the practitioner to withhold antibiotic therapy while awaiting culture results. Most guidelines suggest that throat cultures should be performed when the body temperature is greater than 38.3°C or when the illness is characterized exclusively by a sore throat.[18] The most accurate and cost-effective method to diagnose acute GABHS infection is the use of the rapid strep test. This test is followed by standard throat culture in patients with a negative rapid strep test result and a strong suspicion of streptococcal tonsillitis.

Throat culture have their own flaws: they cannot reliably differentiate acute from chronic infection. There are occasional false-negative results (approximately 10% of cases), although 1 report has found that patients with false-negative results are most likely carriers who do not require treatment.[12] Studies have reported that a single throat culture is 90% to 97% sensitive and 90% specific for GABHS growth.[19] A true infection is shown by a positive throat culture result and at least a two-dilutional increase in the antistreptolysin-O titer.[20] A GABHS carrier without acute infection has a positive culture result with no change in dilution titer.[21] Excluding the diagnosis of group A streptococcal pharyngitis is important because most patients with acute pharyngitis do not have strep throat.

In most cases penicillin is the antibiotic of choice. Anaerobic bacteria contribute significantly in the complications associated with tonsillitis, so they are probably also involved in recurrent tonsillitis. One study has documented the prevalence of *Bacteroides* cultured from chronically inflamed tonsils.[22] Anaerobes also have been implicated in acute tonsillitis.[23] Clinical failure of penicillin should lead to the suspicion of β-lactamase-producing organisms. An alternative to the use of penicillin is to use a penicillin plus a β-lactamase inhibitor such as clavulanic acid (eg, amoxicillin/clavulanic acid).[11] Alternatives include clindamycin and a combination of erythromycin and metronidazole. Antibiotic therapy initiated within 24 to 48 hours of symptom onset results in decreased symptoms associated with sore throat, fever, and adenopathy 12 to 24 hours sooner than without antibiotic administration.[11] Schwartz and colleagues[24] reported that a full 10-day course of antibiotics is necessary. The study showed that children receiving 10 days of therapy have lower clinical and bacteriologic recurrence rates than children receiving only 7 days of therapy.

Peritonsillar and Parapharyngeal Abscess

Secondary complications originating from tonsillitis can be broken down into nonsuppurative and suppurative complications. Scarlet fever, acute rheumatic fever, and poststreptococcal glomerulonephritis are all included in the nonsuppurative category. Suppurative complications are the result of abscess formation and include peritonsillar and parapharyngeal abscess development. For the purpose of this article, only suppurative complications are discussed in detail.

Peritonsillar Infections

Peritonsillar abscess most commonly occurs in patients with recurrent tonsillitis or in those with chronic tonsillitis that has been inadequately treated. The spread of infection is from the superior pole of the tonsil, with pus formation between the tonsil bed and the tonsillar capsule.[25] This infection is usually unilateral and the pain is severe; drooling is caused by odynophagia and dysphagia. Trismus can be present when the pterygoid musculature is irritated by pus and inflammation. There is gross unilateral swelling of the palate and anterior pillar, with displacement of the tonsil downward and medially, with reflection of the uvula toward the opposite side. Cultures of the peritonsillar abscess usually show a polymicrobial infection, both aerobic and anaerobic.[25]

It is critical to differentiate between cellulitis and abscess formation when managing peritonsillar infections. Computed tomography (CT) with contrast enhancement may be indicated to determine the anatomic borders of the infection (**Fig. 4**).

Needle aspiration may be used to obtain a test aspirate and identify the site of the abscess. If pus is found on needle aspiration, the abscess may be opened with a long-handled scalpel to incise the mucosa over the abscess and a blunt-tip hemostat to spread and break up the loculi, draining as much pus as possible.[11]

The traditional management of a peritonsillar abscess consisted of incision and drainage, with tonsillectomy 4 to 12 weeks later. Some surgeons advocate immediate tonsillectomy or Quinsy tonsillectomy as definitive management to ensure complete drainage of the abscess and to alleviate the need for a second hospitalization for an interval tonsillectomy.[26] If incision and drainage or needle aspiration fail to drain an abscess adequately, a tonsillectomy is indicated. Tonsillectomy should be considered in patients with a previous history of recurrent peritonsillar abscess or recurrent severe tonsillitis. Tonsillectomy is favored in children because they are likely to experience further episodes of tonsillitis, and needle aspiration or incision and drainage with a child under local anesthesia is often difficult.[10]

Parapharyngeal Space Abscess

An abscess can develop in the parapharyngeal space if infection or pus drains from either the tonsils or from a peritonsillar abscess through the superior constrictor muscle.[25] The abscess is located between the superior constrictor muscle and the deep cervical fascia and causes displacement of the tonsil on the lateral pharyngeal wall toward the midline.[11] Involvement of the adjacent pterygoid and paraspinal muscle with the inflammatory process results in trismus and a stiff neck. Fluctuance may be difficult to detect because of the thick overlying sternocleidomastoid (**Fig. 5**).

Fever, leukocytosis, and pain are the common characteristics of a patient with parapharyngeal space infection. It is critical to observe a possible progression of the infectious process; the abscess may spread down the carotid sheath into the mediastinum. Parapharyngeal infections are usually polymicrobial and reflect oropharyngeal flora. Intraoral examination reveals swelling of the lateral pharyngeal wall, especially behind the posterior tonsillar

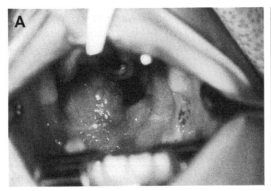
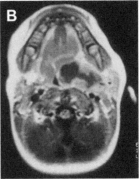

Fig. 4. (*A*) Left peritonsillar abscess in an 18-month-old child. (*B*) Magnetic resonance image of the peritonsillar abscess in the same patient, showing extension of the abscess into the retropharyngeal space. (*From* Flint PW, Haughey BH, Lund VJ, et al. Cummings otolaryngology: head and neck surgery. 5th edition. St Louis (MO): Mosby; 2010. p. 2789; with permission.)

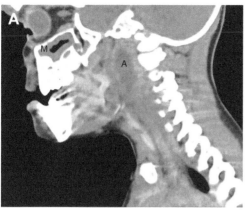
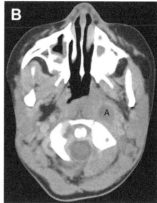

Fig. 5. CT scan of parapharyngeal abscess in a 3-year-old child. (*A*) Sagittal section showing parapharyngeal abscess (A) and mucosal swelling (M) in the maxillary sinus. (*B*) Coronal section of parapharyngeal abscess (A). (*From* Kliegman RM, Stanton BMD, St Geme J, et al. Nelson textbook of pediatrics. 19th edition. Philadelphia: Saunders; 2011. p. 141; with permission.)

pillar. Anteromedial tonsil displacement is present. Clinically, this may be confused with a peritonsillar abscess, so if indicated, a CT scan with contrast enhancement should be obtained.[11]

Lateral pharyngeal space infections should be managed with aggressive antibiotic therapy, fluid replacement, and close observation. Surgical intervention is often required to resolve these infections. Intraoral approaches should be confined to management of peritonsillar abscesses and should not be used in true lateral pharyngeal space abscesses because of inadequate exposure if severe bleeding arises. An external approach to the parapharyngeal space usually consists of a transverse submandibular excision approximately 2 cm inferior to the mandibular margin, which extends from the anterior limits of the submandibular gland just past the angle of the mandible. The submandibular gland is freed inferiorly and posteriorly by sharp, blunt dissection, and access to the space is achieved by dissection between the tail of the submandibular gland and the anterior aspect of the sternocleidomastoid muscle.

REFERENCES

1. Hollinshead WH. The pharynx and larynx. In: Hollinshead WH, editor. Anatomy for surgeons: the head and neck. Philadelphia: JB Lippincott; 1982. p. 389–410.
2. Brodsky L. Modern assessment of tonsils and adenoids. Pediatr Clin North Am 1989;36:1551.
3. Goeringer GC, Vidic B. The embryogenesis and anatomy of Waldeyer's ring. Otolaryngol Clin North Am 1987;20:207.
4. Jeans WD, Fernando DC, Maw AR, et al. A longitudinal study of the growth of the nasopharynx and its contents in normal children. Br J Radiol 1981;54:117.
5. Richtsmeier WJ, Shikhari AM. The physiology and immunology of the pharyngeal lymphoid tissue. Otolaryngol Clin North Am 1987;20:219–28.
6. Siegel G. The influence of tonsillectomy on cell mediated immune response. Arch Otolaryngol Head Neck Surg 1984;239:205.
7. Richtsmeier WJ. Human interferon production in tonsil and adenoid tissue cultures. Am J Otolaryngol 1983;4:325.
8. Brandtzaeg P, Surjan L Jr, Berdal P. Immunoglobulin systems of human tonsils I: control subjects of various ages: quantification of Ig-producing cells, tonsillar morphometry and serum Ig concentration. Clin Exp Immunol 1978;31:367–81.
9. Surjan L, Brantzaeg P, Berdal P. Immunoglobulin system of human tonsils II: patients with chronic tonsillitis or tonsillar hyperplasia: quantification of Ig-producing cells, tonsillar morphometry and serum Ig concentrations. Clin Exp Immunol 1978;31:382.
10. Brook I, Walker RI. Pathogenicity of anaerobic gram-positive cocci. Infect Immun 1984;45:320.
11. Flint PW, Haughey BH, Lund VJ, et al. Cummings otolaryngology–head and neck surgery. 5th edition. St Louis (MO): Mosby; 2010.
12. Bisno AL. Acute pharyngitis: etiology and diagnosis. Pediatrics 1996;97:949.
13. Zalzal GH, Cotton RT. Pharyngitis and adenotonsillar disease. In: Flint PW, Haughey BH, Lund VJ, et al, editors. Otolaryngology–head and neck surgery. St Louis (MO): Mosby; 1986. p. 2782–803.
14. Committee on Infectious Diseases of the American Academy of Pediatrics: 1994 red book: report of the Committee on Infectious Diseases. 23rd edition.

Elk Grove Village (IL): The American Academy of Pediatrics; 1994.

15. Randolph MF, Gerber MA, DeMeo KK, et al. Effect of antibiotic therapy on the clinical course of streptococcal pharyngitis. J Pediatr 1985;106:870–5.

16. Gerber MA. Comparison of throat cultures and rapid strep tests for diagnosis of streptococcal pharyngitis. Pediatr Infect Dis J 1989;8:820.

17. Facklam RR. Specificity study of kits for detection of group A streptococci directly from throat swabs. J Clin Microbiol 1987;25:504.

18. Honikman LH, Massel BF. Guidelines for the selective use of throat cultures in the diagnosis of streptococcal respiratory infections. Pediatrics 1971;48:573.

19. Palumbo FM. Pediatric considerations of infections and inflammations of Waldeyer's ring. Otolaryngol Clin North Am 1987;20:311.

20. Shapiro NL, Cunningham MJ. Streptococcal pharyngitis in children. Curr Opin Otolaryngol Head Neck Surg 1995;3:369.

21. Amir J, Shechter Y, Eilam N, et al. Group A beta-hemolytic streptococcal pharyngitis in children younger than 9 years. Isr J Med Sci 1994;30:619–22.

22. Brook I, Yocum P. Bacteriology of chronic tonsillitis in young adults. Arch Otolaryngol Head Neck Surg 1984;110:803.

23. Brook I. The clinical microbiology of Waldeyer's ring. Otolaryngol Clin North Am 1987;20:259.

24. Schwartz RH, Weintzen RW, Pedreira F. Penicillin V therapy for group A streptococcal pharyngitis. JAMA 1981;246:1790.

25. Zucconi M, Strambi LF, Pestalozza G, et al. Habitual snoring and obstructive sleep apnea syndrome in children: effects of early tonsil surgery. Int J Pediatr Otorhinolaryngol 1993;26:235–43.

26. Christensen PH, Schonsted-Madsen U. Unilateral immediate tonsillectomy as the treatment of peritonsillar abscesses: results with special attention to pharyngitis. J Laryngol Otol 1983;97:1105.

Allergic Rhinitis and the Unified Airway: A Therapeutic Dilemma

Leslie Robin Halpern, MD, DDS, PhD, MPH

KEYWORDS

- Allergic rhinitis • Unified airway • Immunotherapy • Asthma

Within evidence-based clinical medicine/surgery, there has been an increased awareness that inflammatory diseases of the upper and lower airways act not as individual entities but more as an integrated unit. The pathophysiologic mechanisms that activate inflammatory cascades and release of systemic mediators stimulate all components of the respiratory tree, that is, nose, sinuses, and lungs—a unified airway (**Fig. 1**).[1,2] The notion of a unified airway suggests that distinct clinical diseases are not mutually exclusive of one another in a vacuum but act as part of a spectrum of respiratory disequilibrium throughout the upper and lower pulmonary tree.[3,4] An international surgical panel convened several years ago and developed a consensus statement, "…when preparing patients for surgery…considering a diagnosis of allergic rhinitis, rhinosinusitis, or asthma, an evaluation of both the upper and lower airways should be made."[3] Treating the unified airway as an integrated unit may improve overall pulmonary function and health-related quality of life.[3,4]

The oral and maxillofacial surgeon sees patients who present with an array of airway comorbidities concurrently with oral and maxillofacial diseases. Three most frequently seen disease entities are AR, maxillary sinusitis (rhinosinusitis), and asthma. The following scenario is often presented:

A patient has rhinorrhea, sneezing, nasal congestion, and itchy watery eyes in the spring, similar symptoms have occurred annually. Over-the-counter allergy pills have failed to improve symptoms and, when administered, cause dry mouth and somnolence. On physical examination, conjunctivae are injected and nasal mucous membranes are pale, wet, and boggy, and, on auscultation of lungs, there is significant bronchial hyperactivity.

The role/pathogenesis of AR in the unified airway is the focus of this article. The author attempts to provide an overview of AR and its association with upper and lower airway diseases in order to provide a further understanding of how AR acts as a catalyst supporting the unified airway concept. Allergic rhinitis (AR) is described in terms of its epidemiology, pathophysiology, and recent options for successful treatment that can be applied in everyday practice. (Rhinosinusitis and asthma are briefly addressed, and the reader is referred to the references throughout this text for further reading.)

EPIDEMIOLOGY

Within the United States, numerous epidemiologic studies have shown AR to be a significant public health problem.[5] Prevalence rates have ranged between 15% and 40%, and the condition has been estimated to affect 20% of the adult population and 40% of the pediatric population.[5,6] There are approximately 17 million physician office visits annually with prescriptions, either by doctors or over the counter, that cost in excess of $4.5 billion per year.[7] When health-related quality of life is measured, an estimated 3.8 million lost work and school days have been tallied and there is a statistically diminished quality of life when compared with the control, that is, the normal population.[4,8] It is evident that AR has a significant impact on societal production and everyday health in both adults and children.

Center for Cosmetic and Corrective Jaw Surgery, 800-A 5th Avenue, Suite 101, New York, NY 10065, USA
E-mail address: Leslielrbbin@aol.com

Oral Maxillofacial Surg Clin N Am 24 (2012) 205–217
doi:10.1016/j.coms.2012.01.012
1042-3699/12/$ – see front matter © 2012 Elsevier Inc. All rights reserved.

Unified Airway Concept

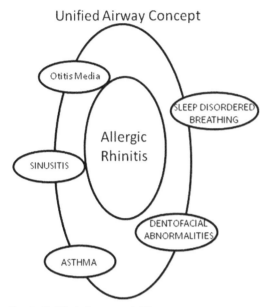

Fig. 1. Unified airway and AR.

There exist epidemiologic links among AR, rhinosinusitis, and asthma—an AR-rhinosinusitis-asthma cascade.[9,10] Rhinosinusitis affects 30 million people in North America. It accounts for an estimated $2 to $3 billion in health care costs annually, and patients spend approximately 150 million for products prescribed or recommended.[11] Yet, sinus infections are among the most frequently misdiagnosed and misunderstood diseases in clinical practice. Studies that have measured immune responses to various allergens and subsequent histopathologic sequelae in the nasal and paranasal sinuses hypothesize a model of pathogenesis of rhinosinusitis to be predicated on previous bouts of AR.[12,13]

The correlation of AR and asthma is significant. Asthma affects approximately 7% of the US population.[6] It has a significant economic impact annually of $16 billion, of which $11.5 billion are in direct costs, with $5 billion as prescriptions. Indirect costs due to lost productivity account for greater than $1.7 billion annually.[14,15] Asthma and AR occur together at a greater rate than each individually. Rates of patients who have both diseases range from 19% to 38%.[11] Multiple clinical studies using retrospective chart reviews have shown that AR is present in 50% to 85% of patients examined with asthma symptoms. In one study of 1245 patients, 52% of patients with asthma also were diagnosed with either seasonal or nonseasonal AR.[9,10] AR as a risk factor for asthma has been further tested within the *United States and globally.[16] A study in Finland using questionnaires over 3 decades found that patients

who reported hay fever in 1975 had a 4-fold increased risk for asthma 15 years later. There was a sexual predilection, with women reporting a 6-fold increased risk for developing asthma 15 years after initial diagnosis with hay fever.[17] Halpern and colleagues[18] studied a claims database (n = 27,398) of patients with asthma and concomitant AR. The presence of rhinitis was associated with more asthma medication and prescription costs. Dixon and colleagues[19] correlated the relationship among AR, sinusitis, and asthma using a database from the American Lung Association—Asthma Clinical Research Center. The investigators found that AR and rhinosinusitis were the 2 most common comorbid associated sequelae observed in patients with poorly controlled asthma. These 2 disease entities significantly influenced the symptoms of asthma as measured by histopathologic markers that were common to both diseases (see the section "Pathophysiology").

It is being examined if clinically diagnosed AR is more common in patients with asthma or if there is a more severe disease complex with both diseases. Although the epidemiologic databases mentioned earlier suggest compelling evidence linking AR to sinusitis and asthma, more prospective studies are needed to support this premise.

PATHOPHYSIOLOGY

The pathophysiology of AR is a result of the immunologic response to 1 or more aeroallergens that interact with genetic factors. This may begin in utero and continue throughout the life of the individual. Shinohara and colleagues[20] suggested that symptoms of AR in women during early pregnancy are associated with a higher prevalence of AR in their offspring. Seasonal AR occurs as such during seasons of pollen production, tree blooming, and ragweed growing. This condition is characterized as hay fever. All 3 incite inflammatory cascades, eliciting specific symptoms (see sections on diagnosis and treatment). Nonseasonal AR or perennial AR is the result of exposure to animal dander, cockroaches, mold, and dust mites. This is the more chronic form of AR occurring annually.

Most aeroallergens are sized between 10 and 100 μm and can be captured by the nasal mucosa.[21,22] The nose provides an effective filtering system for aeroallergens whose particles are 10 μm in size. This effectiveness decreases when particles are between 1 and 2 μm. It is not just the deposition of aeroallergens on the mucosa but the cascade of immunologic events that leads to the clinical expression of AR. Allergic sensitization and subsequent steps occur in a specific cycle. This complex inflammatory cascade occurs in 2 phases, early and late. The allergen first interacts with a specific allergen-presenting cell that presents the allergen to a T-helper cell. The activated T cells then induce B cells to differentiate and produce immunoglobulin class E (IgE). The cornerstone of AR is an IgE-mediated type 1 hypersensitivity reaction to the aeroallergen. The allergen-specific IgE then enters the circulation to initiate the early phase of inflammation.[22] Mast cells and basophils undergo degranulation and release the acute phase inflammatory mediators, such as histamine, cytokines, leukotrienes, and chemokines. There is microvascular leakage, mucosal secretion, and edema and vasodilation. Clinical symptoms include rhinorrhea, lacrimation, sneezing, pruritus, and possible bronchospasm. This early phase occurs 10 to 30 minutes after allergen exposure.

The late phase of AR begins 2 to 6 hours later with the synthesis of new mediators, chemotaxis, and infiltration of eosinophils, neutrophils, basophils, lymphocytes, and macrophages. These cells migrate across the mucosal endothelium into the nasal submucosa. This is clinically expressed as nasal congestion and end organ damage. With repetitive exposure, this condition occurs with a less amount of allergen.[22]

The pathologic similarities of AR, rhinosinusitis, and asthma have their basis in the commonality of the histology of their mucosa. The respiratory lining from the nasal cavity, paranasal cavity, larynx, trachea, and bronchi consists of a pseudostratified ciliated columnar epithelium. The inflammatory infiltrates of mononuclear cells, eosinophils, and other cells appear in both the nasal and bronchial mucosa. The distribution of acute phase reactants, that is, cytokines and other inflammatory mediators, is identical in both AR and asthma, as well as in rhinosinusitis.[23,24] **Box 1** depicts the commonality of histopathology among AR, rhinosinusitis, and asthma.[25] Although these similarities are present, there are morphologic differences on exposures. The vascular engorgement of nasal mucosa is related to changes in capacitance and mucosal edema. The histopathologic condition of asthma is predicated on alterations of the basement membrane and epithelium and hypertrophy of bronchial smooth muscles. A significant similarity between AR and asthma is related to the presence of bronchial hyperactivity in patients with AR who have never been diagnosed with asthma.[26] Forty-eight percent of patients with AR exposed to methacholine during their allergy season exhibited significant bronchial hyperactivity when compared with control groups. A study by the European Community Respiratory health survey

---

Box 1
Common histopathologic conditions of AR, rhinosinusitis, and asthma

Eosinophil infiltration

Basement membrane thickening

Lymphocyte infiltration

Epithelial cytoarchitecture changes

Subepithelial edema

RANTES (regulated on activation, normal T cell expressed and secreted)

Presence of inflammatory mediators: cytokines such as IL-4, IL5, IL-13

Goblet cell hyperplasia/excessive mucous production

Data from Krouse JH, Brown RW, Fineman, et al. Asthma and the unified airway. Otolaryngol Head Neck Surg 2007;136:S75–106.

---

showed self-reporting nasal allergies as an independent predictor of bronchial hyperactivity (odds ratio, 2.2-6.7).[27]

Rhinosinusitis and asthma also have identical histopathologic similarities. Given that the lining of the respiratory epithelium is identical, the remodeling with exposure to allergens is quite similar. However, the smooth muscle changes seen with asthma are unique. Aside from this, there are identical histopathologic cascades between both. The hallmark of chronic inflammation seen is an eosinophil-mediated process. Studies have identified the main effector cell as the eosinophil.[28] Numerous eosinophils are found in the nose of asthmatic patients with or without nasal symptoms. Significant numbers of eosinophils, however, are also seen in patients with rhinosinusitis, AR, and asthma when compared with mild cases of rhinosinusitis.[29]

The pathophysiologic connections discussed here lend support for a commonality of disease cascades among AR, rhinosinusitis, and asthma, supporting a unified airway concept. Further clinical investigations, however, are being done to determine whether a single disease is being manifested or not.

Samter Triad

Many oral/maxillofacial surgeons have seen patients who present with Samter triad. The historic characteristics of bronchial asthma, nasal polyposis, and intolerance to aspirin and related chemicals, recently designated as Samter syndrome, are an inflammatory condition of unknown etiology and pathogenesis.[30] The condition is probably acquired, perhaps secondary to a viral infection, but a hereditary factor may be important in some patients.[30] Most patients with this syndrome are adults, with an occasional case being identified in a teenager or an older child. Although not every patient has the fully developed syndrome, the typical patient has all 3 of the classic features.

The clinical presentation begins initially with nasal congestion and rhinorrhea, often mistaken as a recurrent cold. The rhinitis becomes chronic with new onset of sinusitis, followed by the development of chronic rhinosinusitis and the formation of nasal polyps. These symptoms appear within the fourth decade of life. Sensitivity to aspirin occurs within 1 to 5 years after the onset of symptoms with initial acute asthmatic attacks that may be life threatening, profuse rhinorrhea, orbital edema, and facial flushing.[15,31]

Many patients with Samter syndrome also have a marked eosinophilia of both bronchial and nasal secretions as well as the circulating blood. Approximately 10% of the patients have urticaria and/or angioedema, alone or in combination with respiratory inflammation. The histopathologic condition is similar to that seen for chronic asthma, with a 4-fold increase in eosinophils compared with aspirin-tolerant and normal controls.[31]

The pathophysiology of this sensitivity is not an IgE-mediated pathway but an alteration in arachidonic acid metabolism followed by inhibition of cyclooxygenase and lipoxygenase pathways that decrease the levels of antiinflammatory prostaglandins. The latter mechanism results in high levels of leukotriene, leading to severe inflammation.[31,32]

Avoidance of aspirin-containing products is stressed, as well as other nonsurgical and surgical therapy (see section on treatment later).

DIAGNOSTIC STRATEGIES FOR AR
Diagnosis

As stated earlier, AR poses a significant burden of illness on society. Patients complain of fatigue, headaches, loss of sleep, inability to concentrate, and loss of productivity. The physician must acquire a thorough history of the present illness (HPI).

Important considerations include number of bouts with AR; time of the year, that is, seasonal or perennial; precipitating factors that trigger attacks, whether it occurs at work or in the home; the presence of pets; exposures to new environment; and food.

The HPI should also include a history of contact dermatitis; mucociliary dysfunction, whether acute or associated with systemic manifestations; Kartagener syndrome; or cystic fibrosis in the family.

Autoimmune phenomena should be addressed with conditions such as rheumatoid arthritis, Crohn disease or gastroesophageal reflux disease, adolescent histories of tonsillectomy, adenoidectomy, placement of tubes in the ear, and exacerbations of sinusitis or bronchohyperactiivty.[33]

Physical Examination

There are several physical findings associated with AR. **Box 2** depicts the common symptoms/physical findings. The physical examination includes an intranasal examination with a nasal speculum that reveals mucosa with hyperemia. Auscultation may characterize wheezing, suggestive of associated asthma. Spirometry is useful in detecting subclinical asthma and bronchial hyperactivity.[22,34] Additional laboratory work may be helpful if the diagnosis is uncertain. Blood or nasal eosinophilia suggests an allergic cause, whereas neutrophilia points to an infectious cause. Allergic shiners are often seen, as well as sinus tenderness and pressure on palpation. Computed tomography most reliably reveals sinusitis in patients with symptoms of refractory rhinitis. Otoscopic examinations of the tympanic membranes are judicious because there is recurrent otitis media, as well as perforations, clouding, retraction of the eardrums, and cholesteatomas.[22]

Additional testing may be helpful if the diagnosis is uncertain or equivocal (see later). The severity of AR is assessed by assigning numerical values for eyes symptoms, nasal itching, sneezing, rhinorrhea, and nasal congestion (with 0 denoting none; 1, mild; 2, moderate; and 3, severe), taking into account subjective intensity and whether these symptoms interfere with sleep, leisure, and school or work activities or the duration of symptoms each day (with 0 denoting none, 1, <30 minutes; 2, 30 minutes to 2 hours; and 3, >2 hours).[34,35] These criteria are a valuable sedge way to measure antigen sensitivity objectively.

Additional Workups/Testing

The confirmation of the IgE-mediated type1 Gell and Coombs reaction of AR provides the opportunity for efficiency in treatment strategies, that is, pharmacotherapy, immunotherapy, and avoiding offending environmental allergens.[36] Some current tests confirming allergy sensitivities are described.

Skin testing

Since 1873, the use of skin as a test organ has stood the standard test of time. The skin's abundance, visibility, and accessibility afford numerous therapeutic options/treatment strategies.[37] The use of skin as a bioassay can allow for the option

---

Box 2
Symptoms and physical findings for AR

Symptoms

Nasal

   Sneezing

   Rhinorrhea

   Pruritus

   Impairment of smell

   Congestion

   Eustachian tube dysfunction

Nonnasal

   Lacrimation

   Conjunctivitis

   Fatigue

   Depression

   Headaches

   Midface pressure

   Palatal pruritus

Physical findings

Nasal

   Turbinate hypertrophy/congestion

Ocular

   Allergic shiners due to venous stasis from persistent nasal congestion/lower eyelid edema

   Conjunctivitis

   Dennie lines: creases in the lower eyelids from Mueller muscle spasms

   Allergic lashes

Dental/other

   Crowded teeth/high arch palates

   Dental tooth pain

   Vocal cord edema

   Adenoid hypertrophy

Data from Ahmad N, Zacharek MA. Allergic rhinitis and rhinosinusitis. Otolaryngol Clin North Am 2008; 41(2):267–81.

---

antibodies (**Box 3** depicts examples of the most common tests). These allergens that are tested provide the same antigen extracts that will be used in immunotherapy.[36]

Intradermal testing Intradermal or intracutaneous testing involves the injection of the liquid allergen at specific dilutions into the dermis. A wheal of 4 mm results, just like a tuberculin test. This dilution contacts subepithelial mast cells that form an IgE-mediated reaction. If the patient was previously sensitized, mast cell degranulation occurs and the wheal expands over a period of 10 to 20 minutes. If the measurement increases from 4 to 7 mm or more, the test result is considered positive. Caution must be exerted while interpreting because there can be false-positives and false-negatives due to cross-reactivity with medications that the patient may be taking; skin sensitivity, such as eczema, urticaria, and other dermatologic problems; and glycerin sensitivity because the dilutions contain glycerin.[38] There are single and multidermal intradermal dilution testing.

The benefits of this technique lie in its ability to be qualitative and quantitatively sensitive/specific. Multiple samplings give greater accuracy and safety when evaluating the degree of allergy sensitivity. More importantly, they provide a methodological pathway for a safe starting dose of immunotherapy.[39]

Box 3
Tests for IgE-mediated respiratory allergy sensitivity

Skin tests

Intracutaneous

Intradermal dilution, single/whole

Epicutaneous tests, prick/puncture with single or multiple antigens

End organ provocation

Nasal provocation

Bronchial provocation

Conjunctival provocation

In vitro serologic test: measuring aeroallergen-specific IgE

Radioisotope labeling

Enzyme-linked labeling

Fluorescence labeling

Data from Haydon RC. Allergic rhinitis—current approaches to skin and in vitro testing. Otolaryngol Clin North Am 2008;41(2):331–46.

---

of immunotherapy because allergen-specific immunotherapy can result in significant improvements for allergic nasal, ocular, and bronchial symptoms. Specifically, the clinician can challenge the patient's sensitivity using multiple dosing/strengths to improve sensitivity and specificity, which decreases false-negative findings.

Allergens can be identified by skin or in vitro tests for the presence of allergen-specific IgE

Epicutaneous testing These testing methods were the earliest in determining the sensitivity of allergens. The scratch tests involved placing of the allergen on abraded skin surfaces with equivocal results. Patch testing has been a replacement for chemical sensitivity, and both have been largely replaced by prick/puncture testing.[36,39] The latter approach has become the most often choice for the diagnosis of an IgE-mediated sensitivity. Prick/puncture begins with a drop of allergen on the skin, followed by a puncture through the epidermis only. Multiple antigens can be tested at the same time, and the skin responses are read within 20 minutes.[36] Areas of choice for testing vary from the upper back to volar surfaces of the arms and anterior thighs. Each puncture is about 2 cm from the previous and is compared with controls, which are usually 50% glycerin as a negative control and 50% glycerin with histamine as a positive control. The clinician measures the wheals after 20 minutes, and a positive response is 3 mm or more. The prick/puncture technique is quick, easy, and safe, with good sensitivity and specificity.

In vitro testing In vitro tests for serum IgE antibody to allergens, including varieties of the radioallergosorbent test and enzyme-linked immunosorbent assay, estimate the amount of allergen-specific IgE antibody in a patient's skin. The sensitivity and specificity are equal to that of skin testing.[34,36] The benefits are a single venipuncture, the safety avoidance of cross-reactivity of other medications that the patient may be on, as well as any skin conditions that may exist that can exacerbate the reactions between antigen and IgE-mediated hypersensitivity. The scoring is determined by the intensity of measurements of labeled IgE antibody complexes in the serum. Classes based on 0 to 5 are then interpreted, with class 5 being the most intense reaction, that is, high antibody titers and therefore high allergic sensitivity.[40] These highly sensitive patients can be managed appropriately to avoid any anaphylactic reactions and allow the choosing of appropriate dilution of immunotherapeutic agents.

TREATMENT STRATEGIES FOR AR

The goal of treatment strategies depend on an integrated algorithm based on a cascade of immune responses: (1) an early phase, whereby histamine is released with the resultant acute symptoms of sneezing, itching, rhinorrhea, and congestion, and (2) the late phase, which is mediated by T-cell cytokines of interleukins 4 and 5. This occurs up to 2 hours and involves the infiltration of eosinophils and basophils with more significant rhinorrhea and congestion.[34]

Three main approaches of treatment that are most efficacious against AR are environmental exposure monitoring, pharmacotherapy, and immunotherapy.

Environmental Exposure Monitoring

Environmental control of allergens, both indoors and outdoors, does remain a cornerstone in the preventive therapy for AR. Allergy testing (see earlier) is a valuable place to begin so that both the clinician and the patient can derive a strategy for avoidance/early intervention.[41]

Indoor allergens
Indoor allergens, such as mold, dust mites, and cockroaches, were measured by randomized controlled clinical trials. A trial in 2007 with asthmatic patients showed that eradication of molds significantly reduced attacks.[41] Protocols were developed that included algorithms that were practical and easy to undertake. Limited studies reviewed in a meta-analysis on avoiding house dust mites using high-efficiency particulate air filters (in 1 study), acaricides (in 2 studies), and mattress covers and hot water laundering of bedding (in 1 study) demonstrated that active treatment reduced both levels of house dust mites and rhinitis symptoms.[34,41]

Cockroach sensitization once identified can be eradicated by multiple baits, food monitoring for cleanliness, and traps. Although ventilation is a good way to eradicate indoor allergens, cockroach antigens are not airborne but are heavy and settle into areas that are difficult to keep clean.[41]

Outdoor allergens
It is difficult to perform randomized controlled trials for outdoor allergens, and so a practical approach from wearing protective clothing when gardening to not mowing the lawn during heavy pollen seasons should be adopted. Warm days are associated with high pollen counts, and so outdoor activities need to be monitored.

Pharmacotherapy

Certain classes of drugs have preferential effects against both early- and late-phase symptoms of AR (**Tables 1** and **2**).

Antihistamines
Antihistamines were introduced more than 40 to 50 years ago for the treatment of AR. Their mechanism was to decrease the release of histamine by functioning as a competitive antagonist for the histamine 1 receptor on the target cells of the

Table 1
Pharmacologic agents and their effect on the symptoms of AR

Agent	Sneezing	Itching	Congestion	Rhinorrhea	Ocular Symptoms
Oral antihistamines	+++	+++	±	++	+++
Nasal antihistamines	++	++	++	+	−
Intranasal corticosteroids	++	++	+++	++	+
Leukotriene modifiers	+	+	+	+	+
Oral decongestants	−	−	+++	−	−
Nasal decongestants	−	−	+++	−	−
Mast cell stabilizers	+	+	±	+	−
Topical anticholinergics	−	−	−	+++	−

+++, marked benefit; ++, substantial benefit; +, some mild benefit; ±, questionable benefit; −, no benefit.
Adapted from Krouse JH. Allergic rhinitis—pharmacotherapy. Otolaryngol Clin North Am 2008;41(2):357; with permission.

mucosa of nose, conjunctiva, and lung. The ability to act as a competitive antagonist allowed a decrease in histamine-driven symptoms, that is, rhinorrhea.[34,42] Although clinically effective, antihistamine use was limited by adverse anticholinergic and sedative effects because of the ability of antihistamines to cross the blood-brain barrier, leading to impaired task performance secondary to psychomotor and cognitive impairment. Furthermore, these first-generation agents had significant anticholinergic effects such as xerostomia and blurred vision.

Over the past 30 years, second-generation antihistamines have been developed with better safety profiles. These newer agents do not readily cross the blood-brain barrier and, therefore, lack the

Table 2
Pharmacological agents categorized by their generic and brand names

Agent	Generic Drug Name	Brand Name[R]
Oral Antihistamines	Diphenhydramine	Benadryl
	Hydroxyzine	Atarax
	Chlorpheniramine	Chlor-Trimetron
	Loratadine'	Claritin/Alavert
	Fexofenadine	Allegra
	Cetirizine	Zyrtec
Nasal Antihistamines/	Azelastine	Astelin/Optovar
Opthalmic Anihistamine	Olopatadine	Pataday/Patanol
Intranasal corticosteroids	Beclomethasone diproprionate	Vancenase
	Budesonide	Pulmocort
	Flunisolide	Nasalide
	Fluticasone	Flonase
Leukotriene modifiers	Zileuton	Zyflo
	Montelukast	Singulair
	Zafirlukast	Accolate
Oral decongestants	Pseudoephedrine	Sudafe/Novafed
	Phenylpropanolamine	Accutrim/Propalin
Nasal decongestants	Oxymetazoline	Afrin/Sudafed OM
Mast Cell Stabilizers	Cromolyn sodium	Nasalcrom
Topical anti-cholinergics	Ipratropium bromide	Atrovent/Aepovent
	Ipratropium + Albuterol	Combivent
Mucolytics	Guaifenisin	Mucinex/Humibid

Abbreviation: R, reserved patent drug company.

substantial sedative capability of first-generation drugs. The ability of these agents to significantly interact with central histamine 1 receptors provides for excellent efficacy of the mucosa barrier, which reduces symptoms of nasal itching and watery eyes without impairment of psychomotor function.[42] Terfenadine was the first antihistamine used, although it was withdrawn from the market because of its liver toxicity.[42] Loratadine has been used since the mid-1990s. It is available both as a prescription and an over-the-counter drug. Loratadine is nonsedating at low doses and does not impede liver enzyme activity. Fexofenadine is another agent that has grown in favor since 2005. Although its parent was terfenadine, fexofenadine lacks cardiotoxic capabilities and impediment of liver enzymes. Clinical studies that compared second-generation antihistamines demonstrated equivalence in the reduction of symptoms, with only a small degree of equivocal relationships.[34,42]

The third-generation drugs have been in use since the mid-1990s. Cetirizine, a metabolite of hydroxyzine, has excellent efficacy in allergy-driven symptoms. It has been recently released as an over-the-counter medication safe in doses of 10 mg/d. Over the past few years, desloratadine and levocetirizine have gained favor for the treatment of nasal congestion associated with AR. Clinical studies have shown levocetirizine to have a great efficacy in treating all symptoms of AR, including nasal congestion with minimal sedating effects.[43]

Topical antihistamines, such as azelastine, in conjunction with a topical nasal corticosteroid (see later) are beneficial, rapid, and efficacious in reducing nasal and eye symptoms when compared with oral cetirizine.[44] More studies on the efficaciousness of nasal antihistamines are being evaluated.[34]

Intranasal corticosteroids

Corticosteroids are well known as antiinflammatory medications affecting a variety of cellular mediators in the inflammatory cascade. Topical intranasal corticosteroids are very efficacious in the treatment of moderate to severe AR.[34] The safety profiles of these agents have been evaluated with respect to their systemic effects on growth. A 1-year prospective clinical trial with intranasal mometasone furoate and fluticasone showed no suppression of growth in patients.[34] The bioavailability of nasal corticosteroids is minimal because the amount that is absorbed from the nasal mucosa to the circulation is miniscule.[45] The mechanism of action of nasal corticosteroids occurs mostly during the late phase of AR by acting on T-cell cytokines and eosinophils

as well as during the early phase. Symptoms, including nasal congestion, are better relieved by nasal and oral antihistamines and nasal corticosteroids with respect to symptoms of AR. There was a clinically and statistically significant benefit to nasal corticosteroids over antihistamines for nasal congestion and sneezing.[34,45,46]

Nasal corticosteroids have relatively few adverse effects. The most common effect is epistaxis, which occurs in 10% of cases. Caution is taken when using these agents in terms of timing of doses. They are usually prescribed for 1 to 2 times per day depending on the circumstance. The Food and Drug Administration (FDA) has approved 8 types of medications, beclomethasone, which has grown out of favor because of issues of growth suppression; fluticasone proprionate; and mometasone. Increased intraocular pressure and posterior subcapsular cataracts have been reported in adults. However, these complications are less likely with doses administered intranasally.[34,46,47]

Decongestants

Decongestants are used both topically and orally to decrease nasal vascular congestion and improve nasal airflow. Their mechanism of action is based on α_1-adrenergic and α_2-adrenergic pathways that reduce blood flow within venous capillaries of the nasal and inferior turbinate mucosa. The most commonly prescribed decongestant is pseudoephedrine, which is now restricted because of its ability to be transformed into methamphetamine. The addition of phenylephrine to the formula has helped. In 2001, phenylpropanolamine was also taken off the counter because of the risk of stroke in women. As such, caution must be rendered when prescribing oral decongestants. Even in nonsusceptible patients, side effects such as jitteriness, insomnia, restlessness, and tremulousness must be addressed. Patients who have hypertension and urinary retention are at risk. Topical decongestants are available over the counter, but care must be rendered regarding their efficacy. Hypoxic injury of the nasal mucosa is seen occasionally; rhinitis medicamentosa causes a dependency on nasal medication. These effects may be reversed with nasal corticosteroids if monitored carefully.[42]

Leukotriene receptor antagonists

This group of drugs antagonizes the potent antiinflammatory mediators for the late-phase allergic responses. These antagonists consist of cysteinyl leukotrienes that are released by basophils and mast cells when exposed to antigens, causing an increase in 5-OH-lipoxygenase and the synthesis of active metabolites such as leukotriene D4, E4, and C4. There are a limited number of medications available that are approved by the FDA. Zileuton is used off label for AR and nasal polyps.[42] Another antagonist being used extensively for AR is montelukast. It has been shown to be superior to placebo in relieving nasal symptoms in patients with AR.[48] A meta-analysis demonstrated that, compared with placebo, montelukast induced a moderate but significant reduction in scores for daily symptoms of rhinitis, whereas nasal corticosteroids induced a significant and substantial reduction in symptom scores. This suggests that the role of montelukast is generally as an adjunct in the treatment of a patient who does not have an adequate response to an antihistamine, a nasal corticosteroid, or both.[34,42,48] It can therefore be used in combination therapy.

Mast cell stabilizers, topical anticholinergic, and mucolytics

Mast cell stabilizers Cromolyn sodium is an over-the-counter nasal medication whose mechanism is to decrease calcium influx to mast cells when they bind to antigen. This prevents the degranulation of cells to release histamine. Cromolyn may be more effective when administered just before exposure to an allergen and so is valuable as a prophylactic medication when patients are anticipating an exposure to an antigen.

Topical anticholinergic The one topical agent used is ipratropium bromide. It is used nasally in patients with AR. The drug acts on the parasympathetic tone of the mucosa, with a concomitant decrease in rhinorrhea. It is used with other medications to decrease the nasal discharge when exposed to allergen.

Mucolytics Mucolytics act to decrease the tenacity of nasal secretions. Guaifenesin has been shown to be efficacious because it acts as a vagal stimulant at doses of 2400 mg/d.[49] There is equivocal evidence to support significant improvement in patients with AR, although results may be beneficial for pulmonary secretions.[42]

Monoclonal antibody therapy

There has been much research on the use of monoclonal antibodies for pulmonary diseases refractory to the medications stated earlier. Anti-IgE antibody, omalizumab, has been used to treat asthma refractory to corticosteroids. The mechanism interferes with antigen binding to the mast cell. Although clinical trials show success, it is not a cost-effective treatment $ (10,000 annually) of refractory AR.[50]

The various pharmacotherapeutic options mentioned are predicated on their physiologic ability to alter the mechanisms of action during the early and late phases of AR. **Fig. 2** and see **Table 1** depict the complexity of each phase and the importance of an integrated approach for the most effective management strategies. These options only serve as an adjunct with other treatments to maximize relief from AR.

Immunotherapy for AR

The use of immunotherapy is predicated on patients who are refractory to both environmental control and pharmacotherapy, who require systemic

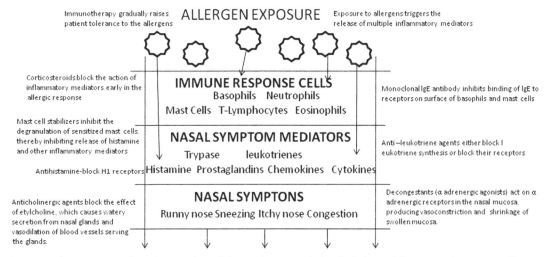

Fig. 2. Mechanisms/cascades of AR and medicine action at each level. (*Adapted from* Marple BF, Fornadley JA, Patel AA, et al. Keys to successful management of patients with allergic rhinitis: focus on patient confidence, compliance, and satisfaction. Otolaryngol Head Neck Surg 2007;136:S112; with permission.)

corticosteroids, who are refractory to the recommended doses of nasal corticosteroids, or who have coexisting conditions such as sinusitis, asthma, or both. This section is divided into 3 units: immunologic mechanisms of immunotherapy, injection immunotherapy, and sublingual immunotherapy (SLIT).

Immunologic mechanisms

A common parameter for investigating how immunotherapy affects immune function is the measurement of serum antibody levels. The predominant class of immunoglobulin is IgG, and, with immunotherapy, there are increases in allergen-specific IgG antibodies. These proteins act as blocking antibodies to prevent allergens from binding to IgE on both mast cells and basophils. Anti-IgG prevents transmembrane signal transduction and degranulation of histamine from mast cells/basophils.[51] The main subset of IgG is IgG1, the levels of which increase rapidly at first when therapy begins but taper off in the first few months of immunotherapy. IgG also inhibits antigen presentation, so a higher concentration of antigen is necessary to induce T-cell proliferation and cytokine release.[52]

Although IgE levels increase in the serum over the first few months of immunotherapy, they decrease to suboptimal levels by 2 years. Symptom change seen in AR seems to be correlated with this increase and decrease. Immunotherapy can also stimulate B cells to increase production of immunoglobulin classes A and M, causing an increase in tolerance to allergen exposure by patients.[51]

The next 2 sections describe the vehicles of immunotherapeutic administration: injection and SLIT.

Injection immunotherapy for AR

Subcutaneous allergen immunotherapy consists of an open-ended schedule of weekly doses of a solution containing the culpable allergens that gradually increase to an optimal maintenance dose.[34,52,53] Maintenance doses are often given at intervals ranging from 2 to 6 weeks; data are lacking to compare various dosing frequencies. Numerous meta-analyses and systematic reviews have been written that support the efficacious effect of subcutaneous injection immunotherapy.[51] A Cochrane systematic review was recently published that scrutinized 51 studies for seasonal allergies. In 15 studies, there were 1645 participants receiving immunotherapy and 1226 receiving placebo. The meta-analyses showed an overall significant reduction in symptom scores as measured by a standard mean difference in all 15 studies after completion of subcutaneous immunotherapy

($P<.0001$).[53] The same systematic review was analyzed for bronchial and ocular symptoms, as well as rhinosinusitis quality-of-life measurements. The results were again significant with reduction in symptom scores.

These reviews support the premise that allergen-specific immunotherapy can decrease allergen symptoms. A systematic review by Calderon and colleagues[53] supports this premise, although, the data lacked samples from pediatric population. This finding suggests that caution must be rendered when applying immunotherapy within this population until more definitive clinical trials are evaluated.[34,44,51,52] Immunotherapy, however, may also confer long-term benefits for AR in that it alters the natural history of the disease. The reviews mentioned reported adverse reactions as local or systemic. The local reactions were analyzed in 30 studies, with approximately 10% requiring treatment: 208 in active treatment and 186 in the placebo group.[51–53]

The systemic reaction was reviewed in 33 studies and graded based on a consensus paper. Reactions are graded from 1 to 4, with 1 being mild to 4 being anaphylactic shock. Although the majority in the sample had mild reactions, the rate of systemic reactions can range for 0.05% to 2.9%, with 1 fatality per 2 million injections.[51,54] Approximately 5% to 10% of patients who receive allergen immunotherapy have systemic reactions, which are moderately to severe in 1% to 3% of patients; rarely, patients have even died of anaphylaxis.[34,51,53]

SLIT for AR

The use of SLIT in the treatment of AR has been researched over the last 2 decades. Meta-analyses on the efficacy/safety of SLIT have been mostly from studies in Europe. Wilson and colleagues[55] published a large meta-analysis on the efficacy of SLIT in AR. Symptom severity scores were measured, and results showed a significant decrease in rhinitis and need for any medications. A meta-analysis done by Penagos and colleagues[56] revealed a significant reduction in symptom severity with SLIT in the pediatric population. The period to 18 months showed the greatest efficacy, suggesting longer treatment of AR when it involves seasons, that is, pollen versus dust mites. The former study by Wilson and colleagues, however, did not see such significance and suggested that it is because of smaller pediatric sample size.[51,56] Although SLIT seems to be very effective as a method for immunotherapy in children and adults, more studies with larger sample sizes are needed.

Box 4
Treatment guidelines for patients with AR

1. Verify the cause of allergic symptoms with the use of history and tests

2. Reduce exposure to allergens

3. Start an inhaled nasal corticosteroid, an oral second-generation antihistamine, or both

4. For resistant nasal symptoms, add a leukotriene receptor antagonist; for resistant itching or tearing eyes, add an ocular antihistamine, mast cell stabilizer, or nonsteroidal antiinflammatory drug

5. Consider immunotherapy if quality of relief with medication is inadequate to forestall progression of disease or if patient is affected by allergy-induced complications, such as sinusitis and asthma

Adapted from Plaut M, Valentine MD. Allergic rhinitis. N Engl J Med 2005;353:1934–44; with permission.

SLIT has been shown to have a good safety profile. Although mild oral and sublingual itching occurs, there have been no reports of systemic reactions to this therapy. The rarity of systemic reactions suggests that this therapy is safer than subcutaneous immunotherapy. There were a few trials that showed adverse events on oral and gastrointestinal sequelae, but none were characterized as anaphylactic.[51] With respect to the pediatric population, SLIT is safer than injection therapy.[51,56] With the evidence presented, it seems that there is a significant role for immunotherapy in preventing the progression of allergen damage. Further studies are being developed to determine whether there is a place for prophylactic immunotherapy in the treatment of AR. In addition, further work is underway to evaluate the efficacy and safety of such therapies and to determine whether the preparation of large numbers of anti-immunoallergens is feasible.[34,56]

SUMMARY/FUTURE DIRECTIONS

Five sets of guidelines for treatment of AR have been developed from expert panels, 2 in the United States and 3 in Europe (**Box 4**). This approach has been used with some success.[57,58] AR, however, only represents one link/catalyst in the spectrum of inflammatory diseases involved in the unified airway. It is an illness of great health expenditure, significantly affecting the health and well-being of those who are susceptible. The clinician must carefully evaluate the symptoms of AR, as well as associated comorbidities throughout the upper and lower airway, to avoid inappropriate

management. There are risk-to-benefit ratios to be weighed when considering therapeutic intervention. The pursuit of further evidence relating to the clinical application of immunotherapy should be a future priority in evidence-based clinical decisions.

REFERENCES

1. Krouse JH. The unified airway—conceptual framework. Otolaryngol Clin North Am 2008;41(2):257–66.
2. Passalaqua G, Ciprandi G, Canonica GW. United airway diseases: therapeutic aspects. Thorax 2000; 55:26–7.
3. Bousquet J, van Cauwenberge P, Khaltaev N, et al. Allergic rhinitis and its impact on asthma (ARIA); executive summary of the workshop report. Allergy 2002;57:841–55.
4. Ahmad N, Zacharek MA. Allergic rhinitis and rhinosinusitis. Otolaryngol Clin North Am 2008;41:267–81.
5. Dykewicz MS, Fineman S, Skoner DP, et al. Diagnosis and management of rhinitis: complete guidelines for the joint Task Force on Practice Parameters in Allergy, Asthma and Immunology. Ann Allergy Asthma Immunol 1998;81:478–518.
6. Meltzer EO. The relationship of rhinitis to asthma. Allergy Asthma Proc 2005;26:336–40.
7. Summary of health statistics for US adults: National Health Interview Survey, 2002. Available at: http://www.cdc.gov/nchc/fastats/allergies.htm. Accessed August, 2008.
8. Kremer B. Quality of life scales in allergic rhinitis. Curr Opin Allergy Clin Immunol 2004;4:171–6.
9. Yawn BP, Yunginger JW, Wollan PC, et al. Allergic rhinitis in Rochester, Minnesota, residents with asthma: frequency and impact on health care changes. J Allergy Clin Immunol 1999;103:54–9.
10. Ryan MW. Asthma and rhinitis: comorbidities. Otolaryngol Clin North Am 2008;41:283–95.
11. Halpern LR, Martin RA, Carter JB. Pharmacotherapeutics of rhinosinusitis: treatment protocols in the adult and pediatric population. Oral and Maxillofacial Surgery Clinics of North America. Philadelphia: W. B. Saunders; 2000.
12. Yaritkas M, Doner F, Demirci M. Rhinosinusitis among the patients with perennial or seasonal allergic rhinitis. Asian Pac J Allergy Immunol 2003;21:75–8.
13. Zacharek M, Krouse J. The role of allergy in chronic rhinosinusitis. Curr Opin Otolaryngol Head Neck Surg 2003;11:196–200.
14. Weiss KB, Sullivan SD, Lyttle CS. Trends in the cost of illness for asthma in the United States, 1985-1994. J Allergy Clin Immunol 2000;106(3):493–9.
15. Joe SA, Thakkar K. Chronic rhinosinusitis and asthma. Otolaryngol Clin North Am 2008;41(2): 297–309.

16. Togias A. Rhinitis and asthma: evidence for respiratory system integration. J Allergy Clin Immunol 2003; 111:1171–83.
17. Huovinen E, Kaprio J, Laitinen LA, et al. Incidence and prevalence of asthma among adult Finnish men and women of the Finnish twin cohort from 1975 to 1990, and their relation to hay fever and chronic bronchitis. Chest 1999;115(4):928–36.
18. Halpern MT, Schmier JK, Richner R, et al. Allergic rhinitis: a potential cause of increased asthmatic medication use, costs, and morbidity. J Asthma 2004;41(1):117–26.
19. Dixon AD, Kaminsky DA, Holbrook JT, et al. Allergic rhinitis and sinusitis in asthma. Chest 2006;130(2): 429–35.
20. Shinohara M, Wakiguchi H, Saito H, et al. Symptoms of allergic rhinitis in women during early pregnancy are associated with higher prevalence of allergic rhinitis in their offspring. Allergol Int 2007;56(4):1–7.
21. Norman P, et al. Allergic rhinitis. In: Frank M, Austen KF, Claman HN, et al, editors. Samter's immunologic diseases, vol. 2, 5th edition. Boston: Little Brown; 1995. p. 1279–82.
22. Eapen RJ, Ebert CS, Pillsbury HC. Allergic rhinitis—history and presentation. Otolaryngol Clin North Am 2008;41(2):325–30.
23. Bachert PG, Vignola AM, Gevaert P, et al. Allergic rhinitis, rhinosinusitis, and asthma: one airway disease. Immunol Allergy Clin North Am 2004;24: 19–43.
24. Pawankar R. Allergic rhinitis and asthma: are they manifestations of one syndrome? Clin Exp Allergy 2006;36:1–4.
25. Krouse JH, Brown RW, Fineman SM, et al. Asthma and the unified airway. Otolaryngol Head Neck Surg 2007;136:S75–106.
26. Townley RG, Ryu UY, Kolotkin BM, et al. Bronchial sensitivity to methacholine in current and former asthmatic and allergic rhinitis patients and control subjects. J Allergy Clin Immunol 1975;56:429–42.
27. The European Community Respiratory Health Survey Steering Committee. The European Community Respiratory Health Survey II. Eur Respir J 2002; 20:1071–9.
28. Benninger MS, Ferguson BJ, Hadley JA, et al. Adult chronic rhinosinusitis: definitions, diagnosis, epidemiology, and pathophysiology. Otolaryngol Head Neck Surg 2003;129(Suppl 3):S1–32.
29. Harlin S, Ansel D, Lane S, et al. A clinical and pathologic study of chronic sinusitis: the role of the eosinophil. J Allergy Clin Immunol 1988;81(5 Pt 1):867–75.
30. Zeitz HJ. Bronchial asthma, nasal polyps and aspirin sensitivity: Samter's syndrome. Clin Chest Med 1988;9(4):567–76.
31. Szczeklik A, Stevenson D. Aspirin-induced asthma: advances in pathogenesis, diagnosis, and management. J Allergy Clin Immunol 2003;127(3):316–21.
32. Sousa A, Parikh A, Scadding G, et al. Leukotriene receptor expression on nasal mucosal inflammatory cells in aspirin-sensitive rhinosinusitis. N Engl J Med 2002;347(19):592–8.
33. Du Buske LS, Sheffer AL. Allergic rhinitis and other disease of the nose. In: Branch W, editor. Office practice of medicine. 3rd edition. Philadelphia: W.B. Saunders; 1994. p. 176–85.
34. Plaut M, Valentine MD. Allergic rhinitis. N Engl J Med 2005;353:1934–44.
35. Bousquet J, Van Cauwenberge P, Khaltaev N. Allergic rhinitis and its impact on asthma. J Allergy Clin Immunol 2001;108(Suppl 5):S147–334.
36. Haydon RC. Allergic rhinitis—current approaches to skin and in-vitro testing. Otolaryngol Clin North Am 2008;41(2):331–46.
37. Blackley CH. Experimental researches on the causes and nature of catarrhus aestivus. London: Balliere, Trindall, Cox; 1873.
38. Mabry RL. Whealing responses. In: Mabry RL, editor. Skin endpoint titration. 2nd edition. New York: Thieme Medical Publishers; 1994. p. 19–25.
39. Smith TF. Allergy testing in clinical practice. Ann Allergy Asthma Immunol 1992;68:293–302.
40. Lockey RF. "ARIA": global guidelines and new forms of allergen immunotherapy. J Allergy Clin Immunol 2001;108(4):497–9.
41. Ferguson BJ. Environmental control of allergies. Otolaryngol Clin North Am 2008;41:411–7.
42. Krouse JH. Allergic rhinitis—current pharmacotherapy. Otolaryngol Clin North Am 2008;41(2): 347–58.
43. Bachert C, Bousquet J, Canonica GW, et al. Levocetirizine improves quality of life and reduces cost in long-term management of persistent allergic rhinitis. J Allergy Clin Immunol 2004;114:838–44.
44. Berger W, Hampel F Jr, Bernstein J, et al. Impact of azelastine nasal spray on symptoms and quality of life compared with cetirizine oral tablets in patients with seasonal allergic rhinitis. Ann Allergy Asthma Immunol 2006;97:375–81.
45. Yanez A, Rodrigo GJ. Intranasal corticosteroids versus topical H1 receptor antagonists for the treatment of allergic rhinitis: a systematic review with meta-analysis. Ann Allergy Asthma Immunol 1997; 79:237–45.
46. Nielsen LP, Dahl R. Comparison of intranasal corticosteroids and antihistamines in allergic rhinitis: a review of randomized, controlled trials. Am J Respir Med 2003;2:55–65.
47. Juniper EF, Stahl E, Doty RL, et al. Clinical outcomes and adverse effect monitoring in allergic rhinitis. J Allergy Clin Immunol 2005;115:S390–413.
48. Wilson AM, O'Byrne PM, Parameswa-ran K. Leukotriene receptor antagonists for allergic rhinitis: a systematic review and meta-analysis. Am J Med 2004;116:338–45.

49. Yuta A, Baraniuk JN. Therapeutic approaches to mucus hypersecretion. Curr Allergy Asthma Rep 2005;5:243–51.

50. Berger WE. Treatment of allergic rhinitis and other immunoglobulin E–mediated diseases with anti-immunoglobulin E antibody. Allergy Asthma Proc 2006;27:S29–32.

51. Leatherman B. Injection and sublingual immuno-therapy in the management of allergies affecting the unified airway. Otolaryngol Clin North Am 2008; 41(2):359–74.

52. van Neerven RJ, Wikborg T, Lund G, et al. Blocking antibodies induced by specific allergy vaccination prevent the activation of CD4+ T cells by inhibiting serum Ig-E facilitated allergen presentation. J Immunol 1999;163:2944–52.

53. Calderon MA, Alves B, Jacobson M, et al. Allergen injection immunotherapy for seasonal allergic rhinitis [see comment]. Cochrane Database Syst Rev 2007;1:CD001936.

54. Tinkelman DG, Cole WQ 3rd, Tunno J. Immuno-therapy: a one year prospective study to evaluate risk factors of systemic reactions. J Allergy Clin Immunol 1995;95:8–14.

55. Wilson DR, Lima MT, Durham SR. Sublingual immuno-therapy for allergic rhinitis: systematic review and meta-analysis [see comment]. Allergy 2005;60:4–12.

56. Penagos M, Compalati E, Tarantini F, et al. Efficacy of sublingual immunotherapy in the treatment of allergic rhinitis in pediatric patients 3 to 18 years of age: a meta- analysis of randomized, placebo controlled, double blinded-trials. Ann Allergy Asthma Immunol 2006;97:141–8.

57. American Academy of Allergy, Asthma, and Immu-nology. The allergy report. Available at: http://www. theallergyreport.org. Accessed October 7, 2005.

58. van Cauwenberge P, Bachert C, Passal-acqua G, et al. Consensus statement on the treatment of allergic rhinitis: European Academy of Allergology and Clinical Immunology. Allergy 2000;55:116–34.

Epistaxis and Hemostatic Devices

Levon Nikoyan, DDS*, Stanley Matthews, DDS

KEYWORDS

- Paranasal sinuses • Nasal anatomy • Sinus anatomy

Epistaxis is a common medical problem that rarely requires surgical intervention.[1] However, when medical or surgical intervention is required, epistaxis can sometimes be difficult to control. Knowledge of nasopharyngeal anatomy is absolutely essential to the proper management of epistaxis. This article begins with a discussion of the essential anatomy of the region and the basic epidemiology of epistaxis, followed by a review of initial treatment as well as devices and procedures specifically designed for the control of epistaxis. Advances and new devices for the control of epistaxis are described.

EPIDEMIOLOGY

Epistaxis is a common reason for hospitalization even though surgical intervention is rarely required.[2] The distribution of epistaxis is largely bimodal: mostly occurring before age 10 years and peaking again much later between ages 45 and 65 years. Estrogen seems to have a protective effect on epistaxis, as males younger than 49 years are more likely to experience the problem. After the age of 49 years, the statistics equalize between male and female populations.[3] Seasonal variation in the frequency of nasal bleeds also exists, with winter being the most common time for epistaxis.[4] Other factors affecting epistaxis include allergic rhinitis, humidity, and upper respiratory tract infections.

ANATOMY

Most nasal bleeds can be broadly classified as either anterior or posterior, based on their origin.

Although anterior bleeds are far more common, posterior epistaxis is occasionally encountered in hospital emergency rooms and is particularly difficult to manage, with a higher chance of patient hospitalizations.[5,6]

The arterial supply of the nose is complex, as it originates from both internal and external carotid arteries. The branches of the internal carotid that supply the nose are branches of the anterior and posterior ethmoid arteries from the ophthalmic artery. The external carotid contributes via the sphenopalatine, greater palatine, superior labial, and angular arteries. The external nose is supplied by the facial artery, which becomes the angular artery coursing over the superomedial aspect of the nose. Internally, the lateral nasal wall is supplied by the sphenopalatine artery posteroinferiorly and by the anterior and posterior ethmoid arteries superiorly. The nasal septum also derives its blood supply from the sphenopalatine and the anterior and posterior ethmoid arteries, with the added contribution of the superior labial artery (anteriorly) and the greater palatine artery (posteriorly).

The anterior nasal septum is the site of an abundant plexus of vessels called the Kiesselbach area, which is supplied by both systems. A summary of particular arteries from both of these systems is presented in **Fig. 1**. Veins in the nose essentially follow the arterial pattern, and are significant for their direct communication with the cavernous sinus and for their lack of valves. These features potentiate the intracranial spread of infection.

The authors have nothing to disclose.
Oral and Maxillofacial Surgery, Department of Dentistry, Woodhull Medical and Mental Health Center, 760 Broadway, Room 2C-320, Brooklyn, NY 11206, USA
* Corresponding author. 7709 Eliot Avenue, Middle Village, NY 11379.
E-mail address: Levon@nyu.edu

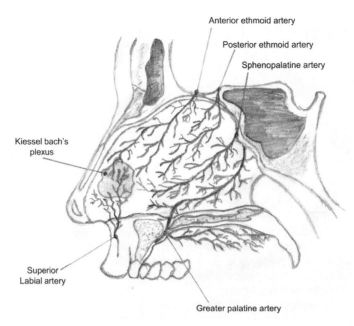

Fig. 1. Kiesselbach plexus. (*Courtesy of* Albert Hakobyan, Queens, NY.)

ETIOLOGY

Just as for the source of the bleed, the primary underlying reason for epistaxis can be divided into local or systemic factors (**Figs. 2** and **3**).[7] A detailed list of local causes is presented in **Fig. 2**, one of the most common of which is digital trauma and reduced humidification during the winter months. Epistaxis is also common after nasal surgery and maxillofacial trauma. Special consideration is given to epistaxis that is recurrent, as it may be a symptom of a benign or malignant neoplasm of the nasal cavity, sinus, or nasopharynx.

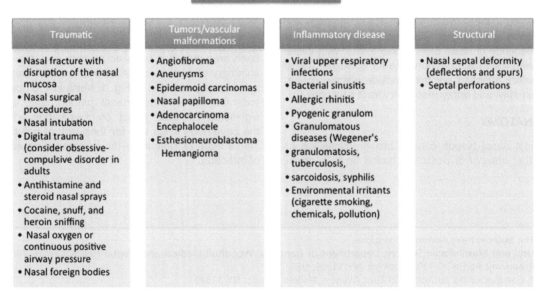

Fig. 2. Local causes of epistaxis. (*Data from* Cummings CW. Otolaryngology—head and neck surgery, vols. 1–4. 4th edition. St Louis (MO): Elsevier Mosby; 2005.)

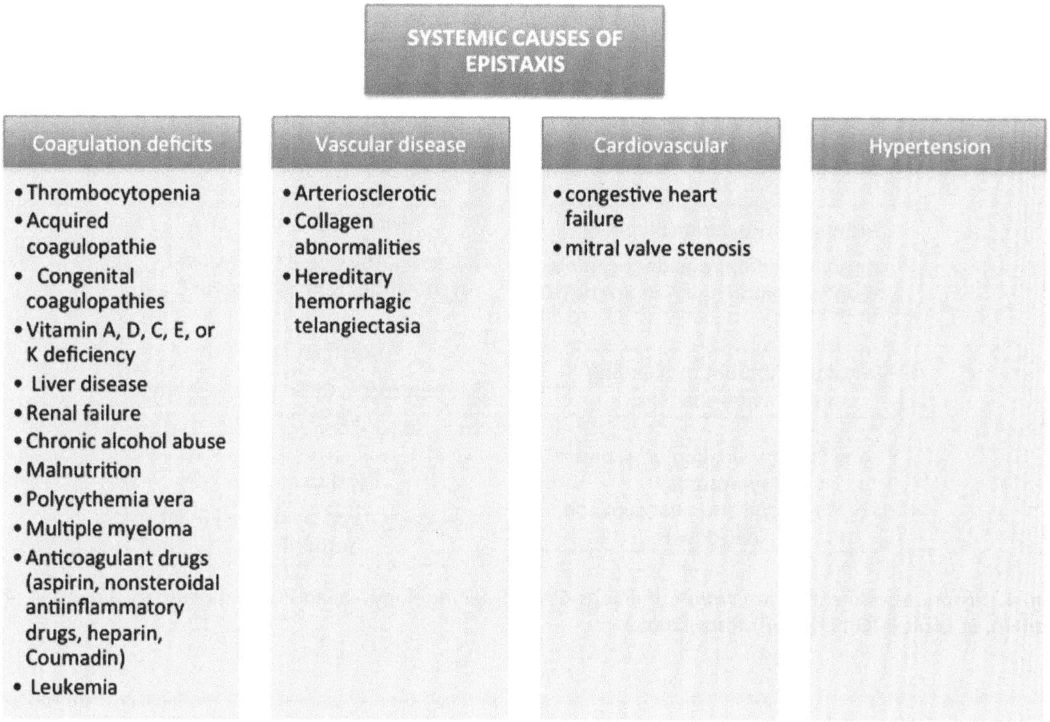

SYSTEMIC CAUSES OF EPISTAXIS			
Coagulation deficits	**Vascular disease**	**Cardiovascular**	**Hypertension**
• Thrombocytopenia • Acquired coagulopathie • Congenital coagulopathies • Vitamin A, D, C, E, or K deficiency • Liver disease • Renal failure • Chronic alcohol abuse • Malnutrition • Polycythemia vera • Multiple myeloma • Anticoagulant drugs (aspirin, nonsteroidal antiinflammatory drugs, heparin, Coumadin) • Leukemia	• Arteriosclerotic • Collagen abnormalities • Hereditary hemorrhagic telangiectasia	• congestive heart failure • mitral valve stenosis	

Fig. 3. Systemic causes of epistaxis. (*Data from* Cummings CW. Otolaryngology—head and neck surgery, vols. 1–4. 4th edition. St Louis (MO): Elsevier Mosby; 2005.)

Systemic causes of epistaxis are far less identifiable, as they may represent problems that arise from multiple systemic conditions and usually remain refractory to local treatment modalities (see the detailed list in **Fig. 3**). A common systemic cause for epistaxis represents a group of coagulation disorders in individuals with prolonged bleeding time from minor cuts or bruises. The most common is von Willebrand disease, which often presents with epistaxis that is frequent and difficult to manage.[8] Other systemic coagulation abnormalities such as low platelet count (<20,000/µL), drug-related acquired bleeding disorders, chronic alcoholism, and vitamin K deficiencies all contribute to the frequency and severity of epistaxis.[9,10] Another relatively rare systemic condition that initially manifests as epistaxis is hereditary hemorrhagic telangiectasia (HHT).[11,12] This condition, also known as Osler-Weber-Rendu disease, is an autosomal dominant disorder affecting blood vessels and resulting in localized vascular malformation.[13] Patients with HHT have normal hemostasis and platelet function, therefore the recurrent hemorrhages are related to the localized abnormality within the blood vessels.[14]

Other logical systemic causes of epistaxis such as hypertension are still debated in the literature, as several studies have failed to show an association with epistaxis.[15,16]

EVALUATION

The initial evaluation of epistaxis should focus on airway assessment and cardiovascular stability, including visual assessment and a review of vital signs and any laboratory studies that may have been obtained. Moreover, assessment of possible compromise of the cardiopulmonary system should be evaluated. After the stability of the patient has been assured, the complete and detailed history should be obtained (**Fig. 4**).

MANAGEMENT

After the initial evaluation of the patient has been completed and all appropriate first steps of treatment have been performed, it is prudent to achieve initial cessation of the bleeding. The initial management should include removal of any poorly coagulated blood clots by blowing the nose, use of intranasal vasoconstrictors such as oxymetazoline, and asking the patient to pinch the nose tightly for 10 minutes. For some patients, 2 sprays of oxymetazoline in each nostril may be the only required treatment.[17] After the initial maneuvers have been

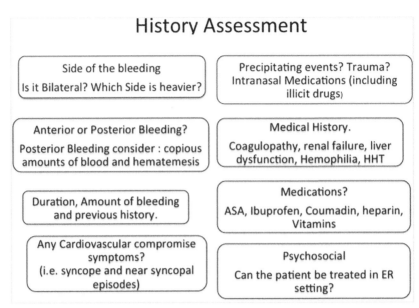

Fig. 4. History assessment. (*Data from* Cummings CW. Otolaryngology—head and neck surgery, vols. 1–4. 4th edition. St Louis (MO): Elsevier Mosby; 2005.)

performed, if the epistaxis has not been brought under control it is reasonable to identify the source of the bleeding; differentiating whether it is an anterior or a posterior bleed is the most crucial step in achieving a positive outcome. On occasion, however, the bleeding has stopped and the source of the bleeding cannot be identified. It is appropriate then to observe the patient for 30 minutes and pack only if the bleeding reoccurs.[18]

ANTERIOR EPISTAXIS

When the source of the bleeding is identified as an anterior epistaxis, it is prudent to properly anesthetize the nasal cavity before any examination. Several anesthetic agents are commonly used to anesthetize the nasal mucosa, and include 2% lidocaine, lidocaine with epinephrine, and 4% cocaine. These agents not only provide anesthesia of the nasal mucosa but also aid in the management of the epistaxis.[19] Such medications can be applied using saturated cotton swabs or cotton pledgets.

When an anterior nasal bleed is identified, the first line of defense should be chemical or electrical cautery. Chemical cautery can be achieved using silver nitrate sticks, which are available in several concentrations. As the concentration of the silver nitrate in the sticks increases, it leads to an increase in the depth of penetration and coagulation properties. However, this can also lead to a potential increase in the complications

associated with chemical cautery.[20] Regardless of the concentration of the silver nitrate applicators, the general principles are the same. The application begins with the proper visualization of the bleeding area; once identified, one should begin at the periphery and slowly move the applicator to the center of the bleed. Care must be exercised not to overcauterize because this might lead to posttreatment rhinorrea.[21]

Any of the currently available electrocautery devices can also be used to cauterize the bleeding sites when the source has been identified. It has been shown that these devices are at least as effective as silver nitrate applicators in the initial management of epistaxis.[22]

NASAL PACKING

When the initial cautery is unsuccessful, the next step in the management of epistaxis is nasal packing. Packing can be achieved with a variety of materials including ribbon gauze (**Fig. 5**), nasal tampons (usually made from newer materials such as Merocel [Medtronic ENT. Jacksonville, FL, USA]), and nasal balloon catheters.[23] Of these devices, Merocel (**Fig. 6**) packing is made of a newer synthetic open-cell foam polymer that seems to provide a less benevolent environment for *Staphylococcus aureus*.[24] The insertion is accomplished quite easily, as follows. Coat the tampon with bacitracin and then insert the tampon by sliding it directly along the floor of the nasal

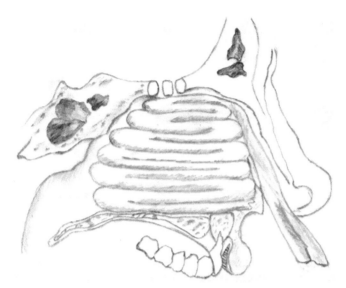

Fig. 5. Ribbon gauze packing. (*Courtesy of* Albert Hakobyan, Queens, NY.)

cavity until it lies within the nasal cavity. As the tampon enters the nasal cavity it should remain almost parallel to the alar-tragal line; this ensures that the tampon will enter the nasal cavity properly. The tampon should then be expanded with approximately 10 mL of saline solution.

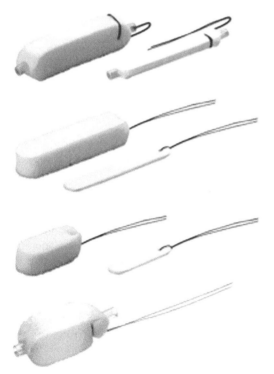

Fig. 6. Merocel epistaxis packing (Medtronic Inc, Jacksonville, FL, USA). (*Courtesy of* Medtronic ENT; with permission.)

Nasal balloon catheters represent a large group of epistaxis devices that are widely available in emergency rooms. These devices are easier to use than gauze, and in several studies have been shown to be as effective as Merocel and gauze packing, but are better tolerated by patients.[25] One such device is the Rapid Rhino (ArthoCare ENT, Austin, TX, USA), a balloon catheter with a large, low-pressure air balloon encased in a carboxymethylated cellulose (CMC) mesh.[26] This catheter is available in several lengths to accommodate anterior and posterior bleeds. A recent addition is the Rapid Rhino 900, a 9-cm long catheter that contains 2 balloons for the tamponade of the sphenopalatine artery (**Fig. 7**).

To use Rapid Rhino, it must be first submerged in sterile water for at least 30 seconds. The catheter will then become soft and lubricated to facilitate the insertion. On contact with blood, the CMC fibers act to promote thrombosis. The placement begins with insertion of the catheter parallel to the nasal floor to the outlined depth (which can vary depending on what length of catheter is used). Once the insertion is satisfactorily achieved, using a 10-mL syringe the balloon is inflated and the pilot cuff is frequently evaluated for the reference pressure.[27] The balloon catheter should remain intact for at least 24 hours and the patient reevaluated before it is removed.

THROMBOGENIC FOAMS AND GELS

There are several new products currently under development and in early use that may change the

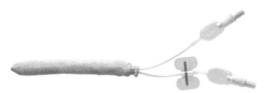

Fig. 7. Rapid Rhino 900 epistaxis device (ArthroCare ENT, Austin, TX, USA). (*Courtesy of* Arthrocare, Austin, TX; with permission.)

initial management of epistaxis. Quixil (Ethicon/Johnson & Johnson, Somerville, NJ, USA) is a fibrin glue and sealant that has been shown to be as effective as nasal packing in the control of epistaxis.[28] The product is supplied as 2 components that, when combined, begin the formation of fibrin, a clotting protein.[28] Another thrombogenic gel is Floseal (Baxter, Hayward, CA, USA) (**Fig. 8**), which is a human-derived thrombin gel that facilitates clotting and can be applied directly to the bleeding site.[29] According to the limited published data to date, Floseal has a much lower rebleeding rate, easier insertion, and better procedure tolerance.[30,31]

POSTERIOR BLEEDING

Posterior nasal bleeding occurs much more rarely than anterior bleeding, and constitutes approximately 5% of all nasal bleeding.[32,33] Moreover, when posterior bleeds do occur, they are generally seen in a much older population with multiple systemic comorbidities. Regardless of the age of the patient, however, posterior epistaxis is challenging to treat, as the definitive source of bleeding is often extremely difficult to identify. Posterior nasal packing has traditionally been the mainstay treatment for initial intervention, and has an isolated success rate of approximately 70%.[33] Recently, successful therapeutic modalities have become available, such as endoscopic arterial ligation or embolization; however, these require the use of special equipment and the expertise of a specialist.[34] The standard of care in an emergency room setting with emergency physicians remains posterior packing to gain primary control of the bleeding and provision of further follow-up with the specialists.[33]

The approach to the patient with a posterior bleed differs somewhat from that for an anterior bleed, and also depends on the principle of pressure. The preferred device for the control of posterior epistaxis is the balloon catheter. Although specific details of application vary, the general

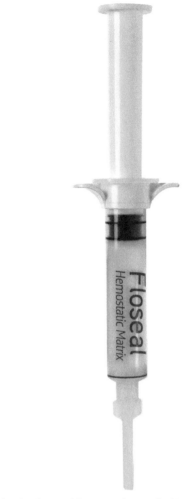

Fig. 8. Flowseal hemostatic matrix (Baxter, Hayward, CA, USA). (*Courtesy of* Baxter, Hayward, CA; with permission.)

principles remain the same. These catheters are generally longer than catheters meant for anterior packing, and may contain 1 or 2 balloon mechanisms.[35] After the initial examination has been completed and the posterior nasal bleed identified, the catheter is advanced along the floor until the retention ring reaches the naris. At this time the posterior balloon should be inflated to 10 mL of sterile water and retracted gently until it reaches the nasopharynx. Once the catheter is seated properly, the anterior balloon can be inflated and the pilot cuff secured to the patient's cheek.

When balloon catheters are not available, a Foley catheter or cotton gauze can be used to manage posterior nasal bleeding (**Fig. 9**). Neither of these techniques is particularly new, and both have been discussed extensively in the literature.[1,36]

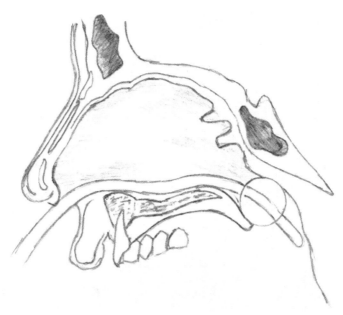

Fig. 9. Foley catheter for posterior epistaxis control. (*Courtesy of* Albert Hakobyan, Queens, NY.)

Regardless of the device used, it should be periodically checked because prolonged pressure resulting from overinflation in the posterior nasal cavity can lead to serious complications, such as palate necrosis. Posterior packing should only remain in place consistently for 48 to 96 hours. When using either the Foley or balloon system, the balloon should be let down occasionally to allow blood flow to the posterior palate, but the pack itself should be left in place. In doing so, the risk of palate necrosis is decreased. After a 24-hour period of no rebleeding, the posterior packing can be removed while the Foley or balloon catheter is deflated. Hospitalization for patients with posterior nasal bleeds should always be a consideration, as it allows close monitoring of effectiveness of the packing and the early detection of nasopulmonary reflex.[37] Other respiratory complications, including hypoxia, hypoxemia, and hypoventilation can also be detected early and treated quickly.[38,39]

Generally speaking, any bleeding that fails to stop after the aforementioned treatment will require surgical intervention, most likely under general anesthesia. The surgical options are broad and range from better visualization of the bleeding, to septal surgery, to ligation of arteries. Ligation of the sphenopalatine artery is perhaps the first step in the surgical procedural ladder and has a very good success rate.[40] Ligation of the sphenopalatine artery has been historically performed with direct laryngoscopy with the patient under general anesthesia in the operating room. In recent years, however, as endoscopic procedures have gained popularity, an increasing number of these procedures are being performed in a minimally invasive fashion via a transnasal endoscope.[41,42]

Occasionally, ligation of other arteries becomes necessary in the case of severe nasal bleeding. Ligation of ethmoidal, maxillary, and external carotid arteries is possible for the treatment of severe and retractable epistaxis.[43] Ethmoidal arteries can be ligated directly via an external ethmoidectomy incision or, as recently described, via an endoscopically assisted external approach.[44] Maxillary artery ligation is now rarely performed, but can be completed via a modified Caldwell-Luc approach.[43,45,46]

For the most severe cases of ligation and as a last resort, ligation of the external artery can be performed.[47]

At certain medical centers where interventional radiologists are readily available, arterial embolization may be an option for the treatment of epistaxis. Embolization is accomplished by cannulation of the external carotid artery and localization of the bleeding by contrast. The artery that is the source of bleeding can then be embolized by coils, gels, or polyvinyl alcohol.[48]

SURGERY

Epistaxis is also common after head and neck surgery. In several studies, epistaxis was the most commonly occurring complication after endoscopic surgery.[49] As a result, many surgeons routinely use techniques such as preoperative nasal packing and sphenopalatine artery ligation before surgery.[50] Of particular interest is epistaxis after orthognathic surgery and more specifically after Lefort I maxillary osteotomy. Although mild and intermittent epistaxis immediately postoperatively and intraoperatively is an easily manageable complication, a severe epistaxis sometimes occurs. There are only a few cases of these life-threatening epistaxis episodes described in the literature, most of which were due to the unique phenomenon of pseudoaneurysms.[51]

False aneurysm (pseudoaneurysm) usually results from an incomplete tear of the artery, leading to continuous bleeding into the adjacent soft tissue while the vessel's blood flow is maintained. The bleeding into the adjacent tissue continues until the pressure between the artery and the periphery equalizes, forming a hematoma. As the hematoma matures, it remains connected with the lumen of the vessel and a sac with an endothelial lining forms around it. This sac continues to increase in size and can rupture at any time, resulting in massive bleeding. The artery most commonly involved in the formation of false aneurysms is the internal maxillary artery and its distal branch the sphenopalatine artery.[52] In the 3 cases described by Lanigan and colleagues[52] and by Solomons and Blumgart,[53] the epistaxis began as late as 2 weeks postoperatively; this may continue intermittently until the pseudoaneurysm ruptures, at which point the epistaxis is generally severely unresponsive to packing.

Epistaxis may also be present in the rupture or false-aneurysm formation of the descending palatine artery (DPA). This artery is a terminal branch of the maxillary artery and lies within the greater palatine canal, which is located in the perpendicular plate of palatine bone and crosses in the anterior-inferior-medial direction with average angulations of 60° in the sagittal plane.[54] The DPA is extremely sensitive to damage as it passes through the pterygopalatine fossa, and it may be severed here by osteotomes (as the maxillary tuberosity is separated from the pterygoid plates) or during down-fracture of the maxilla. Laceration of the DPA leads to heavy bleeding intraoperatively, but this is often controllable by application of direct pressure. At times, the artery will contract into its bony canal and may result in a nosebleed a few days after surgery. Occasionally, however, when using hypotensive anesthesia, laceration of the DPA may be masked, and bleeding may then occur within the first 48 hours after surgery.

The management of postsurgical epistaxis begins with a high index of suspicion as well as patient education. Any patient with postoperative epistaxis after 2 weeks must be suspected to have a false aneurysm, and an angiogram is indicated. Patients must be instructed not to blow their nose because the pressure generated during sneezing will be transmitted to the sinuses, leading to a nosebleed. Keeping the nasal passages free of mucus and blood can prevent sneezing. Common methods include saline or oxymetazoline (Afrin) nasal sprays, use of humidifiers, and frequent showering. Nevertheless, it is common for patients to have light nasal bleeding intermittently 1 or 2 days after surgery. Patients should also be taught to use wire cutters in the event of an emergency outside the hospital; while inpatients, wire cutters should be easily accessible at all times because they may become a life-saving tool.

If arterial bleeding is suspected, large blood clots may be found in the oropharynx, giving the impression of continuous bleeding. However, the initial bleeding usually slows down, allowing for the patient to be transported to the hospital. The definitive treatment in the hospital is end-arterial selective embolization.[55,56] The embolization must be done within all the small vessels feeding the pseudoaneurysm and proximally, as close to the pseudoaneurysm as possible. The advantage of embolization is that vessels distal to the pseudoaneurysm may be occluded without compromising proximal blood supply, which is important after orthognathic surgery, because diminishing the blood supply to the recently traumatized maxilla may result in aseptic necrosis.[57]

SUMMARY

Postoperative treatment and follow-up care are equally important and revolve around prevention. Avoidance of digital trauma, judicious use of certain medications, use of moisturizing saline sprays and gels are of paramount importance. The approach to the patient with epistaxis should begin with basic procedures that can be performed in either clinics or emergency rooms. Recently there has been a considerable expansion in epistaxis management. A myriad of epistaxis control devices is now available in the emergency room, all of which can be used by providers with little or no previous experience. The traditional strategies should also be supplemented with many technologically advanced strategies such as fiberscopes, electrocautery devices, and fibrin glues. As the discipline expands, without doubt numerous new devices will become available to help clinicians treat epistaxis effectively while also avoiding the radical surgical treatment so commonly performed in the past.

REFERENCES

1. Kucik CJ, Clenney T. Management of epistaxis. Am Fam Physician 2005;71(2):305–11.
2. Kotecha B, Fowler S, Harkness P, et al. Management of epistaxis: a national survey. Ann R Coll Surg Engl 1996;78(5):444–6.
3. Tomkinson A, Roblin DG, Flanagan P, et al. Patterns of hospital attendance with epistaxis. Rhinology 1997;35(3):129–31.
4. Nunez DA, McClymont LG, Evans RA. Epistaxis: a study of the relationship with weather. Clin Otolaryngol Allied Sci 1990;15(1):49–51.
5. Schlosser RJ. Epistaxis. N Engl J Med 2009;360(8):784–9.
6. Supriya M, Shakeel M, Veitch D, et al. Epistaxis: prospective evaluation of bleeding site and its impact on patient outcome. J Laryngol Otol 2010;124(7):744–9.
7. Cummings CW. 4th edition. Otolaryngology—head and neck surgery, vols. 1–4. St Louis (MO): Elsevier Mosby; 2005.
8. Mikhail S, Kouides P. von Willebrand disease in the pediatric and adolescent population. J Pediatr Adolesc Gynecol 2010;23(Suppl 6):S3–10.
9. McGarry GW, Gatehouse S, Vernham G. Idiopathic epistaxis, haemostasis and alcohol. Clin Otolaryngol Allied Sci 1995;20(2):174–7.
10. Veldhuizen JA, de Wolf JT, Buiter CT, et al. Epistaxis caused by an acquired thrombocytopathy. Ned Tijdschr Geneeskd 1989;133(12):622–4 [in Dutch].
11. Olitsky SE. Hereditary hemorrhagic telangiectasia: diagnosis and management. Am Fam Physician 2010;82(7):785–90.
12. Aassar OS, Friedman CM, White RI Jr. The natural history of epistaxis in hereditary hemorrhagic telangiectasia. Laryngoscope 1991;101(9):977–80.
13. Peery WH. Clinical spectrum of hereditary hemorrhagic telangiectasia (Osler-Weber-Rendu disease). Am J Med 1987;82(5):989–97.
14. Shah RK, Dhingra JK, Shapshay SM. Hereditary hemorrhagic telangiectasia: a review of 76 cases. Laryngoscope 2002;112(5):767–73.
15. Fuchs FD, Moreira LB, Pires CP, et al. Absence of association between hypertension and epistaxis: a population-based study. Blood Press 2003;12(3):145–8.
16. Lubianca Neto JF, Fuchs FD, Facco SR, et al. Is epistaxis evidence of end-organ damage in patients with hypertension? Laryngoscope 1999;109(7 Pt 1):1111–5.
17. Krempl GA, Noorily AD. Use of oxymetazoline in the management of epistaxis. Ann Otol Rhinol Laryngol 1995;104(9 Pt 1):704–6.
18. Riviello R. Otolaryngologic procedures. In: Roberts J, Hedges JR, editors. Clinical procedures in emergency medicine. 4th edition. Philadelphia: WB Saunders; 2004. p. 1300.
19. Katz RI, Hovagim AR, Finkelstein HS, et al. A comparison of cocaine, lidocaine with epinephrine, and oxymetazoline for prevention of epistaxis on nasotracheal intubation. J Clin Anesth 1990;2(1):16–20.
20. Amin M, Glynn F, Phelan S, et al. Silver nitrate cauterisation, does concentration matter? Clin Otolaryngol 2007;32(3):197–9.
21. Middleton PM. Epistaxis. Emerg Med Australas 2004;16(5–6):428–40.
22. Toner JG, Walby AP. Comparison of electro and chemical cautery in the treatment of anterior epistaxis. J Laryngol Otol 1990;104(8):617–8.
23. Merocel ENT. Merocel epistaxis packing [catalog]. Jacksonville (FL): Medtronic Inc.; 2011. p. 175. Available at: http://www.mcatalogs.com/ent/#/180/. Accessed January 18, 2012.
24. Breda SD, Jacobs JB, Lebowitz AS, et al. Toxic shock syndrome in nasal surgery: a physiochemical and microbiologic evaluation of Merocel and Nu-Gauze nasal packing. Laryngoscope 1987;97(12):1388–91.
25. Moumoulidis I, Draper MR, Patel H, et al. A prospective randomised controlled trial comparing Merocel and Rapid Rhino nasal tampons in the treatment of epistaxis. Eur Arch Otorhinolaryngol 2006;263(8):719–22.
26. ArthroCare ENT. Rapid Rhino 900 epistaxis device. [Image]. 2011; Rapid Rhino 900. Available at: http://www.arthrocareent.com/products/view/74-rapid-rhino-900-epistaxis-device. Accessed July 2, 2011.
27. ENT A. RR900 Epistaxis device technical guide. 2011. Available at: http://www.arthrocareent.com/img/vfsroot/it_1307474404/RR900%20TG%2028709A.pdf. Accessed February 16, 2012.
28. Vaiman M, Segal S, Eviatar E. Fibrin glue treatment for epistaxis. Rhinology 2002;40(2):88–91.
29. Baxter Healthcare Corp. FLOSEAL hemostatic matrix. Instructions for use. 2010. Available at: http://www.baxter.com/healthcare_professionals/products/floseal.html. Accessed July 4, 2011.
30. Mathiasen RA, Cruz RM. Prospective, randomized, controlled clinical trial of a novel matrix hemostatic sealant in patients with acute anterior epistaxis. Laryngoscope 2005;115(5):899–902.
31. Cote D, Barber B, Diamond C, et al. FloSeal hemostatic matrix in persistent epistaxis: prospective clinical trial. J Otolaryngol Head Neck Surg 2010;39(3):304–8.
32. Chiu TW, McGarry GW. Prospective clinical study of bleeding sites in idiopathic adult posterior epistaxis. Otolaryngol Head Neck Surg 2007;137(3):390–3.
33. Schlosser RJ. Clinical practice. Epistaxis. N Engl J Med 2009;360(8):784–9.

34. Douglas R, Wormald PJ. Update on epistaxis. Curr Opin Otolaryngol Head Neck Surg 2007;15(3): 180–3.

35. Gudziol V, Mewes T, Mann WJ. Rapid Rhino: a new pneumatic nasal tamponade for posterior epistaxis. Otolaryngol Head Neck Surg 2005;132(1): 152–5.

36. Garcia Callejo FJ, Munoz Fernandez N, Achiques Martinez MT, et al. Nasal packing in posterior epistaxis. Comparison of two methods. Acta Otorrinolaringol Esp 2010;61(3):196–201 [in Spanish].

37. Frazee TA, Hauser MS. Nonsurgical management of epistaxis. J Oral Maxillofac Surg 2000;58(4): 419–24.

38. Walker TW, Macfarlane TV, McGarry GW. The epidemiology and chronobiology of epistaxis: an investigation of Scottish hospital admissions 1995-2004. Clin Otolaryngol 2007;32(5):361–5.

39. Herkner H, Laggner AN, Mullner M, et al. Hypertension in patients presenting with epistaxis. Ann Emerg Med 2000;35(2):126–30.

40. O'Flynn PE, Shadaba A. Management of posterior epistaxis by endoscopic clipping of the sphenopalatine artery. Clin Otolaryngol Allied Sci 2000;25(5): 374–7.

41. Pothier DD, Mackeith S, Youngs R. Sphenopalatine artery ligation: technical note. J Laryngol Otol 2005;119(10):810–2.

42. Kumar S, Shetty A, Rockey J, et al. Contemporary surgical treatment of epistaxis. What is the evidence for sphenopalatine artery ligation? Clin Otolaryngol Allied Sci 2003;28(4):360–3.

43. Pope LE, Hobbs CG. Epistaxis: an update on current management. Postgrad Med J 2005; 81(955):309–14.

44. Douglas SA, Gupta D. Endoscopic assisted external approach anterior ethmoidal artery ligation for the management of epistaxis. J Laryngol Otol 2003; 117(2):132–3.

45. Matheny KE, Duncavage JA. Contemporary indications for the Caldwell-Luc procedure. Curr Opin Otolaryngol Head Neck Surg 2003;11(1):23–6.

46. Strong EB, Bell DA, Johnson LP, et al. Intractable epistaxis: transantral ligation vs. embolization: efficacy review and cost analysis. Otolaryngol Head Neck Surg 1995;113(6):674–8.

47. Waldron J, Stafford N. Ligation of the external carotid artery for severe epistaxis. J Otolaryngol 1992;21(4): 249–51.

48. Singam P, Thanabalan J, Mohammed Z. Superselective embolisation for control of intractable epistaxis from maxillary artery injury. Biomed Imaging Interv J 2011;7(1):e3.

49. May M, Levine HL, Mester SJ, et al. Complications of endoscopic sinus surgery: analysis of 2108 patients—incidence and prevention. Laryngoscope 1994;104(9):1080–3.

50. Cassano M, Cassano P. Epistaxis after partial middle turbinectomy: the role of sphenopalatine artery ligation. Am J Otolaryngol 2012;33(1):116–20.

51. Steel BJ, Cope MR. Unusual and rare complications of orthognathic surgery: a literature review. J Oral Maxillofac Surg 2011. DOI: 10.1016/j.joms.2011.05.010.

52. Lanigan DT, Hey JH, West RA. Major vascular complications of orthognathic surgery: false aneurysms and arteriovenous fistulas following orthognathic surgery. J Oral Maxillofac Surg 1991;49(6):571–7.

53. Solomons NB, Blumgart R. Severe late-onset epistaxis following Le Fort I osteotomy: angiographic localization and embolization. J Laryngol Otol 1988; 102(3):260–3.

54. O'Regan B, Bharadwaj G. Prospective study of the incidence of serious posterior maxillary haemorrhage during a tuberosity osteotomy in low level Le Fort I operations. Br J Oral Maxillofac Surg 2007; 45(7):538–42.

55. Conner WC 3rd, Rohrich RJ, Pollock RA. Traumatic aneurysms of the face and temple: a patient report and literature review, 1644 to 1998. Ann Plast Surg 1998;41(3):321–6.

56. Hemmig SB, Johnson RS, Ferraro N. Management of a ruptured pseudoaneurysm of the sphenopalatine artery following a Le Fort I osteotomy. J Oral Maxillofac Surg 1987;45(6):533–6.

57. Krempl GA, Noorily AD. Pseudoaneurysm of the descending palatine artery presenting as epistaxis. Otolaryngol Head Neck Surg 1996;114(3): 453–6.

Surgical Management of Nasal Obstruction

Jason A. Moche, MD[a],*, Orville Palmer, MD, MPH, FRCSC[b]

KEYWORDS

- Nasal obstruction • Septoplasty • Turbinates • Nasal valve
- Septorhinoplasty

ANATOMY

The nasal cavity is an epithelial lined passageway bounded by the paranasal sinuses, oral cavity, and intracranial vault. Centrally divided by the nasal septum, the lateral walls of the nose have 3 bony projections known as the superior, middle, and inferior turbinates. Each turbinate, extending the length of the nasal cavity, is covered by respiratory mucosa and is responsible for the filtration, warming, and humidification of the nasal cavity. Below each turbinate lies an associated depression referred to as its meatus.

The nasal septum separates the right and left nasal airways, beginning at the fleshy columella and nostril sill and extending to the nasopharynx. The septum has both an anterior cartilaginous component and a posterior bony structure covered with respiratory nasal mucosa. The anterior quadrangular septal cartilage has direct attachments to the medial crura of the lower lateral cartilages and in this manner contributes to nasal stability and tip support. The quadrangular cartilage posteriorly joins the superior perpendicular plate of the ethmoid bone and the inferior bony vomer at the bony cartilaginous junction. The septum rests securely in the midline maxillary crest completely dividing the right and left nasal cavities. At its anterior extent, insertion of the depressor septi nasi muscle can cause active nasal tip descent with facial animation. The superior aspect of the nasal cavity is bordered by the cribriform plate, which separates the nose from the intracranial vault.

The blood supply of the nasal cavity is robust and derived from branches of both the external and internal carotid systems bilaterally. Although blood flows into the expansive capillary bed of the overlying nasal mucosa, the nasal cavity is physiologically adapted for warming and humidifying inspired air. Primary contributors from the external carotid artery include the facial artery, with peripheral branches, including the superior labial artery, supplying the nasal vestibule and the angular artery investing the skin and soft tissue envelope. Terminal branches of the maxillary artery include the sphenopalatine, which supplies the posterior nasal cavity, lateral nasal walls, and posterior septum, and the greater palatine arteries, which supply the nasal floor and inferior septum. The superior portion of the septum is supplied by the anterior and posterior ethmoid arteries, both direct branches of the ophthalmic artery from the internal carotid system. The Kiesselbach area or plexus is the region of the anteroinferior nasal septum where 4 of the major arteries (anterior ethmoid, sphenopalatine artery, greater palatine artery, and the septal branch of the superior labial artery) anastomose to form a vascular confluence and the site of most epistaxis (**Fig. 1**).

Innervation of the nose is best divided into its internal mucosal component and external skin soft tissue evelope.[1] The upper external nose is innervated by branches of the ophthalmic division (V1), and the inferolateral aspects of the nose are supplied by branches of the maxillary (V2) division. The anterior and posterior ethmoid nerves (V1) and the sphenopalatine nerves (V2) supply the internal

The authors have nothing to disclose.

[a] Division of Otolaryngology, Department of Surgery, Harlem Hospital Center, Columbia University, 506 Lenox Avenue, New York, NY 10037, USA

[b] Otolaryngology-Facial Plastics and Reconstruction, Harlem Hospital Center, Columbia University, 506 Lenox Avenue, New York, NY 10037, USA

* Corresponding author.

E-mail address: jm3583@columbia.edu

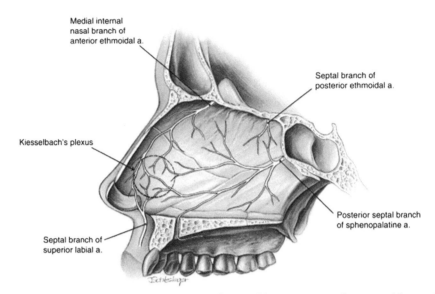

Fig. 1. Arterial supply of the nasal septum. (*Courtesy of* Jaye Schlesinger, Ann Arbor, MI; with permission.)

nasal cavity, including the septum, lateral nasal walls, and cribriform plate. In addition, the cribriform plate holds the special sensory branches of the olfactory or first cranial nerve.

THE NASAL TURBINATES

The inferior turbinate, which is the largest of the turbinates, runs parallel to the floor of the nose. The underlying inferior meatus receives the nasolacrimal duct, which drains the lacrimal tears. The middle turbinate, an extension of the ethmoid bone, rests above the inferior turbinate. Anteriorly, it attaches to the crista ethmoidalis of the maxilla, and extends superiorly and medially to attach to the cribriform plate. Posteriorly, it attaches to the lamina papyracea and medial wall of the maxillary sinus, terminating just anterior to the sphenopalatine foramen. Throughout its course it changes its orientation in a near-coronal plane anteriorly to an almost-horizontal plane more posteriorly, dividing the ethmoid labyrinth into its anterior and posterior components.[2] The shape of the middle turbinate is highly variable, because it can be paradoxically curved or pneumatized. Any pneumatization of the middle turbinate is technically referred to as a concha bullosa. The maxillary sinus, anterior ethmoid sinus, and frontal sinus all drain into the underlying middle meatus. The superior turbinate, also the smallest of the turbinates, lies above the middle turbinate. The posterior ethmoid cells drain into the superior meatus. The space between the superior turbinate, the septum, and the sphenoid sinus anterior wall is known as the sphenoethmoidal recess, where the posterior sphenoid sinus empties.[2] In some patients, a small additional or supreme turbinate exists.

THE NASAL VALVE

The nasal airway, although chiefly responsible for the filtration, warming, and humidification of inspired air, can be the primary site of airway resistance. The nasal valve is an anatomic area that was first described by Mink in 1903.[3] It is the two-dimensional opening formed by the caudal edge of the upper lateral cartilage, the nasal septum, and anterior head of the inferior turbinate, and ideally should be between 15° and 20°. It represents the narrowest part of the nasal cavity and site of maximal resistance.[4] It has also been referred to as a regulator that reacts to pressure changes generated by the act of inspiration and at times it comprises up to 50% of total airway resistance.

Since Mink's original description, which has come to describe the internal nasal valve (INV), the definition has expanded to include an external nasal valve. Current terminology describes the external nasal valve as the region caudal to the internal valve, bounded laterally by the nasal ala and medially by the septum and columella (**Fig. 2**). Disease affecting this area is more often a dynamic collapse of the nasal sidewall during active inspiration. Although less implicated in nasal obstruction than the INV, external nasal valve stenosis is also a primary and surgically treatable cause of nasal airway obstruction.

Nasal valve dysfunction is a well-known cause of nasal obstruction and is often overlooked in patients presenting with nasal congestion. Although several techniques have been described regarding surgical repair of nasal valve dysfunction, there is divergence of evidence and opinion regarding the ideal surgical method.

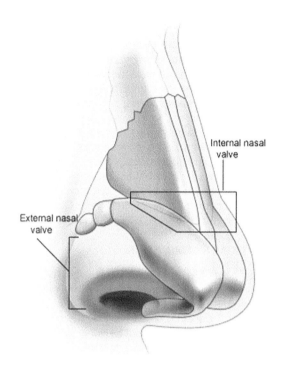

Fig. 2. The INV is formed by the angle between the upper lateral cartilage and nasal septum. The external nasal valve encompasses the lateral nasal wall, as indicated in the figure. (*From* Joe SA. The assessment and treatment of nasal obstruction after rhinoplasty. Facial Plast Surg Clin North Am 2004;12:454; with permission.)

Treatment of nasal valve dysfunction relies on proper identification of the underlying site of disease and the detection of coexistent nasal anomalies. Optimal management of this condition has been hindered by ambiguities in terminology, methods of diagnosis, and selection of treatment options.[5] The purpose of this review is to discuss the various surgical options for improving nasal airflow.

NASAL PHYSIOLOGY

The nasal mucosal lining has several unique functions and properties. Histologically, the entire nasal mucosa is lined by ciliated pseudostratified columnar respiratory epithelium with the exception of a small variable area of 1 to 2 mm of olfactory epithelium at the level of the cribriform plate. Nasal mucosal secretions are composed of 2 elements: glycoprotein and water with associated proteins and ions. The glycoproteins are produced by mucous glands and the water and ions secreted by serous glands and as transudate from the underlying capillary network. The serous glandular cells also produce dense granules containing IgA immunoglobulin, lysozymes, and lactoferrin for innate and adaptive immunity.[6] The nasal mucus film moves in 2 layers: an upper viscous gel layer, and a lower watery sol layer, better allowing the cilia to move efficiently.

CAUSES OF NASAL OBSTRUCTION

The physiologic alternating of vascular congestion and decongestion of the turbinates and nasal mucosa is referred to as the nasal cycle. It is a physiologic process caused by selective autonomic innervation by the hypothalamus. The nasal cycle was first described by the German physician Richard Kayser in 1895.[7] In 1927, Heetderks discussed the alternating turgescence of the inferior turbinates in 80% of a normal population.[8] The turbinates on 1 side filled with blood, whereas the opposite turbinates decongested. This cycle had a mean duration of 2.5 hours, and Heetderks further observed that the turbinates in the dependent nasal cavity filled when the patient was in the lateral decubitus position. Some postulate that this alternating positional obstruction has the purpose of causing a person to turn from 1 side to the other while sleeping.[5] The nasal cycle is an alternating one, with total resistance remaining generally constant. Patients may become aware of this cycle if they have an underlying obstruction, such as a septal deviation.

Nasal obstruction, often referred to as congestion, has several different anatomic and physiologic causes, which may present in isolation or as a combination of events.[9] The varying causes all lead to an objective decreased flow of air primarily through the nasal valve and contiguous nasal cavity. Allergy, environmental irritants, sinus inflammation, anatomic deviations, and pregnancy or hormonal variations can all lead to nasal blockage. Anatomic considerations include congenital or acquired septal deviations, turbinate hypertrophy, or internal/external nasal valve collapse or stenosis. Often, nasal inflammation or rhinitis may exacerbate an already anatomically compromised nose. Although most rhinitis has an allergic cause, several other causes exist, including infectious (both viral and bacterial), and nonallergic or vasomotor-type, including autonomic, hormonal, and environmental causes.[10] Furthermore, medication-induced rhinitis, referred to as rhinitis medicamentosa, is a condition of rebound nasal congestion brought on by extended use of topical decongestants (eg, oxymetazoline, phenylephrine, xylometazoline, and naphazoline nasal sprays), which work by constricting blood vessels in the lining of the nose; chronic atrophic rhinitis results secondary to nasal atrophy of the mucous membrane and glands. Underlying sinus inflammation may affect the nasal passages. Most rhinitis is addressed with medical management including nasal lubricants, oral selective antihistamines, decongestants, and topical nasal steroids. Occasionally, the inflammatory response may be chronic and severe enough such that nasal polyps arise or the inferior turbinates become chronically enlarged secondary to subepithelial deposition, and are refractory to further medical treatment. This review focuses on the surgical correction of nasal obstruction.

HISTORY AND PHYSICAL EXAMINATION

The accurate diagnosis of nasal obstruction begins with a thorough history. Patients often describe a long-standing inability to breathe either through 1 or both nostrils. They may describe an alternating congestion occurring every several hours, which corresponds to exacerbations during the physiologic nasal cycle. It is important to separate what is likely a normal physiologic process from disease. Any history of trauma may signal a fracture or displacement of the nasal septum. Enquiring about purulent nasal drainage or facial pain may indicate an acute or chronic sinusitis. Maxillary tooth pain may suggest an underlying maxillary sinusitis. Patients should be asked about unilateral or bilateral epistaxis. Patients with a caudal septal deflection or deviation may have increased turbulent airflow at the site of deviation, leading to exposed blood vessels on an already thin nasal mucosa. In addition, unilateral nasal bleeding, especially with obstruction, may more ominously signal a nasal or sinus mass. A thorough history should include a history of previous nasal surgeries or medication use as well as environmental irritants. Patients should be asked about underlying inflammatory and collagen vascular disease in themselves and family including Wegener granulomatosis, sarcoidosis, and lupus erythematosus. Patients should also be asked about recreational drug use, especially cocaine abuse, and any history of unprotected sex, indicating possible exposure to syphilis. Patients who have already been taking a nasal steroid for greater than 1 month may signal a more anatomic cause rather than physiologic inflammation or allergy. Occasionally, a patient with rhinitis medicamentosa and total bilateral obstruction may present, confessing that they have been using a topical decongestant for some time, such as oxymetazoline (Afrin) or phenylephrine, and often for longer than they admit.

A common symptom is loss of smell or taste, and these should be determined as well before the start of any intervention. Many surgeons find the use of a validated patient-centered questionnaire to quantify and score symptom severity. We advocate the use of the Nasal Obstruction Symptom Evaluation (NOSE) scale (**Table 1**).

PHYSICAL EXAMINATION

On inspection, a patient with severe nasal obstruction shows mouth open posturing. They may have periorbital congestion, referred to as allergic shiners. A patient with chronic rhinitis may have stigmata of repetitive nasal blowing, with an irritated upper lip and nasal vestibule. The junction of the nasal tip and dorsum may have prominent wrinkles or irritation as well, suggesting an upwards nose wiping called the allergic salute. Take note of the patient's bony nasal pyramid and nasal lateral side walls. Record any deviations along the nasal dorsum or any sidewall depressions at rest and during inspiration, indicating a dynamic collapse. Patients with longer noses from nasion to subnasale and short nasal bones often have an extended cartilaginous middle vault and are more predisposed to internal valve collapse. A narrow nasal base and nostril ostium may limit nasal airflow. It is important to not simply watch the patient at rest but to observe the nose during active respiration. Particularly, a small depression above the nasal alae during inspiration may indicate dynamic external valve collapse. On anterior rhinoscopy with a nasal speculum, take note of the caudal internal valve. Watch the angle formed with the nasal septum. Identify any large

Table 1 The validated NOSE scale					
	Not a Problem	Very Mild Problem	Moderate Problem	Fairly Bad Problem	Severe Problem
Nasal stuffiness	0	1	2	3	4
Nasal blockage or obstruction	0	1	2	3	4
Trouble breathing through my nose	0	1	2	3	4
Trouble sleeping	0	1	2	3	4
Unable to get enough air through my nose during exercise or exertion	0	1	2	3	4

septal irregularities, including spurs or deviations. Signs of erythematous septal inflammation or perforations may indicate an active inflammatory process. Often, patients with large anterior perforations may have the sensation of nasal obstruction secondary to aberrant nasal airflow and inefficient currents circulating through the perforation. Examine the nasal floor and identify the midline. The cartilaginous septum should proceed posteriorly and meet the bony vomer directly. Occasionally, aberrant growth or acquired traumatic or surgical deformities my cause a discrepancy or step-off. Examine the middle turbinate and middle meatus for any signs of purulence or nasal polyps. The inferior turbinates emerging off the lateral nasal wall should generally not be in contact with the nasal septum. A watery and edematous turbinate indicates a degree of rhinitis, which may respond well to a topical nasal steroid. A Cottle maneuver should be performed unilaterally by occluding first the right nostril and with the opposite hand extending the facial soft tissues laterally to open the contralateral internal and largely external valve. A modified Cottle maneuver may also help identify INV collapse by placing the head of a cotton tip applicator in the nasal valve between the upper lateral cartilage and septum. If collapse in either is present, the patient responds to a dramatic improvement in airflow. The combination of these 2 maneuvers can help identify the site of obstruction. The addition of topical decongestant such as oxymetazoline or neosynephrine helps remove any inflammation and allows a large open view of the nasal anatomy.

FIBER-OPTIC EXAMINATION

Often, a fiber-optic examination gives additional information about the patient's nasal anatomy. Careful examination of the middle meatus and posterior nasal cavity in a patient with a longstanding history of sinusitis may augment a good anterior nasal examination. Patients may often have undetected purulence, indicating an active infection or significant nasal polyposis requiring treatment. Often, in patients who have had previous surgery, surgical scarring or synechiae between the nasal septum and turbinates may be present and difficult to appreciate without the use of a fiber-optic scope. Previous surgical septoplasty may reveal sites of resected cartilage, bent or malpositioned septal remnants, or a perforation. Several surgical maneuvers to repair internal and external nasal valve stenosis require cartilage grafting, and it is always a big disappointment to learn in the operating room that your primary donor site for nasal cartilage grafting has already been removed.

IMAGING

A computed tomography (CT) scan of the paranasal sinuses with coronal reconstruction can serve as a useful adjunct to the physical examination and fiber-optic endoscopy. Bony windows show the integrity and straightness of the nasal septum, highlighting any prominent bony or cartilaginous deviations, spurs, or fractures. Evaluation of the inferior and middle turbinates shows large inferior turbinates, or paradoxic middle turbinates that bend medially to obstruct the nasal airway or turbinates that have become pneumatized, also known as concha bullosa. Acute and chronic sinus disease is detected as well as the presence of nasal polyposis. Any obstructing masses are identified with associated changes demanding the need for further investigation and workup. Evaluation with acoustic rhinometry, although useful in the research setting, has not achieved widespread clinical usefulness. We are in the process of publishing our experience with the use of CT scan data for INV evaluation.

SURGICAL MANAGEMENT

After an appropriate evaluation and indicated medical management, a patient may be considered an appropriate surgical candidate. Once underlying physiologic and inflammatory processes have been addressed, the nasal anatomy can be appropriately addressed to provide the patient with more favorable nasal anatomy for air movement. Surgery can largely be divided into the treatment of the nasal septum, the internal and external valves, and the nasal turbinates. Rhee and colleagues[11] and Spielmann and colleagues[12] offered recent systematic reviews of treatment options of nasal valve dysfunction. Although both reviews note a consistent benefit of surgery, they also show that the contribution septoplasty and turbinate reduction could not be extracted from the results attributed to the nasal valve procedure alone.[5,13]

SEPTOPLASTY

Most unilateral nasal airway obstruction can be treated with a well-executed septoplasty. The nasal septum on examination typically shows a large deflection to 1 side or protruding spurs that obstruct the nasal airway. The nasal septum not only provides a substantial amount of support to the nose but also provides stability. It generally determines the symmetry of the nose inside and out, and a poorly performed septal resection not only predisposes the patient to the potential of nasal collapse but also may lead to noticeable external asymmetries and curvature of the nasal dorsum. At least 1.5 cm of dorsal and caudal septum should be maintained at the completion of any planned septal surgery.

Also referred to as a submucous resection, the purpose of a septoplasty is to remove the deviated cartilage and bone obstructing the nasal airway and maintain a straightened midline bilayer of mucous membrane spanning the surgical defect between the residual straightened cartilage. It is important to remove only what is necessary. The procedure is performed using a xenon headlamp, with the patient typically under general anesthesia. The eyes are protected and a sterile headwrap is often applied. Using a small 25-gauge needle, 1% lidocaine with 1:100,000 epinephrine is injected along the septum bilaterally in an anterior to posterior direction beneath the mucoperichondrial layer. An injection in the proper plane shows an appropriate vasoconstrictive blanching of the overlying mucoperichondrium and slight elevation of the layer as it separates from the underlying septal cartilage. After allowing at least 5 minutes for the appropriate vasoconstrictive response, a hemitransfixion is typically performed on the patient's right side at the caudal margin of the septal cartilage or slightly posterior using a number 15 blade. Frequently, this incision is carried along the nasal floor to allow ample exposure for prominent deflections and septal deformities. Careful elevation of the mucoperichondrial flap proceeds posteriorly with a Cottle or Freer elevator. Any septal spurs or deflections are approached prudently above and below the deformity, paying careful attention to not perforate the flap. Once the first side is elevated, attention may be turned toward the contralateral side. Without violating the opposing flap, elevation may proceed along the opposite side of the cartilage separating the mucoperichondrial flap from the underlying septum. Once both flaps are elevated, a 1.5-cm operative ruler is used to measure and preserve the 1.5-cm caudal and dorsal cartilaginous struts. Once the incision is marked, the central cartilage, posterior to the preserved caudal strut, may be incised with the number 15 blade, sharp Freer, or a blunt D knife. Alternatively, the septal swivel knife may be used to perform the submucous resection. The planned resection should encompass the identified deformities preoperatively. Once the segment is removed the mucoperichondrial layers should redrape and lie in the midline. The cartilage at this point may be discarded because a secure caudal and dorsal strut remains for midline nasal support. Often, the resected cartilage may be flattened and crushed in a cartilage press and reinserted between the flaps.

Additional techniques have been used to straighten curved or warped dorsal and caudal cartilages. Occasionally, cartilaginous scoring may be performed on the concave side of curved cartilage to help right bent segments. Mattress suturing may be performed to assist in maintaining the corrected framework.[14] Supporting unilateral or bilateral caudal extension grafts have been used with success to maintain a strong straightened framework. Although auricular or rib cartilage may be used, the best and easiest source of grafting cartilage is frequently the resected septum.

Once the flaps are redraped, and hemostasis ensured, the incision may be closed using 4-0 plain gut in a simple interrupted fashion. A quilting 3-0 mattress suture should then be applied to approximate the mucoepichondrial flaps together, removing the dead space, and decreasing the possibility of latent hematoma formation. Any unilateral flap violations should be closed individually using the 4-0 plain gut suture. In the case of a bilateral opposing perforation, it may be prudent to use bilateral Doyle splints with bacitracin ointment and oral antibiotics for 5 days to decrease the chance of a persistent septal perforation. Patients are typically discharged from recovery, given saline nasal irrigation to be used 3 to 4 times daily, and seen in the office the following week for examination.

Special considerations for septal surgery should be considered in the pediatric patient. Often, children or adolescents present with severe nasal obstruction requiring surgical management. The nasal septum contains what has been described as the growth center of the nose and therefore most procedures are more commonly delayed until adulthood. Any procedure in childhood must be conservative. Goumas and colleagues[15] reported from a small series that children who underwent septoplasty had small noses, retracted columellas, and identical caudal septal nasal deformities at 4-year to 6-year follow-up. In select instances, such as facial trauma, limited septal reconstruction is indicated; however, the literature consistently suggests that any approach to the pediatric septum should be conservative and unequivocally indicated.[16]

SURGICAL TREATMENT OF THE INV

At times, the nasal septum may not be the primary factor contributing to the obstruction, and the site of disease may be the INV. Patients with disease residing at the INV typically respond positively to a modified Cottle maneuver, with improvement in nasal airflow on placement of a cotton tip applicator positioned between the upper lateral cartilage and nasal septum. Patients often report the improvement as dramatic. Since originally described by Sheen in 1984, the mainstay of repair of the INV continues to be spreader grafting.[5,17] In a similar fashion as described earlier, with the use of a xenon headlamp for endonasal visualization, the patient is prepared and draped in a similar fashion as the septoplasty described earlier. One percent lidocaine with 1:100,000 epinephrine is injected along the septum bilaterally in the submucoperichondrial plane. After appropriate time for vasoconstriction, a submucous resection of the nasal septum is performed, paying careful attention to preserve the 1.5-cm caudal and dorsal strut. Classically, spreader grafts are then applied using an external rhinoplasty approach. The soft tissue envelope is injected along the nose in a sub-superficial musculoaponeurotic system (sub-SMAS)/subperiosteal plane along the collumella and nasal vestibule as well. At approximately midway between the nasal lobule and subnasale, a central collumellar gull in flight incision is made. The incision is extended into the nose and along a marginal incision at the caudal aspect of the lower lateral cartilages; the appropriate location typically resides at the termination of the nasal vestibule along the junction of the small nasal vibrissae and nasal mucosa. The nose is elevated in a sub-SMAS plane, exposing first the lower lateral cartilages and then the upper lateral cartilages and underlying nasal back toward the nasal bones. At this point, the upper lateral cartilages can be isolated and freed from their attachments to the dorsal septum sharply. It is important that the mucoperichondrial flaps are raised bilaterally, as noted earlier for the septoplasty, or alternatively, they may be dissected from above through the open rhinoplasty approach. Once the upper lateral cartilages are divided sharply from the nasal septum, using an operative ruler, the distance from the nasal bones to the caudal aspect of the upper lateral cartilages should be measured. Typically, adequate spreader grafts should be at least 20 mm in length, and it is important that enough septal cartilage is available for grafting. The interposition of the spreader grafts should span the length of the upper lateral cartilages and frequently measures between 20 and 25 mm long and 5 and 7 mm high. The width of the graft varies depending on the width of the harvested septum, but ideally it should measure at least 4 mm. The grafts are then inserted and the upper lateral cartilages reapproximated to the septum and spreader grafts, creating a sandwich that comprises upper lateral cartilages on the outside, septum in the center, and bilateral spreader grafts on either side in between (**Fig. 3**). Often, they are beveled at the ends to maximize the nasal airway. They can be held in place with 25-gauge needles while they are secured with 4-0 polydioxanone (PDS) suture in a mattress fashion. This procedure stents the internal valve. The nasal mucoperichondrial flaps can be closed as described earlier and the nasal soft tissue envelope should be closed with 4-0 plain gut at the marginal alar incisions and 6-0 prolene at the columellae. The columellar sutures should be removed in 6 days.

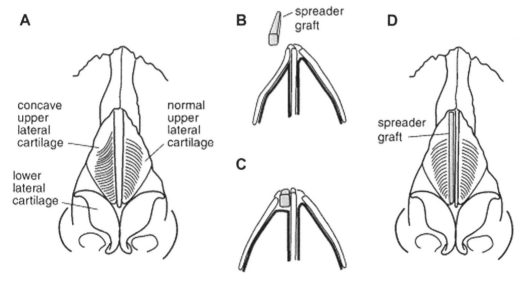

Fig. 3. The right upper lateral cartilage and resultant INV is corrected with placement of a unilateral spreader graft. (*A*) Demonstrates right sided middle vault collapse. (*B*) Unilateral interposition spreader graft is sutured between the nasal septum and collapsed upper lateral cartilage as shown in (*C*). (*D*) Illustrates restoration of the middle vault concavity. (*From* Quatela VC, Deirdre L, Sabini P. Surgical management of concavities of the distal nose. Facial Plast Surg Clin North Am 2004;12:139; with permission.)

SURGICAL TREATMENT OF THE EXTERNAL NASAL VALVE

Treatment of the external nasal valve primarily involves supporting a dynamic collapse of the nasal sidewall during active inspiration. The nasal septum is harvested as described earlier, and an external rhinoplasty approach is performed. The principle behind improving this deformity is creating batten grafts from the harvested septum to support the nasal sidewall.[18] Once the nose is elevated, a batten overlay of cartilage is typically fashioned, which can vary from 3 to 5 mm wide by 15 to 20 mm long. Often, patients have associated weakening of the lower lateral cartilages, presenting with thin, flimsy, or bent lower lateral cartilages. The batten grafts can be used to help bolster the lower lateral cartilages as well, and span a gap between them, the upper lateral cartilages, and the lateral bony pyriform aperture. The batten grafts can be placed superficial or deep to the lower lateral cartilages. Although placement below can help camouflage their presence in a thin-skinned individual, they can take longer to place given the careful dissection of the thin nasal vestibular skin and mucosa required. Once positioned, they can be secured above the underlying nasal pyriform aperture and to lower lateral cartilages with 4-0 PDS suture. The nasal soft tissue envelope and mucoperichondrial septal flaps are returned and closed as described earlier. Nostril silicone stents may be used for 1 to 2 weeks to assist while healing. Patients are reviewed within the week for columellar suture removal and follow-up examination.

TURBINATE SURGERY

As our understanding of nasal airflow and its relation to the paranasal sinuses has evolved over the past several decades, so has turbinate surgery changed.[19–21] After evaluation and adequate management of hypertrophied turbinates, the patient may be an appropriate candidate for turbinate resection. Historically, large inferior and middle turbinates were aggressively removed to enhance nasal airflow. Long-term follow-up has shown that an overly resected lateral nasal wall can predispose the patient to chronic infections, exacerbation of sinus disease, and atrophic rhinitis; paradoxically, with the absence of precious sensate nasal mucosa patients may complain of diminished airflow when it has increased. Emphasis is now placed on the preservation of nasal mucosal, decreasing the volume of primarily the inferior turbinate.[22–29] Several instruments have been evaluated, from radiofrequency ablation to small microcutting powered blades. In some patients, the submucous

venous tissue comprising the turbinate may cover an overly large conchal bony structure. Typically performed in the operative setting under general anesthesia, the procedure is initiated with 1% lidocaine with 1:100,000 epinephrine injection. Once the mucosa is well infiltrated, and appropriate time has passed for adequate vasoconstriction, the anterior turbinate mucosa in incised with a number 15 blade. The venous erectile submucosa of the inferior turbinate is circumferentially raised off the bone. The premise is to disrupt the venous channels and prevent the vasomotor and inflammatory response typically associated with turbinate hypertrophy. The tissue can be elevated with a Freer or Cottle elevator. The bone can then be approached with a small Rongeur or 2-mm osteotome. The hypertrophied bone should then be partially removed to allow the turbinate mucosa to redrape. Alternatively, in patients in whom the bone itself is not excessively large but extends further into the nasal airway, the turbinate can be outfractured using a Goldman displacer to improve nasal patency. Radiofrequency electrocautery is often used to decrease the residual submucous channels and decrease recurrence. Sutured closure is generally not necessary and patients can be placed on saline irrigations and reviewed within the week for evaluation and removal of any overlying crusting.

A narrow nasal airway with underlying nasal obstruction is frequently encountered in patients undergoing orthognathic surgery. The tight pyriform aperture and elevated nasal floor often follows a narrow maxillary arch and anterior vertical excess. These findings are typical in patients undergoing LeFort I (downfracture) osteotomies. In addition, patients may present with enlarged inferior turbinates requiring simultaneous management of chronic nasal obstruction. Posnick[26] conducted a prospective clinical study using the NOSE scale questionnaire to prospectively assess a consecutive series of patients (N = 43) who reported both chronic nasal obstruction and dentofacial deformity. Patients treated with simultaneous septoplasty and inferior turbinate reduction along with Le Fort I osteotomy showed a significant improvement in nasal breathing without an associated risk of increased complication.[27] The LeFort I downfracture provides ample exposure and an opportune time for simultaneous septoplasty and inferior turbinate reduction.

SUMMARY

The surgical management of nasal airway obstruction relies on the proper identification of the site of obstruction. Once a patient has failed medical management, recognizing the nasal septum, nasal valve, and turbinates as possible sites of obstruction and addressing them accordingly dramatically improves a patient's nasal breathing. Patients presenting for orthognathic surgery often have simultaneous nasal obstruction, requiring surgical management at the time of LeFort osteotomy. Conservative resection of septal cartilage, and structural grafting of the nasal valve when appropriate, provide the optimal improvement in nasal airflow and allow for the most stable results over time.

REFERENCES

1. Hornung DE. Nasal anatomy and the sense of smell. Adv Otorhinolaryngol 2006;63:1–22.

2. Bolger WE. Anatomy of the paranasal sinuses. In: Kennedy DW, Bolger WE, Zinreich SJ, editors. Diseases of the sinuses diagnosis and management. Ontario (Canada): BC Decker; 2001. p. 1–9.

3. Mink PJ. Le nez comme voie respiratorie. Belgium: Presse Otolaryngol; 1903. p. 481–96 [in French].

4. Apaydin F. Nasal valve surgery. Facial Plast Surg 2011;27(2):179–91.

5. Yarlagadda BB, Dolan RW. Nasal valve dysfunction: diagnosis and treatment. Curr Opin Otolaryngol Head Neck Surg 2011;19(1):25–9. Review. Comprehensive discussion on identifying and treating pathology affecting the nasal valve.

6. Stierna P. Physiology, mucociliary clearance, and neural control. Anatomy of the paranasal sinuses. In: Kennedy DW, Bolger WE, Zinreich SJ, editors. Diseases of the sinuses diagnosis and management. Ontario (Canada): BC Decker; 2001. p. 36–44.

7. Kayser R. Die exacte Messung der Luftdurchgangigkeit der Nase. Arch Laryngol Rhinol 1895;3: 101–20 [in German].

8. Heetderks DL. Observations on the reactions of normal mucous membrane. Am J Med Sci 1927;174:231–44.

9. Patou J, De Smedt H, van Cauwenberge P, et al. Pathophysiology of nasal obstruction and meta-analysis of early and late effects of levocetirizine. Clin Exp Allergy 2006;36(8):972–81.

10. Kimmelman CP, Ali GH. Vasomotor rhinitis. Otolaryngol Clin North Am 1986;19(1):65–71.

11. Rhee JS, Weaver EM, Park SS, et al. Clinical consensus statement: diagnosis and management of nasal valve compromise. Otolaryngol Head Neck Surg 2010;143:48–59.

12. Spielmann PM, White PS, Hussain SS. Surgical techniques for the treatment of nasal valve collapse: a systematic review. Laryngoscope 2009;119:1281–90.

13. Dolan RW. Advances in rhinoplasty: nasal valve and nasal alar dysfunction. Facial Plast Surg Clin North Am 2000;8:447–64.

14. Pastorek NJ, Becker DG. Treating the caudal septal deflection. Arch Facial Plast Surg 2000; 2(3):217–20.

15. Goumas P, Strambis G, Antonakopoulos L, et al. Long-term results of nasal surgery in children. Ear Nose Throat J 1988;67:294–6.

16. Derkay CS. A conservative role for septoplasty in young children. Arch Otolaryngol Head Neck Surg 1999;125(6):702–3.

17. Sheen J. Spreader graft: a method of reconstructing the roof of the middle nasal vault following rhinoplasty. Plast Reconstr Surg 1984;73(2):230–9.

18. Toriumi DM, Ries WR. Innovative surgical management of the crooked nose. Facial Plast Surg Clin North Am 1993;1:63–78.

19. Grymer LF, Illum P, Hilberg O. Bilateral inferior turbinoplasty in chronic nasal obstruction. Rhinology 1996;34(1):50–3.

20. Elwany S, Harrison R. Inferior turbinectomy: comparison of four techniques. J Laryngol Otol 1990;104(3): 206–9.

21. Kizilkaya Z, Ceylan K, Emir H, et al. Comparison of radiofrequency tissue volume reduction and submucosal resection with microdebrider in inferior turbinate hypertrophy. Otolaryngol Head Neck Surg 2008;138(2):176–81.

22. Carrie S, Wright RG, Jones AS, et al. Long-term results of trimming of the inferior turbinates. Clin Otolaryngol Allied Sci 1996;21(2):139–41.

23. Joinau S, Wong I, Rajapaksa S, et al. Long-term comparison between submucosal cauterization and powered reduction of the inferior turbinates. Laryngoscope 2006;116:1612–6.

24. Liu CM, Tan CD, Lee FP, et al. Microdebrider-assisted versus radiofrequency-assisted inferior turbinoplasty. Laryngoscope 2009;119(2):414–8.

25. Quine SM, Aitken PM, Eccles R. Effect of submucosal diathermy to the inferior turbinates on unilateral and total nasal airflow in patients with rhinitis. Acta Otolaryngol 1999;119(8):911–5.

26. Posnick JC. Managing chronic nasal airway obstruction at the time of orthognathic surgery: a twofer. J Oral Maxillofac Surg 2011;69(3):695–701.

27. Posnick JC, Fantuzzo JJ, Troost T. Simultaneous intranasal procedures to improve chronic obstructive nasal breathing in patients undergoing maxillary (le fort I) osteotomy. J Oral Maxillofac Surg 2007; 65(11):2273–81.

28. Quatela VC, Deirdre L, Sabini P. Surgical management of concavities of the distal nose. Facial Plast Surg Clin North Am 2004;12:133–56.

29. Wright WK. Principles of nasal septum reconstruction. Trans Am Acad Ophthalmol Otolaryngol 1969; 73:252–5.

Oroantral Communication

Harry Dym, DDS[a],*, Joshua C. Wolf, DDS[b]

KEYWORDS

- Oroantral communication • Oroantral fistula
- Soft tissue closure • Buccal sliding flap

Oroantral communication (OAC) is the space created between the maxillary sinus and the oral cavity, which, if not treated, will progress to oroantral fistula (OAF) or chronic sinus disease.[1] The most common precipitating factor of an OAC is the extraction of posterior maxillary teeth, usually the first or second molar. This post-extraction complication occurs more likely if there is pre-existing periapical abnormality associated with the offending tooth near the maxillary sinus or extraction of maxillary molar teeth with widely divergent roots. If these teeth are not carefully removed by surgically sectioning the roots, the floor of the sinus may be removed along with the tooth. In patients with healthy sinuses, after an extraction, most maxillary sinus perforations less than 5 mm close spontaneously after the development of a blood clot in the socket.[2] If the sinus communication is between 2 and 6 mm, a collagen plug can be placed into the socket and secured in place with figure-of-eight sutures across the socket; larger openings do not heal spontaneously and require a surgical procedure to close the resulting oroantral opening.

OACs can also occur as a result of implant surgery, cyst and tumor enucleations, orthognathic surgeries (Le Fort osteotomies), osteomyelitis, trauma, and pathologic entities. To avoid problems secondary to OACs (eg, infections of the sinus), surgical closure is advisable within the first 48 hours.[3] If the larger OACs are left untreated and allowed to stay patent, 50% of the patients will experience sinusitis after 48 hours and 90% after 2 weeks.[4]

OAF may result from either a known or an unknown perforation of the maxillary sinus. Primary epithelial fusion of the schneiderian membrane to the oral epithelium may occur before the closure of the defect by the cells of its own origin. Thus, a permanent epithelialized tract forms, allowing a persistent communication between the oral cavity and the sinus. On postoperative follow-up, the patient may complain of fluids entering the nasal cavity while eating or drinking, nasal congestion, or sanguineous discharge. The patient may also report poorly localized discomfort around the extraction site that radiates to the orbital area and is often perceived as an adjacent toothache.

Decision on how to treat an OAC should be based on the size of communication, time of diagnosis, and presence of an infection. Furthermore, the selection of treatment strategy is influenced by the amount and condition of tissue available for repair and the possible placement of dental implants in the future.[5] Consequently, to close a long-standing OAF, the maxillary sinusitis present should be evaluated and treated first before closing the defect; otherwise the rotational flap will fail. Imaging studies must be performed, preferably a computed tomography or cone beam study, to evaluate the degree of sinus disease and also accurately measure the size of bone opening. That the bone defect is always significantly larger than the soft tissue defect visualized in the oral cavity is a well-established clinical finding. If sinusitis is diagnosed, prospectively, the patients should be treated with Augmentin 875 mg twice daily, Clindamyicn 300 mg 4 times daily, or Avelox 400 mg

[a] Department of Dentistry/Oral and Maxillofacial Surgery, The Brooklyn Hospital, 121 DeKalb Avenue, Box 187, Brooklyn, NY 11201, USA
[b] Department of Oral and Maxillofacial Surgery, The Brooklyn Hospital Center, 121 DeKalb Avenue, Brooklyn, NY 11201, USA
* Corresponding author.
E-mail address: hdymdds@yahoo.com

Oral Maxillofacial Surg Clin N Am 24 (2012) 239–247
doi:10.1016/j.coms.2012.01.015
1042-3699/12/$ – see front matter © 2012 Elsevier Inc. All rights reserved.

once daily for at least 10 days. Culture and sensitivity tests should be performed if purulent discharge is present, and the patients are also treated with a decongestant and mucolytic agent.

The affected sinus should also be irrigated copiously through the fistula with physiologic saline solution 3 times a week until the lavage fluid does not contain any inflammatory exudates.

Once acute sinusitis is cleared, closure of the OAC should be attempted. The Caldwell-Luc procedure is performed to remove all maxillary sinus polyps and infected antral mucosa before closure of the OAC based on the diagnostic imaging studies.

WHAT IS THE BEST SURGICAL TREATMENT OF AN OAC?

Several alternative techniques have been presented throughout the years. An overview of these treatment modalities is given in **Fig. 1**. Most investigators maintain that soft tissue closure of OACs is more than adequate to achieve the intended goal of sealing the maxillary sinus from the oral cavity in cases of most OAC defects, and it still seems to be the treatment of choice for OACs.

SOFT TISSUE CLOSURES
The Buccal Sliding Flap

The most common and oldest surgical technique used for the treatment of OACs is the buccal sliding flap designed by Rehrmann (**Fig. 2**).[6,7]

Oral surgeons should be familiar with this flap design to close the OACs in a safe, efficient, and predictable manner. The flap is developed by making 2 buccal divergent vertical incisions extending into the buccal vestibule from the extraction socket. The trapezoidal buccal flap is elevated and brought across the defect and sutured to the palatal margins of the defect. A technique to help ensure flap survivability by decreasing tension on the flap and ease of advancement is to horizontally score the buccal periosteum high in the vestibule with a new number 15 blade, which allows the rotational flap to fit passively into the site. Disadvantages of the Rehrmann method include the risk of decreasing the depth of buccal sulcus, postoperative pain, and swelling.[7] This procedure when performed in a shallow vestibule can cause a further decrease in the depth of buccal vestibule, but in the author's clinical experience, this is not often the case. If needed, a procedure can be performed to help deepen the vestibule 6 to 8 months after complete healing. The overall success rate of the buccal sliding flap has been 87.2% in a retrospective study, making it a straightforward and reliable method for repair of OACs, which is practical in most situations.

Palatal-Based Rotational Flap

The palatal-based rotational flap for the closure of large OAFs is a well-established and another often-performed successful technique (**Fig. 3**).[7]

The technique involves excision of the fistula tract, if present, and development of a broad-based full-thickness flap, ensuring the inclusion of the greater palatine artery for adequate blood supply and then rotating the flap to cover the

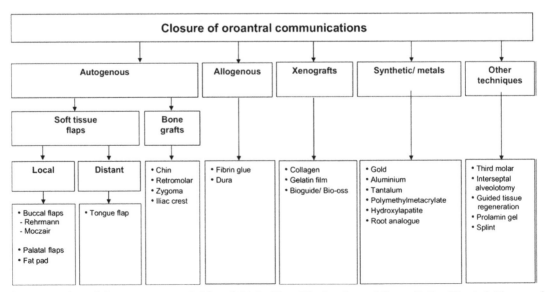

Fig. 1. Overview of the treatment modalities of OACs. (*From* Visscher S, von Minnen B, Bos RR, et al. Closure of oroantral communications: a review of the literature. J Oral Maxillofac Surg 2010;68:1384–91; with permission.)

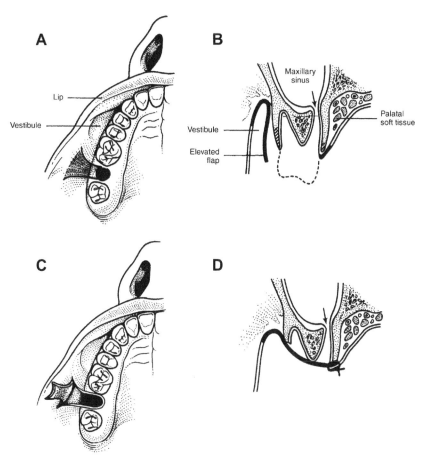

Fig. 2. (*A*) Development of a broad-based buccal flap to achieve primary closure of large sinus exposure or after excision of an OAF tract. (*B*) Undermining of the mucoperiosteal flap, horizontal scoring of the periosteum, and removal of bone to allow tension-free closure. (*C*) Advancement of flap into position of defect to ensure that margins are supported by the underlying bone. (*D*) Cross section demonstrating closure. (*From* Schow SR. Odontogenic diseases of the maxillary sinus. In: Peterson LJ, Ellis E, Hupp JR, et al, editors. Contemporary oral and maxillofacial surgery. 2nd edition. St Louis (MO): CV Mosby; 1993. p. 477; with permission.)

communication. The exposed palatal bone will heal by secondary epithelialization. If the palatal flap does not reach the lateral alveolus, a smaller buccal flap is used to complete the closure. The palatal flap can be either anteriorly or posteriorly based. The anteriorly based flap is ideal for the closure of large tuberosity defects.[8] Palatal flaps are preferred to the buccal (cheek) advancement flaps because it does not lead to any reduction in the depth of the maxillary buccal vestibule, and it is less vulnerable to breaking down than a buccal flap because of the thickness of the palatal mucosa and because inclusion of the artery prevents vascular compromise. The technique leaves an area of palatal denudation that can be left exposed or closed with a bolster sutured in place or with some plastic palatal stent, and a bulge of tissue is created at the axis of rotation.

Buccal Fat Pad

Another surgical technique recommended for closing small- to medium-sized intraoral defects is the pedicled buccal fat pad, which was first described by Egyedi[9] in 1977 for the closure of OAC and oronasal communication, but before Egyedi's description, buccal fat pad grafts were used but only as free nonvascularized grafts.

Closure of iatrogenic OAC during or after maxillary molar extractions is the most common use of the buccal fat pad in oral and maxillofacial surgeries.

Buccal fat pad anatomy

Traditional anatomic descriptions state that the buccal fat pad has a central body and 4 processes: buccal, pterygoid, pterygopalatine, and superficial and deep temporal (**Fig. 4**).[10] The blood supply to

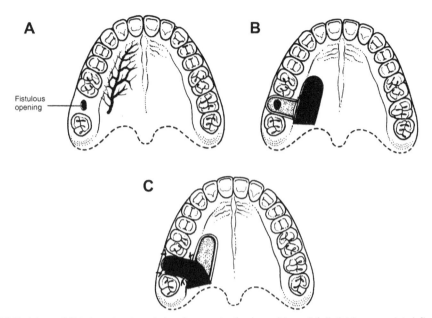

Fig. 3. (*A, B*) Excision of fistulous tract and development of a broad-based full-thickness palatal flap, ensuring inclusion of the greater palatine artery for adequate blood supply. (*C*) Rotation of the flap into position over the opening, where it is sutured. Exposed palatal bone will heal by secondary epithelialization. (*From* Schow SR. Odontogenic diseases of the maxillary sinus. In: Peterson LJ, Ellis E, Hupp JR, et al, editors. Contemporary oral and maxillofacial surgery. 2nd edition. St Louis (MO): CV Mosby; 1993. p. 477; with permission.)

the buccal fat pad originates from the buccal and deep temporal branches of the maxillary artery, the transverse branch of the superficial temporal artery, and branches of the facial artery.

Surgical technique

After a vestibular incision is made in the distobuccal depth of the maxillary tuberosity, the buccal flap and periosteum are raised (**Fig. 5**).[10] A sharp scissors is used to cut through the periosteum, and with pressure applied to the zygomatic arch region, the buccal fat pad should easily extrude into the operative side. Blunt dissection with a Metzenbaum scissors helps to mobilize as much fat pad as needed to obtain a tension-free closure across the communication. The tissue is fixed into bone with bur holes or screws and into adjacent palatal and buccal mucosa with resorbable sutures. The exposed buccal fat pad epithelializes in 4 to 6 weeks.[10] A surgical splint can be secured to the dentition to protect the flap during the healing phase.

Complications

According to the literature, the buccal fat pad graft procedure has a low failure rate and low morbidity associated with it. A possible partial necrosis of the flap has been reported often, in case of which the dehiscence should be treated conservatively, and if the defect is small, spontaneous closure

will probably occur. If the area of necrosis is large and fails to close, the other flap techniques should be attempted (such as palatal and tongue) rather than reattempting a buccal fat pad technique. A rare visible change in facial contour has been reported in patients only when the buccal fat pad is used for reconstruction of large defects.

Dr Egyedi recommended securing the fat pad with catgut sutures and then covering the graft with a split-thickness skin graft. He also recommended securing a prosthesis to the maxilla to help keep the skin adapted to the underlying fatty tissue. Tideman and colleagues[11] used the fat pad as an uncovered pedicled graft with no skin graft or other covering and saw complete epithelialization in approximately 2 weeks. Tideman and colleagues advised that to help minimize the incidence of postoperative complications, the fat pad graft should adequately cover the surgical defect and that it not be sutured under tension. The investigators also recommended that the patient receive a liquid or soft non-chewy diet until soft tissue healing has taken place.

Tongue Flaps

An alternative soft tissue flap procedure to use when buccal or palatal flaps have failed is the pedicled tongue flap (**Fig. 6**).[12] The use of tongue flaps has been reserved for cases in which the defect

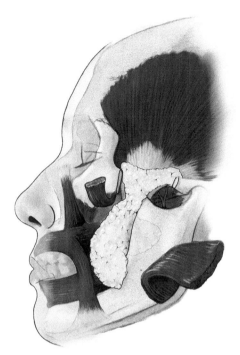

Fig. 4. Traditional description of buccal fat pad with its central body and 4 processes: buccal, pterygoid, pterygopalatine, and superficial and deep temporal. (*From* Arce K. Buccal fat pad in maxillary reconstruction. Atlas Oral Maxillofac Surg Clin North Am 2007;15:23–32; with permission.)

has been more than 1.5 cm and in which conservative methods have failed.[12,13] Because of its rich blood supply and pliability, the tongue flap has become a versatile procedure for reconstructing lip, cheek, oroantral, oronasal, or palatal defects.[14]

Tongue flaps can be created from the ventral, dorsal, or lateral parts of the tongue and can be anteriorly or posteriorly based. One difficulty associated with tongue-based flaps is the constant mobility of the flap because of speech and swallowing. This issue has been addressed by some investigators that the patients be placed in intermaxillary fixation simultaneously with the flap procedure. Some investigators argue that the anteriorly based tongue flap is better tolerated by patients and allows for the greatest degree of tongue mobility, decreasing the risk of tearing the flap from its palatal insertion.

Posteriorly based tongue flaps are recommended in the treatment of defects of the soft palate and posterior buccal mucosa and anteriorly based flaps in the treatment of defects of the hard palate, anterior-based buccal mucosa, and lips.[7] The tongue flaps are allowed to stay in place for 14 to 21 days to permit adequate healing after which the pedicle is severed and the tongue tissue is reinserted. In some cases, a third procedure is needed to debulk the recipient site but should not be performed for 3 months after the separation of the pedicle.

The success of the tongue flap is largely attributable to its favorable vasculature. The lingual artery and its branches are mainly responsible for the rich vascular supply to the tongue. Potential complications from this procedure are similar to those from performing any tongue flap procedure and may include flap failure, bleeding, swelling, pain, infection, hematoma, contour deformities, temporary loss of tongue sensation, and gustatory changes.

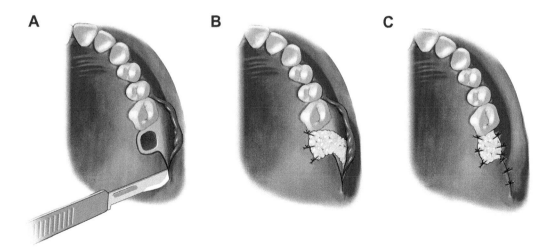

Fig. 5. (*A*) Full-thickness mucoperiosteal flap elevated to expose the OAC and allow access to the buccal fat pad. (*B*) Buccal fat pad mobilized and secured to the palatal soft tissue. (*C*) Mucoperiosteal flap closure with preservation of buccal vestibule. The exposed buccal fat pad will epithelialize in 4 to 6 weeks. (*From* Arce K. Buccal fat pad in maxillary reconstruction. Atlas Oral Maxillofac Surg Clin North Am 2007;15:23–32; with permission).

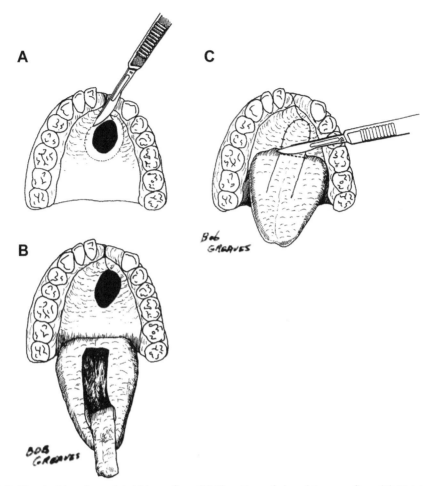

Fig. 6. (*A*) Outline incision for palatal hinge flap. (*B*) Elevation of dorsal tongue flap. (*C*) Division of lingual pedicle graft from the base of tongue. (*From* Smith TS, Siegrfried JS, Collins JT, et al. Repair of a palatal defect using a dorsal pedicle tongue flap. J Oral Maxillofac Surg 1982;40:670–73; with permission.)

The principles of sound flap design are well illustrated in the use of lingual flaps. The tissue is richly vascularized, can provide a broad-based pedicle, is extremely pliable, and can be placed free of tension in most areas of the hard palate. The pedicled tongue flap is, therefore, recommended for the repair of oroantral defects that cannot be successfully treated by palatal or buccal mucosa grafts because of size and/or position.[15]

Bone Grafts

In large OAC defects or in cases in which multiple attempts at soft tissue closure have failed previously, some investigators recommended the placement of an autologous solid bone graft into the OAC site to seal the bony defect before attempting soft tissue closure.[16] Because of the continued need for implant rehabilitation and the necessity of preimplant surgical procedures, such as sinus floor elevation, the routine soft tissue

closure of OAFs has become a major problem. The source of the bone most often can be intraoral donor sites, such as the symphysis, tuberosity, or anterior ramus; however, extraoral sites, such as the iliac crest, may be needed if the maxillary defect is extremely large. Harvesting bone from the intraoral donor areas significantly reduces the stress on the patients and involves less donor-site morbidity but does not provide the quantity of bone as available in the iliac crest. Alternative donor areas have been investigated, including bone grafts from the retromolar area and zygoma.

Hass and colleagues[16] have proposed using monocortical block grafts harvested intraorally for closing OAFs (**Fig. 7**).[17] Irregular bony defects of the sinus floor were standardized to a round shape using a round trephine bur. A monocortical block graft would then be harvested using the same trephine size to create a graft that can be press-fit into the defect. If the press-fit graft is unstable, mini plates or screws can be inserted for internal

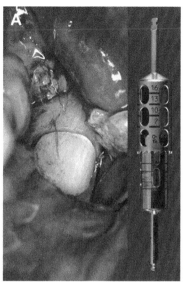
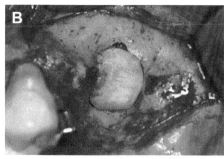

Fig. 7. (*A*) Intraoperative view of left retromolar donor site (*left*) and trephines of matching sizes (*right*). (*B*) Intraoperative view showing press-fit of monocortical bone graft in the molar region on the left side. (*From* Watzack G, Tepper G, Zechner W, et al. Bony press-fit closure of oro-antral fistulas: a technique for pre-sinus lift repair and secondary closure. J Oral Maxillofac Surg 2005;63:1288–94; with permission.)

fixation. Soft tissue closure can be established using a Rehrmann flap. Care must be taken not to accidentally force the graft into the maxillary sinus during graft placement. Watzack and colleagues[17] recommended creating 2 small holes in the center of the block graft and pulling through a thread to ensure that the graft does not fall into the sinus. As with any patient with an OAC, the patient should follow postoperative sinus precautions including treatment with antibiotics, decongestant and antihistamine therapy, and no nose blowing or sneezing for 3 weeks. The patient should be closely followed up for signs of sinusitis. Although previous studies have recommended waiting for sinus lift elevation following the closure of sinus lift elevation, there have been reports that simultaneous procedures can be performed assuming an aseptic environment at the time of treatment.[18]

CLOSURE OF OROANTRAL DEFECTS
Alloplastic Material to Close OACs

In 1992, Zide and Karas[19] reported on the use of nonporous hydroxylapatite (HA) blocks to close chronic fistula and OAF. The technique requires that the acute sinusitis be resolved after appropriate treatment with antibiotics, irrigation, and decongestants as is the usual regimen before the procedure. A nonporous HA block is then cut to fit the bony ostium with diamond burs under irrigation and securing the block through holes in the maxillary alveolar bone using a 26-gauge wire. Advantages include the ability to have a press-fit graft closure without the

morbidity associated with a second-site surgery and the ability to allow exposure of the block if soft tissue closure cannot be achieved.

Resorbable Collagen Membranes

The use of a resorbable collagen membrane for the closure of a large OAC has been reported in the literature.[20] The investigators positioned a resorbable collagen membrane over the OAC and secured it into position with resorbable pins. A buccal flap was raised but could not fully cover the OAC, leaving the collagen membrane exposed to the oral cavity. Complete coverage of the membrane was achieved in 14 days.

The membrane provides support for the blood clot in the defect so that it will organize and be replaced by bone and epithelium on the oral surface. This procedure offers an easy alternative for large openings that may have required bone grafting before OAC closure. Ogunsalu[21] used Bio-Gide (porcine collagen membrane) and Bio-Oss (bovine bone grafting material) to close an OAC in 1 patient. An advantage is that seemingly bony and soft closures are accomplished without donor-site surgery.

Gold Foil

Several studies have reported on the use of gold foil or gold plate for the closure of OACs (**Fig. 8**).[22] The procedure entails raising mucoperiosteal flaps to expose the bony margins of the defect. The gold foil is burnished into place with its edges around on a healthy bone, thus acting

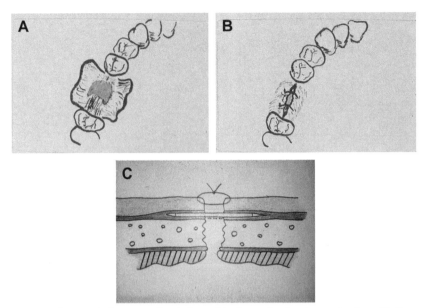

Fig. 8. (A) Placement of a metal plate over fistula in an ideal case for barrier protection. (B) Flaps repositioned over the metal without tension. The metal is visible at all times. (C) Inner layer of periosteum is still present to initiate proliferation of the tissue. (*From* Steiner M, Gould AR, Madion DC, et al. Metal plates and foils for closure of oroantral fistulae. J Oral Maxillofac Surg 2008;66:1551–55; with permission.)

as a bridge for overgrowing sinus mucosa. The elevated tissue is sutured across the gold foil without attempting to realize primary closure. In general, the gold foil exfoliates after a period of 6 weeks. The value of the gold foil technique depends on the closure of large OACs that failed in previous attempts and on the unaltered intraoral anatomy. A disadvantage of this expensive technique is the relatively long period needed for complete closure and healing of the defect. An alternative to a gold foil is the aluminum foil found in dental film packages cut to cover the OAC.

Alternative Approaches for the Closure of OAC

The use of laser light in low-dose applications has been reported for the closure of OACs. Laser light in low doses has also been used successfully in the prevention and/or healing of chemotherapy-induced oral mucositis. Grzesiak-Janas and Janas[23] used a biostimulative laser of 30 mW power for 3 cycles of extraoral and intraoral irradiation. Patients were exposed to the laser light for 10.5 minutes for 4 consecutive days.

The disadvantages of this technique include the cost of laser therapy and the need for large number of visits to accomplish complete closure.[23] Logan and Coates[24] proposed a treatment strategy for OACs in immunocompromised patients. The OAC was first de-epithelialized under local anesthesia followed by the placement of an acrylic surgical

splint fitted to cover the fistula and edentulous area, including the hard palate. The patient wears the splint continuously for 8 weeks, removing it only for cleaning. The technique be a very useful option when a surgical intervention is contraindicated because of immunosuppression.

SUMMARY

The practicing oral and maxillofacial surgeon treating patients with OAC/OAFs should be familiar and competent with the various treatment options available. Multiple techniques are available from purely soft tissue flaps, which have proved to be successful over time, to a combination of hard tissue grafts (autologous, alloplastic, or allograft), which can be useful with the increased demand for implant restorations. Although different procedures have proved to be successful, all are premised on the treatment of any underlying sinusitis, which is associated with a higher risk of recurrent OAC.

REFERENCES

1. Abuabara A, Cortez AL, Passeri LA, et al. Evaluation of different treatments for oroantral/oronasal communications: experience of 112 cases. Int J Oral Maxillofac Surg 2006;35:155.
2. von Wowern N. Correlation between the development of an oroantral fistula and the size of the corresponding bony defect. J Oral Surg 1973;31:98.

3. von Wowern N. Frequency of oro-antral fistulae after perforation to the maxillary sinus. Scand J Dent Res 1970;78:394.

4. Del Junco R, Rappaport I, Allison GR. Persistent oral antral fistulas. Arch Otolaryngol 1998;114:1315–6.

5. Visscher S, von Minnen B, Bos RR, et al. Closure of oroantral communications: a review of the literature. J Oral Maxillofac Surg 2010;68:1384–91.

6. Rehrmann A. Eine methode zur schliessung von kieferhöhlenperforationen. Dtsch Zahnärztl Wschr 1936;39:1136 [in German].

7. Wells DL, Capes JO. Complications of dentoalveolar surgery. In: Fonseca RJ, editor. Oral and maxillofacial surgery, vol. 1. Philadelphia (PA): WB Saunders Co; 2000. p. 432.

8. Salins PC, Kishore SK. Anteriorly based palatal flap for closure of large oroantral fistula. Oral Surg Oral Med Oral Pathol Oral Radiol Endod 1996;82:253.

9. Egyedi P. Utilization of the buccal fat pad for closure of oro-antral and/or oro-nasal communication. J Maxillofac Surg 1977;5:241–4.

10. Arce K. Buccal fat pad in maxillary reconstruction. Atlas Oral Maxillofac Surg Clin North Am 2007;15:23–32.

11. Tideman H, Bosanquet A, Scott J. Use of the buccal fat pad as a pedicled graft. J Oral Maxillofac Surg 1986;44(6):435–40.

12. Smith TS, Siegrfried JS, Collins JT, et al. Repair of a palatal defect using a dorsal pedicle tongue flap. J Oral Maxillofac Surg 1962;40:670–3.

13. Jackson IT. Use of tongue flaps to resurface lip defects and close palatal fistulae in children. Plast Reconstr Surg 1972;49:537.

14. Steinhauser E. Experience with dorsal tongue flaps for closure of defects of the hard palate. J Oral Maxillofac Surg 1982;40:787.

15. Smith TS, Schaberg SJ. Repair of a palatal defect using a dorsal pedicle tongue flap. J Oral Maxillofac Surg 1982;40(10):670–3.

16. Hass R, Watzak G, Baron M, et al. A preliminary study of monocortical bone grafts for oroantral fistula closure. Oral Surg Oral Med Oral Pathol Oral Radiol Endod 2003;96:263.

17. Watzack G, Tepper G, Zechner W, et al. Bony press-fit closure of oro-antral fistulas: a technique for pre-sinus lift repair and secondary closure. J Oral Maxillofac Surg 2005;63:1288–94.

18. Cortes D, Rafael MC. Simultaneous oral antral fistula closure and sinus floor augmentation to facilitate dental implant placement or orthodontics. J Oral Maxillofac Surg 2010;68:1148–51.

19. Zide MF, Karas ND. Hydroxylapatite block closure of oroantral fistulas: report of cases. J Oral Maxillofac Surg 1992;50:71–5.

20. Markovic A, Colic S, Drazk R, et al. Closure of large oroantral fistula with resorbable collagen membrane: case report. Serbian Dent J 2009;56:4.

21. Ogunsalu C. A new surgical management for oroantral communication: the resorbable guided tissue regeneration membrane—bone substitute sandwich technique. West Indian Med J 2005;54:261.

22. Steiner M, Gould AR, Madion DC, et al. Metal plates and foils for closure of oroantral fistulae. J Oral Maxillofac Surg 2008;66:1551–5.

23. Grzesiak-Janas G, Janas A. Conservative closure of antro-oral communications stimulated with laser light. J Clin Laser Med Surg 2001;19:181.

24. Logan RM, Coates EA. Non-surgical management of an oroantral fistula in a patient with HIV infection. Aust Dent J 2003;48:255.

Benign Cysts and Tumors of the Paranasal Sinuses

Joseph E. Pierse, DMD, MA*, Avichai Stern, DDS

KEYWORDS

- Benign • Cysts • Tumors • Paranasal sinuses • Treatment

BENIGN CYSTS OF THE PARANASAL SINUSES

Cysts of the paranasal sinuses may be categorized as intrinsic, which originate in the mucosa of the paranasal sinuses, or extrinsic, which originate in the adjacent structures, such as the dental tissues.

INTRINSIC CYSTS
Mucous Retention Cyst (Salivary Duct Cyst)

The most common intrinsic sinus cysts do not produce bone destruction.[1–7] They can be appreciated on routine sinus films and are often asymptomatic. The major concern is in differentiating them from malignant disease. The mucous retention cyst is found frequently within the maxillary antrum. This cyst results from the obstruction of the minor seromucinous glands and is visible radiographically as a dome-shaped, homogeneous, sharply defined mass outlined by the air of the paranasal sinus. The mucous retention cyst commonly involves the floor of the maxillary sinus, but may sometimes manifest in the lateral wall or roof of the sinus. A large cyst may fill the sinus and cause complete opacification, thereby obscuring its cystic nature on radiographic analysis. However, a small cyst may be hidden by the surrounding intrasinus fluid.

The salivary duct cyst is an epithelium-lined cavity that arises from salivary gland tissue. The cause of such cysts is uncertain. Some cases may represent ductal dilatation secondary to obstruction, which creates intraluminal pressure, whereas other cases seem to represent true developmental salivary duct cysts that are separate from the adjacent normal salivary ducts.

Salivary duct cysts usually occur in adults and can arise within either the major or minor salivary glands. Cysts of the major glands are most common within the parotid gland, presenting as slowly growing, asymptomatic edema. Intraoral cysts can occur at any minor salivary gland. Although these cysts may manifest in the paranasal sinuses, they most frequently develop in the floor of the mouth, buccal mucosa, and lips. They mimic the appearance of mucoceles and are characterized by a soft, fluctuant swelling that may appear bluish, depending on the depth of the cyst below the surface, whereas some cysts may feel relatively firm to palpation.

The lining of the mucous retention cyst is variable and may consist of cuboidal, columnar, or atrophic squamous epithelium surrounding thin or mucoid secretions in the lumen. In some cases, especially those in ductal obstruction, the epithelium may undergo malignant transformation, showing papillary folds into the cystic lumen reminiscent of a small Warthin tumor but without the prominent lymphoid stroma. If this proliferation is extensive, these lesions are sometimes diagnosed as papillary cystadenomas. The individual lesions of patients with multiple mucous retention cysts also show prominent oncocytic metaplasia of the epithelial lining.

Isolated salivary duct cysts are treated by conservative surgical excision. For cysts in the major glands, partial or total gland excision may be necessary. This lesion has a low percentage of recurrence.

The authors have nothing to disclose.
Department of Dentistry/Oral Maxillofacial Surgery, The Brooklyn Hospital Center, 121 Dekalb Avenue, Box 187, Brooklyn, NY 11201, USA
* Corresponding author.
E-mail address: drjoenyhq@yahoo.com

Oral Maxillofacial Surg Clin N Am 24 (2012) 249–264
doi:10.1016/j.coms.2012.01.007

oralmaxsurgery.theclinics.com

Serous Cyst

Less common then the mucous retention cyst is the serous cyst.[8–12] It may be found within any of the paranasal sinuses but has a predilection for the maxillary sinus floor. These cysts are not lined with epithelium and are loculated collections of serous fluid within the loose stroma of the submucosa. Serous cysts, mucous cysts, mucosal polyps, loculated pus, granulomas, and dental and neoplastic lesions may mimic each other radiographically. A blowout fracture of the floor of the orbit with downward orbital soft tissue herniation may be simulated by a mucous retention cyst of the antral roof. These cysts are treated similarly to mucous retention cysts, with minimal recurrence.

Mucocele (Mucus Extravasation Phenomenon)

The mucocele is a cystic lesion that commonly produces bone destruction within the paranasal sinuses.[13–28] It is an expanding lesion that results from the continued accumulation of secretion within an obstructed sinus cavity. The ostial obstruction may be the result of inflammation, trauma, or osteoma. This lesion has a definite predilection for the frontal and ethmoidal sinuses, because of the dependent position of the ostia. Approximately 60% of all mucoceles involve the frontal sinus: most of the remainder involves the ethmoid labyrinth. Maxillary and sphenoidal mucoceles are rare. However, the sphenoidal mucocele may cause serious neurologic symptoms by intracranial extension.

Occasionally infection may convert a mucocele into a pyocele. Radiographically, the sinus is initially opacified by retained secretions, which displaces all the air content. Pressure erosion of the surrounding bony walls by the mucocele decalcifies the mucoperiosteal cortical plate and destroys the normal scalloped borders of the frontal sinus. With progression of the lesion, the sinus appears more radiolucent radiographically. There may be a zone of reactive osteitis and bone sclerosis about the margins of the mucocele. In approximately 5% of the mucoceles, peripheral calcification is evident radiographically. This calcification may be large enough to stimulate the growth of an osteoma. With extensive intracranial extension by a frontal mucocele, a segment of the posterior wall of the frontal sinus may be displaced as a bony fragment deeply into the frontal lobe. A view of the optic foramen may be valuable in the diagnosis of a mucocele of the frontal sinus as well as of the posterior ethmoidal cells. The sphenoidal mucocele presents radiographically as a destructive expanding cystic or mass lesion.

The maxillary sinus mucocele may stimulate a carcinoma of the antrum both clinically and radiographically.

On microscopic examination, inflammation usually includes an abundance of histiocytes. In some cases, ruptured salivary ducts may be identified supplying the area. The adjacent minor salivary glands often contain a chronic inflammatory cell infiltrate and dilated ducts.

Most mucoceles are self-limiting. They rupture and resolve on their own. However, other lesions are chronic in nature, and local surgical excision is necessary. To minimize the risk of recurrence, when the area is excised, the surgeon should remove any adjacent salivary glands that may be supplying the lesion. The specimen should be submitted for pathologic examination to confirm the diagnosis and rule out the possibility of a salivary gland malignancy. The prognosis is excellent, although occasional mucoceles recur, necessitating reexcision, especially if the associated glands are not removed.

Cholesteatoma (Keratoma; Epidermoidoma)

A rare expansile cystic lesion of the paranasal sinuses that produces bone destruction,[29–35] this keratin-filled cyst is believed to arise from squamous epithelium through an oral-antral fistula. A cholesteatoma occurring within the sinus cannot be differentiated radiographically from a mucocele or a dermoid cyst. In some instances, a primary cholesteatoma of the cranial vault arising from congenital epithelial cell rests in the diploë or meninges may involve the paranasal sinuses by secondary extension. Surgical excision is the treatment of choice. Recurrence is rare.

Extrinsic Cysts

The most common group of extrinsic cysts involving the paranasal sinuses are of dental origin.[36–45] The pathologic and radiographic nature of a dental cyst can best be understood in relation to dental embryogenesis.

Dentigerous Cyst (Follicular Cyst; Primordial Cyst)

The term follicular or primordial cyst is applied to a cyst that forms in the tooth bud before the ectodermal enamel and mesenchymal dentin have formed.[46–63] Radiographically this cyst appears as an expanded radiolucent area with a well-circumscribed mucoperiosteal border, usually in the maxillary canine area, or maxillary/mandibular third molar area. The dentigerous cyst causing sinus involvement is usually seen in the piriform region and involves one of the canines. As the cystic lesion extends into the maxillary sinus, secondary bone deformity or infection may result.

The dentigerous cyst is defined as a cyst that originates by the separation of the follicle from around the crown of an unerupted tooth. This is the most common type of developmental odontogenic cyst; approximately 20% of all epithelium-lined cysts of the jaws are developmental odontogenic cysts. The dentigerous cyst encloses the crown of an unerupted tooth and is attached to the tooth at the cementoenamel junction. The pathogenesis of this cyst is uncertain, but often develops by accumulation of fluid between the reduced enamel epithelium and the tooth crown.

Although dentigerous cysts may occur in association with any unerupted tooth, they are most commonly involved with mandibular third molars. Other relatively frequent sites include maxillary canines, maxillary third molars, and mandibular second premolars. Dentigerous cysts rarely involve unerupted deciduous teeth. Occasionally, they are associated with supernumerary teeth or odontomas.

Although dentigerous cysts may be encountered in patients across a wide age range, they manifest most frequently in patients 10 to 30 years of age, and are more prominent in white males. Small dentigerous cysts are usually asymptomatic and are discovered only on routine radiographic examination. Dentigerous cysts can proliferate to a considerable size, and large cysts may be associated with a painless expansion of the bone in the involved area. Extensive lesions may result in facial asymmetry. Large dentigerous cysts are uncommon, and most lesions that are considered to be large dentigerous cysts on radiographic examination are odontogenic keratocysts (OKCs) or ameloblastomas. After pathologic examination, dentigerous cysts may become infected and be associated with localized pain and edema. Such infections may arise in a dentigerous cyst that is associated with a partially erupted tooth or by extension from a periapical or periodontal lesion that affects an adjacent tooth.

Radiographically, the dentigerous cyst shows a unilocular radiolucent area that is associated with the crown of an unerupted tooth. The radiolucency usually has a well-defined sclerotic border, whereas an infected cyst may show ill-defined borders. Although a large dentigerous cyst may give the impression of a multilocular process because of bone trabeculae within the radiolucency, dentigerous cysts are grossly and histopathologically unilocular processes.

The cyst-to-crown relationship shows multiple radiographic variations. In central lesions, which are the most common, the cyst surrounds the crown of the tooth and the crown projects into the cyst. The lateral cyst is often associated with distoangular maxillary third molars that are completely impacted, or mesioangular mandibular third molars that are partially erupted. The lesion grows laterally along the root surface and partially surrounds the crown. In the circumferential variant, the cyst surrounds the crown and extends a particular distance along the root so that most of the root lies within the cyst. Rarely, a third molar may be displaced to the inferior border of the mandible or superior and posterior along the ascending ramus. Maxillary anterior teeth are displaced into the floor of the nose, and maxillary posterior teeth may be moved through the maxillary sinus to the floor of the orbit. Dentigerous cysts may displace the involved tooth for a considerable distance. Root resorption of adjacent erupted teeth can also occur.

Radiographic distinction between a small dentigerous cyst and an enlarged follicle surrounding the crown of an unerupted tooth is difficult. For the lesion to be considered a dentigerous cyst, some clinicians believe that the radiolucent space surrounding the tooth crown should be at least 3 to 4 mm in diameter. Radiographic findings are not pathoneumonic for a dentigerous cyst. OKCs, unilocular ameloblastomas, and other odontogenic and nonodontogenic tumors may have radiographic features that are essentially identical to those of a dentigerous cyst and warrant further investigation.

The histologic features of dentigerous cysts vary, depending on whether or not the cyst is inflamed. In the noninflamed dentigerous cyst, the fibrous connective tissue wall is loosely arranged and contains considerable glycosaminoglycan ground substance. Small islands or cords of inactive odontogenic epithelial rests may be appreciated in the fibrous wall. These rests may be numerous at times, and the lesion may be misdiagnosed as an ameloblastoma. The epithelial lining consists of approximately 2 to 4 layers of flattened nonkeratinizing cells, and the epithelium and connective tissue interface is flat.

In an inflamed dentigerous cyst, the fibrous wall has a marked collagen component with a variable infiltration of chronic inflammatory cells. Hyperplasia may be evident in the epithelium, with the development of rete ridges and more definitive squamous features. A keratinized surface may also be evident; however, these changes must be differentiated from those observed in OKCs. Focal areas of mucous cells may be found in the epithelial lining of dentigerous cysts. Rarely, ciliated columnar cells are present. Small groups of sebaceous cells may be noted within the fibrous cyst wall. These mucous, ciliated, and sebaceous elements represent the multipotentiality of the odontogenic epithelial lining in the dentigerous cyst.

Examination of the wall of a dentigerous cyst may reveal 1 or several areas of nodular thickening on the luminal surface. These areas must be evaluated microscopically to rule out the presence of early oncotic change. Because a thin layer of reduced enamel epithelium normally lines the dental follicle surrounding the crown of an unerupted tooth, it can be difficult to distinguish a small dentigerous cyst from a normal or enlarged dental follicle based on microscopic features alone. The most important factor is ensuring that the lesion does not represent a more significant malignant process (eg, OKC or ameloblastoma).

Treatment of a dentigerous cyst is enucleation with concomitant extraction of the unerupted tooth. Large dentigerous cysts may be treated by marsupialization. This treatment permits decompression of the cyst, with a resulting reduction in the size of the bone defect. The cyst can then be excised at a later date, with a less extensive surgical procedure.

The prognosis for dentigerous cysts is excellent, and recurrence is minimal after complete enucleation. However, several potential complications must be considered. According to the literature, the lining of a dentigerous cyst has the potential to undergo neoplastic transformation into an ameloblastoma. Although this transformation can occur, the frequency of malignant transformation is low. Rarely, a squamous cell carcinoma may arise in the lining of a dentigerous cyst. Furthermore, some intraosseous mucoepidermoid carcinomas may develop from mucous cells in the lining of dentigerous cysts.

Lateral Periodontal Cyst (Radicular Cyst)

This cyst evolves after the eruption of a tooth and usually reflects continued inflammatory stimulation of the epithelial cells in the periodontal membrane (the Hertwig sheath) and accounts for less than 2% of all epithelium-lined jaw cysts.[64–75] As these cells are stimulated, a cystic lesion develops, which can appear as a small radiolucent area about the dental root resulting from bone absorption. These cysts may enlarge and erode into the maxillary sinus and become secondarily infected. Dental extraction of a tooth associated with a radicular cyst often results in an oral-antral communication.

The lateral periodontal cyst is most often an asymptomatic lesion that is detected during a radiographic examination. It most frequently occurs in patients in the fifth to the seventh decades of life; rarely does it occur in patients younger than 30 years of age. Although 75% to 80% of cases occur in the mandibular premolar-canine-lateral incisor area, these cysts may also occur in their maxillary counterparts.

Radiographically, the cyst appears as a well-circumscribed radiolucent area located laterally to the root or roots of vital teeth. Most of these cysts are less than 10 mm in diameter. Occasionally, the lesion may have a polycystic appearance. Such examples have been termed botryoid odontogenic cysts. Grossly and microscopically, they appear as grapelike clusters of small individual cysts. These lesions represent a variant of the lateral periodontal cyst, resulting from cystic degeneration and subsequent fusion of adjacent foci of dental lamina rests. The botryoid variant has a multilocular radiographic appearance but also may appear unilocular.

The radiographic features of the lateral periodontal cyst are not pathoneumonic (ie, an OKC that develops between the roots of adjacent teeth may show identical radiographic findings). An inflammatory radicular cyst that occurs laterally to a root in relation to an accessory foramen or a cyst that arises from periodontal inflammation may also simulate a lateral periodontal cyst radiographically.

The lateral periodontal cyst has a thin, noninflamed, fibrous wall, with an epithelial lining that is predominantly 1 to 3 cells thick. This epithelium usually consists of flattened squamous cells, but may also be cuboidal in shape. Foci of glycogen-rich clear cells may be interspersed among the lining epithelial cells. Some cysts show focal nodular thickenings of the epithelial lining, which are composed chiefly of clear cells. Clear cell epithelial rests may be appreciated within the fibrous wall. Rarely, botryoid odontogenic cysts show focal areas that histopathologically are suggestive of a glandular odontogenic cyst.

Conservative enucleation of the lateral periodontal cyst is the treatment of choice. This treatment can be accomplished without damage to the adjacent teeth. Recurrence is rare, although it has been reported with the botryoid variant because it is polycystic. Although rare, lateral periodontal cysts have the potential to develop into squamous cell carcinoma.

Neurogenic Cysts

Two types of neurogenic cystic lesions involve the paranasal sinuses: the encephalocele and the meningocele. Both are the result of congenital herniation of intracranial meningeal and neural tissue, or meninges alone into the paranasal sinuses.[76–80] The more common of the 2, the encephalocele, contains primitive neural and supporting tissue, whereas the meningocele contains arachnoid and dural tissue and cerebrospinal fluid. The encephalocele has also been referred to as a nasal glioma. This is not a neoplastic lesion but rather a sequestered gliomatous mass with or without an intracranial connection. The encephalocele may herniate through the suture lines between the nasal, frontal, ethmoid, sphenoid, or lacrimal bones and disrupt the cribriform plate, expanding into the nasal cavity medial to the middle turbinate. The rare frontal meningocele usually appears before the development of the frontal sinuses.

Radiographically these neurogenic cysts are seen as bony dehiscences in the base of the skull or cranial vault associated with a soft tissue mass extending into the nose or paranasal sinuses. The bone defect may be obvious or very small and may be evident only on computed tomography (CT) analysis or may remain undetectable. The meningoencephalocele may be well outlined by air either in the frontal or sphenoid sinuses. When treating these lesions, careful clinical and radiographic differential diagnosis is important to avoid aggressive nasal surgery and subsequent meningeal infection; tomograms, cerebral angiograms, and pneumoencephalograms may be required in the differential diagnosis before surgical enucleation can commence.

FISSURAL CYSTS

The fissural group of extrasinus cysts result from the sequestration of ectoderm within the lines of fusion of the bony facial skeleton during development.[25,28,81–85] The embryonic fissural nonodontogenic cysts are classified as follows: the medial group, which includes cysts of the incisive canal and papilla palatina but does not involve the maxillary sinus, and the lateral group, which includes bony and soft tissue cysts. The soft tissue cyst is a neuroalveolar cyst, which arises in the lateral half of the nasal floor anterior to the inferior turbinate, and may produce appreciable deformity of the nasoantral wall. The lateral bony inclusion cyst, also known as the globulomaxillary cyst, commonly appears between the roots of the upper lateral maxillary incisor and canine teeth; these cysts can encroach on the paranasal sinuses similar to nasopalatine duct cysts, and median palatal cysts.

Globulomaxillary Cysts (Lateral Bony Inclusion Cyst)

This cyst was purported to be a fissural cyst that developed from entrapped epithelium during

fusion of the medial nasal process with the maxillary process.[86–94] Virtually all cysts between the lateral incisor and canines can be explained on an odontogenic basis. They are lined by inflamed stratified squamous epithelium and are consistent with periapical cysts. Some show specific histopathologic features of an OKC or a lateral periodontal cyst. According to the literature, these lesions may also arise from inflammation of the reduced enamel epithelium at the time of eruption of the teeth. On rare occasions, cysts in the globulomaxillary region may be lined by pseudostratified, ciliated, columnar epithelium. Such cases may lend credence to their fissural origin. However, this epithelium may be appreciated because of the close proximity of the sinus lining. In addition, transitional epithelium also has been reported in periapical cysts, dentigerous cysts, and glandular odontogenic cysts found in other locations. When a radiolucency between the maxillary lateral incisor and canine is encountered, the clinician should first consider an odontogenic origin for the lesion. Treatment is surgical enucleation. If the lesion is related to an adjacent nonvital tooth, then root canal therapy may be indicated. Prognosis depends on histopathology, and recurrence potential is low.

Nasopalatine Duct Cyst (Incisive Canal Cyst)

The nasopalatine duct cyst is the most common nonodontogenic cyst of the oral cavity, occurring in about 1% of the population.[95–105] It develops from remnants of the nasopalatine duct, an embryologic structure connecting the oral and nasal cavities in the area of the incisive canal. At the seventh week, the developing palate consists of the primary palate, which is formed by the fusion of the medial nasal processes. Posterior to the primary palate, down-growth of the nasal septum produces 2 communications between the oral and nasal cavities: the primitive nasal choanae. Formation of the secondary palate begins during the eighth week of gestation, with downward growth of the palatine processes to a location on either side of the tongue.

As the mandible develops and the tongue is displaced inferiorly, these palatine processes grow horizontally, fusing with the nasal septum in the midline and with the primary palate at the premaxilla. Two passages persist in the midline between the primary and secondary palates (the incisive canals). These canals house the nasopalatine ducts. These ducts degenerate in humans during development but epithelial remnants may be left behind in the incisive canals. The incisive canals begin on the floor of the nasal cavity on either side of the septum, coursing inferior and anterior to exit the palate via a common foramen at the incisive papilla. In addition to the nasopalatine ducts, these canals contain the nasopalatine nerve, and anastomosing branches of the descending palatine and sphenopalatine arteries. Occasionally, 2 smaller foramina (the canals of Scarpa) carrying the nasopalatine nerves can be found within the incisive foramen.

The nasopalatine duct cyst can develop at any age, but is most prevalent in men in the fourth to sixth decades of life. The most common presenting symptoms include edema of the anterior palate, drainage, and pain. However, many lesions can be asymptomatic and are discovered only on routine radiographs. Although rare, a large cyst may produce a through-and-through fluctuant expansion involving the anterior palate and labial alveolar mucosa.

Radiographs show a well-circumscribed radiolucency in or near the midline of the anterior maxilla, interproximal and apical to the central incisors. There is no root resorption. The lesion presents as round or oval with a sclerotic border. Some cysts may have an inverted pear shape, whereas other lesions may show a classic heart shape as a result of superimposition of the nasal spine or because they are notched by the nasal septum. The radiographic diameter of nasopalatine duct cysts can range from 6.0 mm to 6.0 cm, with a mean size of 1.0 to 2.5 cm and a diameter of 1.5 to 1.7 cm. It may be difficult to distinguish a small nasopalatine duct cyst from a large incisive foramen. It is generally accepted that a diameter of 6 mm is the upper limit of normal size for the incisive foramen.

The epithelial lining of nasopalatine duct cyst is highly variable, and may be composed of stratified squamous epithelium, pseudostratified columnar epithelium, simple columnar epithelium, or simple cuboidal epithelium. More than 1 epithelial type is frequently found in the same cyst. Stratified squamous epithelium is the most common, present in approximately 75% of all cysts. Pseudostratified columnar epithelium has been reported in 30% to 75% of all cases. Simple cuboidal and columnar epithelium are discovered less frequently. Cilia and goblet cells can be found in association with columnar linings. The type of epithelium may be related to the vertical position of the cyst within the incisive canal. Cysts developing within the superior aspect of the canal near the nasal cavity are more likely to show respiratory epithelium, whereas those in an inferior position near the oral cavity show squamous epithelium. The contents of the cyst wall may be variable in diagnosis. Because the nasopalatine duct cyst arises within the incisive canal, moderate-sized nerve capillaries and veins are found in the cyst wall. Small mucous glands have been reported in approximately 30% of cases. Occasionally, small islands of hyaline cartilage may also be present. Frequently, an inflammatory response is noted in the cyst wall. This inflammation is often chronic in nature and is composed of lymphocytes, plasma cells, and histiocytes.

Nasopalatine duct cysts are treated by conservative enucleation. Biopsy is recommended because the lesion is not diagnostic radiographically; other benign and malignant lesions have been known to mimic the nasopalatine duct cyst. Recurrence and malignant transformation are rare.

Median Palatal (Palatine) Cyst

The median palatal cyst is a rare fissural cyst that develops from the epithelium entrapped along the embryonic line of fusion of the lateral palatal shelves of the maxilla.[106–111] This cyst may be difficult to distinguish from a nasopalatine duct cyst because of its anatomic position. Because the nasopalatine ducts course posteriorly and superiorly as they extend from the incisive canal into the nasal cavity, a nasopalatine duct cyst that arises from the posterior remnants of this duct near the nasal cavity might be mistaken for a median palatal cyst. However, if a true median palatal cyst were to develop toward the anterior portion of the hard palate, then it could easily be mistaken for a nasopalatine duct cyst.

The median palatal cyst presents as a firm or fluctuant swelling of the midline of the hard palate posterior to the palatine papilla. It predominantly manifests in young adults. It is asymptomatic, but some patients may complain of pain or expansion. The average size of this cyst is between 2 mm and 2 cm, but sometimes it can encompass 70% of the hard palate. Occlusal radiographs show a well-circumscribed radiolucency in the midline of the hard palate. Some cases have been associated with divergence of the central incisors, although it may be difficult to rule out a nasopalatine duct cyst in these instances.

To differentiate the median palatal cyst from other cystic lesions of the maxilla, diagnostic criteria should include: symmetry along the midline of the hard palate; a location posterior to the palatine papilla; it should appear ovoid or circular radiographically; it should not be intimately associated with a nonvital tooth; it does not communicate with the incisive canal; and it shows no microscopic evidence of large neurovascular bundles, hyaline cartilage, or minor salivary glands in the cyst wall. A true median palatal cyst should show clinical enlargement of the palate. A midline radiolucency without clinical evidence of expansion is probably a nasopalatine duct cyst.

Histopathologic examination shows a cyst that is usually lined by stratified squamous epithelium. Areas of ciliated pseudostratified columnar epithelium can also be present. Chronic inflammation may be appreciated in the cyst wall.

The median palatal cyst is treated by complete enucleation. Recurrence is low.

BENIGN TUMORS OF THE PARANASAL SINUSES

Excluding inflammatory and allergic polyps, benign epithelial tumors within the paranasal sinuses are infrequent.

EPITHELIAL TUMORS
Sinonasal Papillomas

Papillomas of the sinonasal tract are benign, localized proliferations of the respiratory mucosa of this region.[112–136] The mucosa develops into 3 histomorphologically distinct papillomas: fungiform, inverted, or cylindrical cell lesions showing features of both the inverted and the cylindrical cell types that may be termed mixed or hybrid papillomas.

In addition, a keratinizing squamous papilloma, similar to the oral squamous papilloma, may rarely occur in the nasal vestibule. Collectively, sinonasal papillomas represent 10% to 25% of all tumors of the nasal and paranasal regions. Fifty percent of the sinonasal papillomas arise from the mucosa of the lateral nasal wall, whereas the other half predominantly involve the maxillary, ethmoid sinuses, and the nasal septum. Multiple lesions may be present.

The cause of sinonasal papillomas remains controversial. Some clinicians believe that these lesions represent neoplasms, whereas others consider them to be a reactive hyperplasia secondary to a variety of environmental stimulants, such as allergy, chronic bacterial or viral (human papillomavirus [HPV] type 11) infection, and tobacco smoking. Molecular and genetic research have shown that inverted papillomas arise from a single progenitor cell, suggesting that these lesions can be neoplastic and recurrence may result from growth of residual transformed cells.

Fungiform (septal; squamous; exophytic) papilloma

The fungiform papilloma is similar to the oral squamous papilloma, although it possesses a more aggressive biologic behavior, and more variability in the epithelium.[112–136] It represents 18% to 50% of all sinonasal papillomas. Almost all variants are positive for HPV type 6 or 11.

This papilloma develops almost exclusively on the nasal septum and is more prevalent in men. It occurs in patients 20 to 50 years of age. It shows unilateral nasal obstruction or epistaxis and appears as a pink or tan, broad-based nodule with papillary or verrucous surface projections.

The fungiform papilloma has a microscopic appearance similar to that of the oral squamous papilloma, although the stratified squamous epithelium covering the fingerlike projections is seldom keratinized. Transitional epithelium may be seen in some lesions. Goblet cells and intraepithelial microcysts containing mucus are often present. Mitoses are rare, and dysplasia is uncommon. The underlying connective tissue consists of delicate fibrous tissue with a minimal inflammatory component, unless it is irritated.

Complete surgical excision is the treatment of choice. Recurrence is common, developing in approximately one-third of all cases, although this may be caused by incomplete excision. According to the literature, this lesion has minimal or no potential for malignant transformation.

Inverted papilloma (inverted schneiderian papilloma)

The most common sinonasal papilloma, the inverted papilloma, is also the variant with the greatest potential for local destruction and malignant transformation.[112–136] HPV types 6, 11, 16, and 18 have been identified, with considerable variability in the reported proportion of cases positive for HPV.

The inverted papilloma occurs in patients older than 20 years of age, with an average age of 55 years. There is a strong male predilection. This lesion predominantly arises from the lateral nasal cavity wall or a paranasal sinus, usually the maxillary antrum or the ethmoid labyrinth. Typically, the inverted papilloma results in unilateral nasal obstruction; additional symptoms include pain, epistaxis, purulent discharge, or local deformity. The papilloma appears as a soft, pink or tan, polypoid or nodular growth. Multiple lesions may be present. Pressure erosion of the underlying bone is usually present and may be visible radiographically as an irregular radiolucency. Primary sinus lesions may be distinguishable only as a soft tissue radiodensity or mucosal thickening on radiographs; sinus involvement generally represents extension from the nasal cavity. Magnetic resonance imaging (MRI) is used to identify the extent of the lesion.

Microscopically, the inverted papilloma is characterized by squamous epithelial proliferation into the submucosal stroma. The basement membrane remains intact, and the epithelium appears to be invading into underlying connective tissue. Goblet cells and mucin-filled microcysts are appreciated within the epithelium. Keratin production is rare, but thin surface keratinization may be seen. Mitoses often are noted within the basilar or parabasilar cells, as well as varying degrees of dysplasia. Papillary surface projections are present, and deep clefts may be seen between projections. The stroma consists of dense fibrous or loose myxomatous connective tissue with or without inflammatory cells.

Destruction of underlying bone is often appreciated. Immunohistochemical expression of specific cell adhesion molecules (CD44) are increased in this papilloma, which helps to distinguish it from invasive papillary squamous cell carcinoma, which lacks this marker. Although hyperkeratosis has been suggested, prominent epithelial hyperplasia and high mitotic index are negative prognostic indicators, and no histopathologic parameters have been found to be reliably predictive of recurrence or malignant transformation among inverted papillomas.

The inverted papilloma has a significant growth potential and, if left untreated, may extend into the nasopharynx, middle ear, orbit, or cranial base. According to the literature, recurrence after conservative surgical excision has occurred in nearly 75% of all cases. However, with more aggressive surgical therapy, consisting of medial maxillectomy via a lateral rhinotomy or midfacial degloving, recurrence rates of less than 14% have been reported. Although an open surgical approach historically has been regarded as the standard of care, advances in transnasal endoscopic surgery have led to wider acceptance of this method as an alternative. Recurrences are usually noted within 2 years of surgery but can occur later after the procedure. Thus, long-term follow-up is essential. Continued tobacco use is associated with an increased risk of multiple recurrences. The inverted papilloma is a premalignant lesion, which has the potential to develop into squamous cell carcinoma in 3% to 24% of cases. In such an event, the lesion is treated as a malignancy, typically by performing more radical surgery, with or without adjunctive radiotherapy.

Cylindrical cell papilloma (oncocytic schneiderian papilloma)

The cylindrical cell papilloma accounts for less than 7% of sinonasal papillomas.[112–136] This lesion is considered to be a variant of the inverted papilloma because of the similarity in clinical and histopathologic features and a similarly low frequency of HPV.

Cylindrical cell papilloma typically occurs in adults 20 to 50 years of age. It is more common in men, with a predilection for the maxillary antrum, lateral nasal cavity wall, and ethmoid labyrinth. The presenting symptom is usually unilateral nasal obstruction, and it appears as a robust-red or brown mass with a multinodular surface.

Microscopically, the cylindrical cell papilloma shows both endophytic and exophytic growth. Surface papillary projections have a fibrovascular connective tissue core and are covered by a multi-layered epithelium of tall columnar cells with small, dark nuclei and eosinophilic, occasionally granular, cytoplasm. The lesional epithelial cell is similar to an oncocyte. Cilia may be seen on the surface, and there are numerous intraepithelial microcysts filled with mucin, neutrophils, or a combination of the 2.

Cylindrical cell papilloma is treated in the same manner as inverted papilloma. However, the potential for recurrence and malignant transformation is lower than that of the inverted papilloma.

MESENCHYMAL TUMORS

The most common mesenchymal tumors that may develop in the paranasal sinuses include osteomas, angiofibromas, and hemangiomas.

Osteoma

Is the most common mesenchymal tumor.[137–147] It arises at the junction of the periosteum of membranous bone and endochondral bone in the region of the frontoethmoidal suture. The 2 histologic types are the hard cortical osteoma and the soft cancellous osteoma. They are characterized by different radiologic findings. The hard osteoma has lobulated densities, whereas the soft osteoma is less dense and may be mistaken for a soft tissue sinus mass. The osteoma can cause bone erosion and deformity as well as intracranial, intraorbital, and intranasal extension. If a sinus osteum is obstructed, the lumen of the sinus may be opacified. Signs of secondary infection may also be present clinically. Surgical excision is the treatment of choice. Recurrence is low.

Angiofibroma

The angiofibroma frequently involves the paranasal sinuses and is usually an extension from a primary juvenile angiofibroma of the nasopharynx.[148–154] Most often, the angiofibroma extends into the sphenoidal and ethmoidal sinuses. According to the literature, this tumor can occur within the maxillary sinus, without naso-pharyngeal involvement. Tomography and carotid angiography are valuable diagnostic tools because angiofibromas usually contain tumor vessels fed by a hypertrophied internal maxillary artery. Conservative surgical excision is the preferred treatment. Recurrence is low.

Hemangioma

Hemangiomas are the most common tumors of infancy, occurring in 5% to 10% of 1-year-old children.[155–167] They are more common in white females. The most frequent location is the head and neck, which accounts for 60% of all cases. Eighty percent of hemangiomas occur as single lesions, but 20% of affected patients have multiple tumors. Periocular tumors often result in amblyopia, strabismus, or astigmatism. Tumors in the neck and laryngeal region can sometimes lead to airway embarrassment.

Large, segmental cervicofacial hemangiomas can be a component of PHACE(S) syndrome, which stands for posterior fossa brain anomalies (usually Dandy-Walker malformation; hemangioma (usually cervical segmental hemangioma); arterial anomalies; cardiac defects and coarctation of the aorta; eye anomalies; and sternal cleft or supraumbilical Raphe Kasabach-Merritt phenomenon, which is a serious coagulopathy that has been associated with 2 rare vascular tumors known as tufted hemangioma and kaposiform hemangioendothelioma. This disorder is characterized by severe thrombocytopenia and hemorrhage because of platelet trapping within the tumor. The mortality is as high as 20% to 30%.

Intrabony hemangiomas may also occur and represent either venous or arteriovenous malformations. In the jaws, such lesions are detected most often during the first 3 decades of life. There is a slight prevalence to females, often occurring in the mandible rather than the maxilla. The lesion may be completely asymptomatic, although some examples are associated with pain and edema. Mobility of teeth or bleeding from the gingival sulcus may occur. A bruit or pulsation may be apparent on auscultation and palpation.

The radiographic appearance of intrabony vascular malformations is variable. Most commonly, the lesion shows a multilocular radiolucent defect. The individual loculations may be small, taking on a honeycomb appearance, or large, simulating a soap bubble appearance. In other cases the lesion may present as an ill-defined radiolucent area or a well-defined, cystic radiolucency. Large malformations may cause cortical expansion, and occasionally a sunburst radiographic pattern is produced. Angiography aids in showing the vascular nature of the lesion.

Hemangiomas of infancy are characterized by multiple rounded endothelial cells and often-indistinct vascular lumina. At this stage, such lesions are often known microscopically as juvenile or cellular hemangiomas. Because of their cellular nature, these lesions also have been called juvenile hemangioendotheliomas. As the lesion matures, the endothelial cells become flattened, and the small, capillary-sized vascular spaces become more evident. As the hemangioma undergoes involution, the vascular spaces become less prominent and are replaced by fibrous connective tissue.

Because most hemangiomas of infancy undergo involution, management often consists of watchful neglect. Surgical resection is rarely warranted during infancy. For life-threatening hemangiomas, pharmacologic therapy may be indicated. Systemic corticosteroids may help to reduce the size of the lesion and are associated with a 70% to 90% response rate. Intralesional and topical corticosteroids also have been used for smaller localized, problematic lesions. Intravenous vincristine is used for complicated tumors that are unresponsive to systemic corticosteroid therapy. The management of venous malformations depends on the size, location, and associated complications of the lesion. Small stable malformations may not require treatment. Larger, symptomatic lesions may be treated with a combination of sclerotherapy, which involves injection of the lesion with 95% ethanol to induce fibrosis, and surgical excision. Sclerotherapy alone may be sufficient for smaller lesions; for larger lesions, subsequent surgical resection can be accomplished with less risk of bleeding after sclerotherapy.

ODONTOGENIC TUMORS AND CYSTS
Ameloblastoma

Ameloblastomas are odontogenic tumors of epithelial origin.[168,169] Because metastasis is rare, ameloblastomas are considered benign and are locally invasive. Overall only 20% of ameloblastomas occur in the maxilla, although 45% of the desmoplastic type occur in the maxilla. Although they are most often identified as oral tumors, ameloblastomas that do occur in the maxilla can easily encroach on the nasal cavity, paranasal sinuses, and even the skull base. Tumor location has no bearing on the histopathology. Ameloblastomas occur most commonly in 30-year-olds to 50-year-olds, with an early female predilection and later-age male predilection.

Clinically, ameloblastomas present as they would in the oral cavity, either as cystic lesions or as solid neoplasms, both of which cause local bony expansion. They may present later than they would otherwise in the oral cavity because they are asymptomatic and have more space to expand into before they become clinically noticeable to the patient. Radiographically, ameloblastomas appear radiolucent unilocular or multilocular and may displace teeth. Surgical management principles are unchanged as well. Unicystic lesions may be enucleated if there is no transmural component. Solid and multicystic lesions should be resected with 1.0-cm margins when possible and an uninvolved anatomic barrier when not. Although the surgical principles are the same, these extensive midface tumors often require wide exposure using a Weber-Ferguson or transoral degloving approach and the resulting defect may be disfiguring. Incisions and expectations for postoperative appearance, including asymmetry, scar management, and options for facial and dental reconstruction, should be discussed in advance with the patient. The recurrence rate approaches 90% up to 10 years after treatment.

Ameloblastic Fibroma

The ameloblastic fibroma is a mixed epithelial and mesenchymal benign odontogenic tumor.[168] It occurs most commonly in late childhood and presents most commonly as an asymptomatic cortical expansion. These lesions are typically encapsulated and can often be enucleated. Large destructive lesions may need to be resected. Postsurgical recurrence is rare.

OKC

The OKC is an aggressive benign cyst of odontogenic origin.[170–172] When present in the maxilla, the lesion often infiltrates the maxillary sinus, and the cyst lining may become adherent to the sinus membrane and can sometimes even replace it. Treatment of sinus-infiltrating OKCs is similar to other OKCs and can range from marsupialization to enucleation with curettage to resection with margins. Recurrence of OKC, which can range from 5% to 70%, is more difficult to detect in the maxilla with plain films, and consideration should be given to annual CT scans for follow-up evaluation.

Benign Fibro-osseous Tumors

Fibrous dysplasia and ossifying fibroma are both fibro-osseous lesions histologically; however, although ossifying fibroma is considered a true neoplasm, fibrous dysplasia is considered a disorder of bone maturation.[172] They can be differentiated easily with CT. Fibrous dysplasia appears homogeneous from cortex to cortex, and ossifying fibroma has clear cortices and a more heterogeneous appearance. Clinically both present as bony expansions of the jaws and both can involve the maxillary sinuses. The treatment between the 2 differs as well. Ossifying fibromas are treated with resection with 5-mm margins. Fibrous dysplasia is typically not treated unless the patient desires osseous recontouring for aesthetic purposes or the expansion affects function. Osseous recontouring is best performed after growth completion.

Calcifying Epithelial Odontogenic Tumor (Pindborg Tumor)

Calcifying epithelial odontogenic tumors (CEOTs) are rare neoplasms; less than 1% of odontogenic tumors are CEOTs.[173,174] They generally appear in the fourth to sixth decades of life, with no gender tendency. Comparable with ameloblastomas, CEOTs are considered benign and their associated morbidity is caused by local bony expansion. Despite their benign behavior, CEOTs are prone to local recurrence but at a lower rate than ameloblastomas (15% vs up to 90%). Clinically, they may not be detectable early in the maxilla because of expansion into the sinus space and later may be detectable with facial asymmetry or palpable bony expansion. They generally present as painless. Radiographically, the lesion appears well circumscribed, with local soft tissue attenuation and scattered hyperdensity on CT. Recommended treatment is excision with a clean anatomic margin. Large margins are not recommended. The approach depends on the size and extent of the tumor.

SUMMARY

Differential diagnosis is sometimes complex because some of the benign cysts and tumors can sometimes be premalignant. Therefore, surgeons must have a thorough understanding of oral pathology to render an accurate diagnosis and course of treatment to properly inform and care for their patients.

REFERENCES

1. Eversole LR. Oral sialocysts. Arch Otolaryngol 1987;113:51–6.
2. Takeda Y, Yamamoto H. Salivary duct cyst: its frequency in a certain Japanese population group (Tohoku districts), with special reference to

adenomatous proliferation of the epithelial lining. J Oral Sci 2001;43:9–13.

3. Tal H, Altini M, Lemmer J. Multiple mucous retention cysts of the oral mucosa. Oral Surg Oral Med Oral Pathol 1984;58:692–5.

4. Bell GW, Joshi BB, Macleod RI. Maxillary sinus disease: diagnosis and treatment. Br Dent J 2011;3:113–8.

5. Ng YH, Sethi DS. Isolated sphenoid sinus disease: differential diagnosis and management. Curr Opin Otolaryngol Head Neck Surg 2011;1:16–20.

6. Weber RK, Werner JA, Hildenbrand T. Endonasal endoscopic medial maxillectomy and preservation of the inferior turbinate. Am J Rhinol Allergy 2010;6: 132–5.

7. Habesoglu TE, Habesoglu M, Surmeli M, et al. Unilateral sinonasal symptoms. J Craniofac Surg 2010;6:2019–22.

8. Weireb I, Gnapp DR, Laver NM, et al. Seromucinous hamartomas: a clinicopathological study of a sinonasal glandular lesion lacking myoepithelial cells. Histopathology 2009;2:205–13.

9. Kadymova MI, Bogomilskii MR. On the differential diagnosis of antrum Highmore cysts from serous forms of chronic sinusitis. Vestn Otorinolaringol 1963;25:21–4 [in Russian].

10. Berg O, Carenfelt C, Sobin A. On the diagnosis and pathogenesis of intramural maxillary cysts. Acta Otolaryngol 1989;108(5–6):464–8.

11. Som PM, Schatz CJ, Flaum EG, et al. Aneurismal bone cyst of the paranasal sinuses associated with fibrous dysplasia: CT and MR findings. J Comput Assist Tomogr 1991;3:513–5.

12. Moskow BS. A histomorphologic study of the effects of periodontal inflammation on the maxillary sinus mucosa. J Periodontol 1992;8:674–81.

13. Baurmash HD. Mucoceles and ranulas. J Oral Maxillofac Surg 2003;61:369–78.

14. Campana F, Sibaud V, Chauvel A, et al. Recurrent superficial mucoceles associated with lichenoid disorders. J Oral Maxillofac Surg 2006;64:1830–3.

15. Cataldo E, Mosadomi A. Mucoceles of the oral mucous membrane. Arch Otolaryngol 1970;91: 360–5.

16. Chi A, Lambert P, Richardson M, et al. Oral mucoceles: a clinicopathologic review of 1,824 cases including unusual variants, Abstract No. 19. Paper presented at the annual meeting of the American Academy of Oral and Maxillofacial Pathology. Kansas City (MO), May 5–9, 2007.

17. Eveson JW. Superficial mucoceles: pitfall in clinical and microscopic diagnosis. Oral Surg Oral Med Oral Pathol 1988;66:318–22.

18. Jensen JL. Superficial mucoceles of the oral mucosa. Am J Dermatopathol 1990;12:88–92.

19. Jinbu Y, Kusama M, Itoh H, et al. Mucocele of the glands of Blandin-Nuhn: clinical and histopathologic

20. Jinbu Y, Tsukinoki K, Kusama M, et al. Recurrent multiple superficial mucocele on the palate: histopathology and laser vaporization. Oral Surg Oral Med Oral Pathol Oral Radiol Endod 2003;95:193–7.

21. Standish SM, Shafer WG. The mucous retention phenomenon. J Oral Surg 1959;17:15–22.

22. Sugerman PB, Savage NW, Young WG. Mucocele of the anterior lingual salivary glands (glands of Blandin and Nuhn): report of 5 cases. Oral Surg Oral Med Oral Pathol Oral Radiol Endod 2000;90:478–82.

23. Hu P, Zhu G, Lai R, et al. Clinical diagnosis and treatment of nasal sinus mucoceles with visual loss. Lin Chung Er Bi Yan Hou Tou Jing Wai Ke Za Zhi 2011;25(5):217–9 [in Chinese].

24. Babinski D, Skorek A, Stankiewicz C, et al. Intracranial mucocele of the frontal sinus. Otolaryngol Pol 2011;1:62–5.

25. Bahadir O, Arslan S, Arslan E, et al. Sphenoid sinus mucocele presenting with unilateral visual loss: a case report. B-ENT 2011;1:65–8.

26. Gupta S, Goyal R, Shahi M. Frontal sinus mucopyelocele with intracranial and intraorbital extension. Nepal J Opthalmol 2011;5:91–2.

27. Kriukov AI, Artem'ev ME, Arzhimatova GSh, et al. A case of chronic pyopolypous pansinusitis with mucopyelocele of the frontal sinus. Vestn Otorinolaringol 2011;(2):66–7 [in Russian].

28. Chong AW, Prepageran N, Rahmat O, et al. Bilateral asymmetrical mucoceles of the paranasal sinuses with unilateral orbital complications. Ear Nose Throat J 2011;2:E13.

29. Hammami B, Mnejja M, Chakroun A, et al. Cholesteatoma of the frontal sinus. Eur Ann Otorhinolaryngol Head Neck Dis 2010;6:213–6.

30. Hansen S, Sorensen CH, Stage J, et al. Massive cholesteatoma of the frontal sinus: case report and review of the literature. Auris Nasus Larynx 2007;3:387–92.

31. Barnett FC, Barnett JC Jr. Massive bifrontal epidermoid tumor. Surg Neurol 1992;6:437–40.

32. Storper IS, Newman AN. Cholesteatoma of the maxillary sinus. Arch Otolaryngol Head Neck Surg 1992;9:975–7.

33. Hartman JM, Stankiewicz JA. Cholesteatoma of the paranasal sinuses: case report and review of the literature. Ear Nose Throat J 1991;70(10):719–25.

34. Salf E, Rigaud A. Cholesteatoma of the maxillary sinus. Apropos of a case. Ann Otolaryngol Chir Cervicofac 1991;8:469–71.

35. Cobarro J, Valles H, Blach JL, et al. Cholesteatoma of the paranasal sinuses. Apropos of 2 cases. Ann Otolaryngol Chir Cervicofac 1991;5:307–10 [in French].

36. Barnes L, Eveson JW, Reichart P, et al. World Health Organization classification of tumours: pathology

and genetics of head and neck tumours. Lyon (France): IARC Press; 2005.

37. Jones AV, Craig GT, Franklin CD. Range and demographics of odontogenic cysts diagnosed in a UK population over a 30-year period. J Oral Pathol Med 2006;35:500–7.

38. Kramer IR, Pindborg JJ, Shear M. Histological typing of odontogenic tumors. 2nd edition. New York: Springer-Verlag; 1992.

39. Kramer IR, Pindborg JJ, Shear M. The World Health Organization histological typing of odontogenic tumours: introducing the second edition. Eur J Cancer B Oral Oncol 1993;29B:169–71.

40. Kreidler JF, Raubenheimer EJ, van Heerden WF. A retrospective analysis of 367 cystic lesions of the jaw–the Ulm experience. J Craniomaxillofac Surg 1993;21:339–41.

41. Nakamura T, Ishida J, Nakano Y, et al. A study of cysts in the oral region: cysts of the jaws. J Nihon Univ Sch Dent 1995;37:33–40.

42. Neville BW, Damm DD, Allen CM. Odontogenic cysts and tumors. In: Gnepp D, editor. Diagnostic surgical pathology of the head and neck. Philadelphia: WB Saunders; 2001. p. 785–839. Chapter 10.

43. Philipsen HP, Reichart PA. The development and fate of epithelial residues after completion of the human odontogenesis with special reference to the origins of epithelial odontogenic neoplasms, hamartomas and cysts. Oral Biosci Med 2004;1:171–9.

44. Shear M. Developmental odontogenic cysts. An update. J Oral Pathol Med 1994;23:1–11.

45. Shear M, Speight P. Cysts of the oral and maxillofacial regions. 4th edition. Oxford (United Kingdom): Blackwell; 2007.

46. Ackermann G, Cohen MA, Altini M. The paradental cyst: a clinicopathologic study of 50 cases. Oral Surg Oral Med Oral Pathol 1987;64:308–12.

47. Adelsperger J, Campbell JH, Coates DB, et al. Early soft tissue pathosis associated with impacted third molars without pericoronal radiolucency. Oral Surg Oral Med Oral Pathol Oral Radiol Endod 2000;89:402–6.

48. Benn A, Altini M. Dentigerous cysts of inflammatory origin: a clinicopathologic study. Oral Surg Oral Med Oral Pathol Oral Radiol Endod 1996;81:203–9.

49. Clauser C, Zuccati G, Barone R, et al. Simplified surgical-orthodontic treatment of a dentigerous cyst. J Clin Orthod 1994;28:103–6.

50. Craig GT. The paradental cyst: a specific inflammatory odontogenic cyst. Br Dent J 1976;141:9–14.

51. Curran AE, Damm DD, Drummond JF. Pathologically significant pericoronal lesions in adults: histopathologic evaluation. J Oral Maxillofac Surg 2002; 60:613–7.

52. Daley TD, Wysocki GP. The small dentigerous cyst: a diagnostic dilemma. Oral Surg Oral Med Oral Pathol Oral Radiol Endod 1995;79:77–81.

53. Delbem AC, Cunha RH, Afonso RL, et al. Dentigerous cysts in primary dentition: report of 2 cases. Pediatr Dent 2006;28:269–72.

54. Gorlin RJ. Potentialities of oral epithelium manifest by mandibular dentigerous cysts. Oral Surg Oral Med Oral Pathol 1957;10:271–84.

55. Kusukawa J, Irie K, Morimatsu M, et al. Dentigerous cyst associated with a deciduous tooth: a case report. Oral Surg Oral Med Oral Pathol 1992;73:415–8.

56. Lustmann L, Bodner L. Dentigerous cysts associated with supernumerary teeth. Int J Oral Maxillofac Surg 1988;17:100–2.

57. Motamedi MH, Talesh KT. Management of extensive dentigerous cysts. Br Dent J 2005;198:203–6.

58. Takeda Y, Oikawa Y, Furuya I, et al. Mucous and ciliated cell metaplasia in epithelial linings of odontogenic inflammatory and developmental cysts. J Oral Sci 2005;47:77–81.

59. Ziccardi VB, Eggleston TI, Schneider RE. Using fenestration technique to treat a large dentigerous cyst. J Am Dent Assoc 1997;128:201–5.

60. Buyukkurt MC, Omezli MM, Miloglu O. Dentigerous cyst associated with an ectopic tooth in the maxillary sinus: a report of 3 cases and review of the literature. Oral Surg Oral Med Oral Pathol Oral Radiol Endod 2010;1:67–71.

61. Ray B, Bandyopadhyay SN, Das D. A rare cause of nasolacrimal duct obstruction: dentigerous cyst in the maxillary sinus. Indian J Opthalmol 2009;6:465–7.

62. Litvin M, Caprice D, Infranco L. Dentigerous cyst of the maxilla with impacted tooth displaced into the orbital rim and floor. Ear Nose Throat J 2008;3:160–2.

63. Christmas DA, Mirante JP, Yanagisawa E. Endoscopic view of the maxillary dentigerous cyst. Ear Nose Throat J 2008;6:316.

64. Altini M, Shear M. The lateral periodontal cyst: an update. J Oral Pathol Med 1992;21:245–50.

65. Baker RD, D'Onofrio ED, Corio RL. Squamous-cell carcinoma arising in a lateral periodontal cyst. Oral Surg Oral Med Oral Pathol 1979;47:495–9.

66. Carter LC, Carney YL, Perez-Pudlewski D. Lateral periodontal cyst: multifactorial analysis of a previously unreported series. Oral Surg Oral Med Oral Pathol Oral Radiol Endod 1996;81:210–6.

67. Cohen D, Neville B, Damm D, et al. The lateral periodontal cyst: a report of 37 cases. J Periodontol 1984;55:230–4.

68. Fantasia JE. Lateral periodontal cyst: an analysis of forty-six cases. Oral Surg Oral Med Oral Pathol 1979;48:237–43.

69. Greer RO, Johnson M. Botryoid odontogenic cyst: clinicopathologic analysis of ten cases with three recurrences. J Oral Maxillofac Surg 1988; 46:574–9.

70. Gurol M, Burkes EJ Jr, Jacoway J. Botryoid odontogenic cyst: analysis of 33 cases. J Periodontol 1995;66:1069–73.

71. Kerezoudis NP, Donta-Bakoyianni C, Siskos G. The lateral periodontal cyst: aetiology, clinical significance and diagnosis. Endod Dent Traumatol 2000;16:144–50.

72. Ramer M, Valauri D. Multicystic lateral periodontal cyst and botryoid odontogenic cyst: multifactorial analysis of previously unreported series and review of literature. N Y State Dent J 2005;71:47–51.

73. Rasmusson LG, Magnusson BC, Borrman H. The lateral periodontal cyst: a histopathological and radiographic study of 32 cases. Br J Oral Maxillofac Surg 1991;29:54–7.

74. Wysocki GP, Brannon RB, Gardner DG, et al. Histogenesis of the lateral periodontal cyst and the gingival cyst of the adult. Oral Surg Oral Med Oral Pathol 1980;50:327–34.

75. Sheehan DJ, Potter BJ, Davis LS. Cutaneous draining sinus tract of odontogenic origin: unusual presentation of a challenging diagnosis. South Med J 2005;2:250–2.

76. Cappabianca P, Cavallo LM, Esposito F, et al. Extended endoscopic endonasal approach to the midline skull base: the evolving role of transsphenoidal surgery. Adv Tech Stand Neurosurg 2008; 33:151–99.

77. Gurkanlar D, Akyuz M, Acikbas C, et al. Difficulties in treatment of CSF leakage associated with a temporal meningocele. Acta Neurochir (Wien) 2007;12:1239–42.

78. Abe T, Ludecke DK, Wada A, et al. Transsphenoidal cephaloceles in adults. A report of two cases and review of the literature. Acta Neurochir (Wien) 2000;4:397–400.

79. Clyde BL, Stechison MT. Repair of temporosphenoidal encephalocele with a vascularized split calvarial cranioplasty: technique case report. Neurosurgery 1995;1:202–6.

80. Buchfelder M, Fahlbusch R, Huk WJ, et al. Intrasphenoidal encephaloceles–a clinical entity. Acta Neurochir (Wien) 1987;89:10–5.

81. Han MH, Chang KH, Lee CH, et al. Cystic expansile masses of the maxilla: differential diagnosis with CT and MR. AJNR Am J Neuroradiol 1995;2:333–8.

82. Bodner L, Shohat S, Ulmansky M. Unusual cyst of the zygoma. J Oral Maxillofac Surg 1982;4:229–31.

83. Bassichis BA, Thomas JR. Foreign-body inclusion cyst presenting on the lateral nasal sidewall 1 year after rhinoplasty. Arch Facial Plast Surg 2003;6:530–2.

84. Johnston WC, Stoopack JC. Globulomaxillary cyst invading the maxillary antrum. Report of case. Oral Surg Oral Med Oral Pathol 1966;5:675–81.

85. Hertz J. Globulomaxillary cyst invading the maxillary sinus. Report of two cases. Oral Surg Oral Med Oral Pathol 1963;16:392–6.

86. Christ TF. The globulomaxillary cyst: an embryologic misconception. Oral Surg Oral Med Oral Pathol 1970;30:515–26.

87. D'Silva NJ, Anderson L. Globulomaxillary cyst revisited. Oral Surg Oral Med Oral Pathol 1993;76:182–4.

88. Ferenczy K. The relationship of globulomaxillary cysts to the fusion of embryonal processes and to cleft palates. Oral Surg Oral Med Oral Pathol 1958;11:1388–93.

89. Little JW, Jakobsen J. Origin of the globulomaxillary cyst. J Oral Surg 1973;31:188–95.

90. Steiner DR. A lesion of endodontic origin misdiagnosed as a globulomaxillary cyst. J Endod 1999; 25:277–81.

91. Vedtofte P, Holmstrup P. Inflammatory paradental cysts in the globulomaxillary region. J Oral Pathol Med 1989;18:125–7.

92. Wysocki GP. The differential diagnosis of globulomaxillary radiolucencies. Oral Surg Oral Med Oral Pathol 1981;51:281–6.

93. Wysocki GP, Goldblatt LI. The so-called "globulomaxillary cyst" is extinct. Oral Surg Oral Med Oral Pathol 1993;76:185–6.

94. Ide F, Mishima K, Saito I, et al. Diagnostically challenging epithelial odontogenic tumors: a selective review of 7 jawbone lesions. Head Neck Pathol 2009;1:18–26.

95. Abrams AM, Howell FV, Bullock WK. Nasopalatine cysts. Oral Surg Oral Med Oral Pathol 1963;16: 306–32.

96. Allard RH, van der Kwast WA, van der Waal I. Nasopalatine duct cyst: review of the literature and report of 22 cases. Int J Oral Surg 1981;10:447–61.

97. Anneroth G, Hall G, Stuge U. Nasopalatine duct cyst. Int J Oral Maxillofac Surg 1986;15:572–80.

98. Brown FH, Houston GD, Lubow RM, et al. Cyst of the incisive (palatine) papilla: report of a case. J Periodontol 1987;58:274–5.

99. Chapple IL, Ord RA. Patent nasopalatine ducts: four case presentations and review of the literature. Oral Surg Oral Med Oral Pathol 1990;69:554–8.

100. Hisatomi M, Asaumi J, Konouchi H, et al. MR imaging of nasopalatine duct cysts. Eur J Radiol 2001;39:73–6.

101. Swanson KS, Kaugars GE, Gunsolley JC. Nasopalatine duct cyst: an analysis of 334 cases. J Oral Maxillofac Surg 1991;49:268–71.

102. Takagi R, Ohashi Y, Suzuki M. Squamous cell carcinoma in the maxilla probably originating from a nasopalatine duct cyst: report of case. J Oral Maxillofac Surg 1996;54:112–5.

103. Vasconcelos RF, de Aguiar MF, Castro WH, et al. Retrospective analysis of 31 cases of nasopalatine duct cyst. Oral Dis 1999;5:325–8.

104. Suter VG, Sendi P, Reichart PA, et al. The nasopalatine duct cyst: an analysis of the relation between clinical symptoms, cyst dimensions, and involvement of neighboring anatomical structures using cone beam computed tomography. J Oral Maxillofac Surg 2011;69(10):2595–603.

105. Nonaka CF, Henriques AC, de Matos FR, et al. Nonodontogenic cysts of the oral and maxillofacial region: demographic profile in a Brazilian population over a 40-year period. Eur Arch Otorhinolaryngol 2011;6:917–22.

106. Courage GR, North AF, Hansen LS. Median palatine cysts. Oral Surg Oral Med Oral Pathol 1974;37:745–53.

107. Donnelly JC, Koudelka BM, Hartwell GR. Median palatal cyst. J Endod 1986;12:546–9.

108. Gingell JC, Levy BA, DePaola LG. Median palatine cyst. J Oral Maxillofac Surg 1985;43:47–51.

109. Gordon NC, Swann NP, Hansen LS. Median palatine cyst and maxillary antral osteoma: report of an unusual case. J Oral Surg 1980;38:361–5.

110. Queiroz TP, Scartezini GR, de Souza Carvalho AC, et al. Median palatal cyst. J Craniofac Surg 2011;2:737–40.

111. Bacci C, Valente ML, Quadrio M, et al. Is the median palatine cyst a distinct entity? J Oral Maxillofac Surg 2011;5:1385–9.

112. Batsakis JG, Suarez P. Schneiderian papillomas and carcinomas: a review. Adv Anat Pathol 2001;8:53–64.

113. Bawa R, Allen GC, Ramadan HH. Cylindrical cell papilloma of the nasal septum. Ear Nose Throat J 1995;74:179–81.

114. Busquets JM, Hwang PH. Endoscopic resection of sinonasal inverted papilloma: a meta-analysis. Otolaryngol Head Neck Surg 2006;134:476–82.

115. Califano J, Koch W, Sidransky D, et al. Inverted sinonasal papilloma: a molecular genetic appraisal of its putative status as a precursor to squamous cell carcinoma. Am J Pathol 2000;156:333–7.

116. Eggers G, Mühling J, Hassfeld S. Inverted papilloma of paranasal sinuses. J Craniomaxillofac Surg 2007;35:21–9.

117. Holzmann D, Hegyi I, Rajan GP, et al. Management of benign inverted sinonasal papilloma avoiding external approaches. J Laryngol Otol 2007;121:548–54.

118. Hyams VJ. Papillomas of the nasal cavity and paranasal sinuses: a clinicopathological study of 315 cases. Ann Otol Rhinol Laryngol 1971;80:192–206.

119. Kaufman MR, Brandwein MS, William L. Sinonasal papillomas: clinicopathologic review of 40 patients with inverted and oncocytic Schneiderian papillomas. Laryngoscope 2002;112:1372–7.

120. Lane AP, Bolger WE. Endoscopic management of inverted papilloma. Curr Opin Otolaryngol Head Neck Surg 2006;14:14–8.

121. Lawson W, Kaufman MR, Biller HF. Treatment outcomes in the management of inverted papilloma: an analysis of 160 cases. Laryngoscope 2003;113:1548–56.

122. Maitra A, Baskin LB, Lee EL. Malignancies arising in oncocytic Schneiderian papillomas: a report of 2 cases and review of the literature. Arch Pathol Lab Med 2001;125:1365–7.

123. Mansell NJ, Bates GJ. The inverted Schneiderian papilloma: a review and literature report of 43 new cases. Rhinology 2000;38:97–101.

124. Melroy CT, Senior BA. Benign sinonasal neoplasms: a focus on inverting papilloma. Otolaryngol Clin North Am 2006;39:601–17.

125. Minovi A, Kollert M, Draf W, et al. Inverted papilloma: feasibility of endonasal surgery and long-term results of 87 cases. Rhinology 2006;44:205–10.

126. Mirza S, Bradley PJ, Acharya A, et al. Sinonasal inverted papillomas: recurrence, and synchronous and metachronous malignancy. J Laryngol Otol 2007;1:1–8.

127. Pasquini E, Sciaretta V, Farneti G, et al. Inverted papilloma: report of 89 cases. Am J Otolaryngol 2005;25:178–85.

128. Sauter A, Matharu R, Hörmann K, et al. Current advances in the basic research and clinical management of sinonasal inverted papilloma (review). Oncol Rep 2007;17:495–504.

129. Sulica RL, Wenig BM, Debo RF, et al. Schneiderian papillomas of the pharynx. Ann Otol Rhinol Laryngol 1999;108:392–7.

130. Weiner JS, Sherris D, Kasperbauer J, et al. Relationship of human papillomavirus to Schneiderian papillomas. Laryngoscope 1999;109:21–6.

131. Yang YJ, Abraham JL. Undifferentiated carcinoma arising in oncocytic Schneiderian (cylindrical cell) papilloma. J Oral Maxillofac Surg 1997;55:289–94.

132. Yoskovitch A, Braverman I, Nachtigal D, et al. Sinonasal schneiderian papilloma. Otolaryngology 1998;27:122–6.

133. Vayisoglu Y, Unal M, Apa DD, et al. Schneiderian carcinoma developing in an inverted papilloma of the palatine tonsil: an unusual case. Ear Nose Throat J 2011;5:E32–4.

134. Nakamaru Y, Furuta Y, Takagi D, et al. Preservation of the nasolacrimal duct during endoscopic medial maxillectomy for sinonasal inverted papilloma. Rhinology 2010;4:452–6.

135. Weinreb I. Low grade glandular lesions of the sinonasal tract: a focused review. Head Neck Pathol 2010;1:77–83.

136. Sham CL, Lee DL, Van Hasselt CA, et al. A case study of the risk factors associated with sinonasal inverted papilloma. Am J Rhinol Allergy 2010;1:E37–40.

137. Cutilli BJ, Quinn PD. Traumatically induced peripheral osteoma: report of case. Oral Surg Oral Med Oral Pathol 1992;73:667–9.

138. Kondoh T, Seto K, Kobayashi K. Osteoma of the mandibular condyle: report of a case with a review of the literature. J Oral Maxillofac Surg 1998;56:972–9.

139. Ortakoglu K, Gunaydin Y, Aydintug YS, et al. Osteoma of the mandibular condyle: report of a case with 5-year follow-up. Mil Med 2005;170: 117–20.

140. Richards HE, Strider JW Jr, Short SG, et al. Large peripheral osteoma arising from the genial tubercle area. Oral Surg Oral Med Oral Pathol 1986;61:268–71.

141. Schneider LC, Dolinski HB, Grodjesk JE. Solitary peripheral osteoma of the jaws: report of a case and review of the literature. Oral Surg Oral Med Oral Pathol 1980;38:452–5.

142. Woldenberg Y, Nash M, Bodner L. Peripheral osteoma of the maxillofacial region. Diagnosis and management: a study of 14 cases. Med Oral Patol Oral Cir Bucal 2005;10(Suppl 2):E139–42.

143. Yassin OM, Bataineh AB, Mansour MJ. An unusual osteoma of the mandible. J Clin Pediatr Dent 1997; 21:337–40.

144. Xing Y, Zhao J, Wang T. A case of paranasal sinuses osteoma detected on bone SPECT/CT. Clin Nucl Med 2011;3:224–6.

145. Guedes Bde V, Da Rocha AJ, Da Silva CJ, et al. A rare association of tension pneumocephalus and a large frontoethmoidal osteoma: imaging features and surgical treatment. J Craniofac Surg 2011;1:212–3.

146. Daneshi A, Jalessi M, Heshmatzade-Behzadi A. Middle turbinate osteoma. Clin Exp Otorhinolaryngol 2010;4:226–8.

147. Edmond M, Clifton N, Khalil H. A large atypical osteoma of the maxillary sinus: a report of a case and management challenges. Eur Arch Otorhinolaryngol 2011;2:315–8.

148. Lee LN, Shin JJ, Kunst MM, et al. Radiology quiz case 3. Organizing hematoma of the maxillary sinus (OHMS). Arch Otolaryngol Head Neck Surg 2011;4:406.

149. Gallia GL, Ramanathan M Jr, Blitz AM, et al. Expanded endonasal endoscopic approach for resection of a juvenile nasopharyngeal angiofibroma with skull base involvement. J Clin Neurosci 2010;11:1423–7.

150. Ardehali MM, Samimi Ardestani SH, Yazdani N, et al. Endoscopic approach for excision of juvenile nasopharyngeal angiofibroma: complications and outcomes. Am J Otolaryngol 2010;5:343–9.

151. Margalit N, Wasserzug O, De-Row A, et al. Surgical treatment of juvenile nasopharyngeal angiofibroma with intracranial extension. Clinical article. J Neurosurg Pediatr 2009;2:113–7.

152. Harvey RJ, Sheahan PO, Schlosser RJ. Surgical management of benign sinonasal masses. Otolaryngol Clin North Am 2009;2:353–75.

153. Tosun F, Onerci M, Durmaz A, et al. Spontaneous involution of nasopharyngeal angiofibroma. J Craniofac Surg 2008;6:1686–9.

154. Biswas D, Saha S, Bera SP. Relative distribution of the tumors of ear, nose and throat in the pediatric patients. Int J Pediatr Otorhinolaryngol 2007;5: 801–5.

155. Adams DM, Lucky AW. Cervicofacial vascular anomalies. I. Hemangiomas and other benign vascular tumors. Semin Pediatr Surg 2006;15: 124–32.

156. Bunel K, Sindet-Pederson S. Central hemangioma of the mandible. Oral Surg Oral Med Oral Pathol 1993;75:565–70.

157. Chang MW. Updated classification of hemangiomas and other vascular anomalies. Lymphat Res Biol 2003;1:259–65.

158. Drolet BA, Esterly NB, Frieden IJ. Hemangiomas in children. N Engl J Med 1999;341:173–81.

159. Elluru RG, Azizkhan RG. Cervicofacial vascular anomalies. II. Vascular malformations. Semin Pediatr Surg 2006;15:133–9.

160. Ethunandan M, Mellor TK. Haemangiomas and vascular malformations of the maxillofacial region–a review. Br J Oral Maxillofac Surg 2006; 44:263–72.

161. Fishman SJ, Mulliken JB. Hemangiomas and vascular malformations of infancy and childhood. Pediatr Clin North Am 1993;40:1177–200.

162. Greene LA, Freedman PD, Friedman JM, et al. Capillary hemangioma of the maxilla. A report of two cases in which angiography and embolization were used. Oral Surg Oral Med Oral Pathol 1990; 70:268–73.

163. Kaban LB, Mulliken JB. Vascular anomalies of the maxillofacial region. J Oral Maxillofac Surg 1986; 44:203–13.

164. MacArthur CJ. Head and neck hemangiomas of infancy. Curr Opin Otolaryngol Head Neck Surg 2006;14:397–405.

165. Gupta N, Kaur J, Srinivasan R, et al. Fine needle aspiration cytology in lesions of the nose, nasal cavity and paranasal sinuses. Acta Cytol 2011;2: 135–41.

166. Goel AK, Yadav SP, Goel R. Hemangioma of a posterior ethmoid sinus: report of a rare case. Ear Nose Throat J 2010;12:E18.

167. Holsinger FC, Hafemeister AC, Hicks MJ, et al. Differential diagnosis of pediatric tumors of the nasal cavity and paranasal sinuses: a 45-year multi-institutional review. Ear Nose Throat J 2010; 11:534–40.

168. Press SG. Odontogenic tumors of the maxillary sinus. Curr Opin Otolaryngol Head Neck Surg 2008;16:47–54.

169. Sun ZJ, Wu YR, Cheng N, et al. Desmoplastic ameloblastoma–a review. Oral Oncol 2009;45:753–9.

170. Houpis C, Konstantinos TI, Merkourea S, et al. Unusual odontogenic keratocyst of the maxillary sinus. J Craniofac Surg 2011;22(2):721–3.

171. Gupta A, Rai B, Nair MA, et al. Keratocystic odontogenic tumor with impacted maxillary third molar involving the right maxillary antrum: an unusual case report. Indian J Dent Res 2011;22(1):157–60.

172. Marx R, Stern D. Oral and maxillofacial pathology: a rationale for diagnosis and treatment. Hanover Park (IL): Quintessence Publishing Co, Inc; 2003.

173. Angadi PV, Rekha K. Calcifying odontogenic tumor (Pindborg tumor). Head Neck Pathol 2011;5:137–9.

174. Bridle C, Visram K, Piper K, et al. Maxillary calcifying epithelial odontogenic (Pindborg) tumor presenting with abnormal eye signs: case report and literature review. Oral Surg Oral Med Oral Pathol Oral Radiol Endod 2006;102:e12–5.

Management of Frontal Sinus Fractures

Ladi Doonquah, MD, DDS[a,b,*], Phillip Brown, MBBS[a],
Warren Mullings, MBBS[a]

KEYWORDS

- Frontal sinus • NFOT • Fractures • Endoscopic • Stents

The treatment of frontal sinus fractures has been an ongoing source of controversy. There are distinct international and regional variations to the approach of management of these patients. Despite the introduction of new technologies and surgical methods in the last 20 years, there is still no broad-based unanimity in the surgical management of frontal sinus trauma. A plethora of factors contribute to this dilemma, such as the relatively low incidence of occurrence compared with other skeletal fractures, the small number of subjects in most studies, the long length of follow-up that is required to ascertain results, and the devastating sequelae that can develop despite different treatment methodologies. This article seeks to review current thoughts on the treatment of frontal sinus fractures and develop updated guidelines on how to manage these injuries.

ANATOMY OF THE FRONTAL SINUS

A thorough knowledge of frontal sinus anatomy is critical for the proper management of frontal sinus trauma. The frontal sinus is absent at birth and does not develop until after age 2 years.[1] It develops from the second frontal pit, which becomes pneumatized into the frontal bone. The other pits become the anterior ethmoidal cells. The frontal sinus is therefore originally an anterior ethmoidal cell and communicates with the mature anterior ethmoidal cells via an inverted funnel-shaped space.[2] The frontal sinus is radiographically identifiable at age 8 years and matures to full size at approximately age 15 years.[3] The final shape of the frontal sinus is asymmetrical, with multiple incomplete septations, and the septum between the sinuses usually deviates from the midline plane.[1,4,5] Approximately 12% of normal adults may possess a rudimentary frontal sinus or completely lack pneumatization of the frontal bone on one side.[6] The frontal sinus is absent in 4% of the population.[6]

The sinus cavity lies between the anterior and posterior tables (**Fig. 1**). The thicker anterior table has cancellous bone between its cortical plates. The thinner posterior table lies in direct contact with the dura.[6] Whereas the posterior table is only 0.1 to 4.8 mm thick, offering little protection to the anterior cranial fossa and its contents, the anterior table requires a force of 800 to 2,200 pounds of force for a fracture to occur.[7] Of all the facial bones, the anterior table can resist the greatest force, and therefore a fracture is likely associated with orbital and nasoethmoidal complex fractures. The anterior to posterior depth is relatively constant at 8.0 to 9.3 mm to the left or right of the midline, and the height of the frontal sinus is greatest at midline at 24.5 mm and progressively decreases laterally.[8] The floor of the frontal sinus is the roof of the orbit laterally, and the nasofrontal outflow tract (NFOT) lies medially. The frontal recess, which is the outflow tract pathway of the frontal sinus, is bounded posteriorly by the skull base, anteriorly by the anterior

The authors have nothing to disclose.
a Department of Surgery, University Hospital of the West Indies, Mona, Jamaica
b Faculty of Medicine, University of the West Indies, Mona, Jamaica
* Corresponding author. Department of Surgery, University Hospital of the West Indies, Mona, Jamaica.
E-mail address: ldoonquah@hotmail.com

Oral Maxillofacial Surg Clin N Am 24 (2012) 265–274
doi:10.1016/j.coms.2012.01.008
1042-3699/12/$ – see front matter © 2012 Elsevier Inc. All rights reserved.

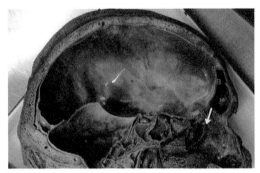

Fig. 1. Sagittal view of the frontal sinus. A, anterior table; B, posterior table; 10, frontal sinus; yellow arrow, NFOT. (*Courtesy of* Michael Gardener, University of the West Indies [Mona].)

wall of the agger nasi or middle meatus, laterally by the lamina papyracea/superior medial orbital wall, and medially by the vertical attachment of the middle turbinate to the skull base.[9] Obstruction to the NFOT may lead to mucoceles or mucopyoceles, recurrent sinusitis, meningitis, and even fatal brain abscesses.[10,11] The frontal sinus is lined by respiratory-type mucosa. Along the posterior table are the foramina of Breschet, through which there is direct venous drainage between the sinus and the subdural venous system. Therefore, there is a potential for spread of infection intracranially.

A distinct nasofrontal duct is not present most of the time, and, as such, the cavity may drain through the duct or via other structures such as the anterior ethmoid cells. The duct is identifiable in only 15% of patients.[12] Thus the designation NFOT is indeed appropriate.

MECHANISMS OF INJURY

There has been a significant decrease in the incidence of frontal sinus fractures in the last 20 years because of the increased prevalence of motor vehicles with various restraint devices.[13] Fractures involving the frontal sinus are sustained primarily from forces that are applied directly to the anterior aspect of the skull in the glabellar region. Most fractures are the result of blunt trauma directed to this region.[14]

The most common cause of frontal sinus fractures is motor vehicle accidents (57.6%).[15] These accidents are associated with high-velocity blunt trauma to the head resulting in various fracture patterns. Penetrating injuries from gunshot wounds and industrial accidents are associated with greater concentration of force to a smaller area. These injuries are therefore associated with a greater risk of damage to both tables of the frontal sinus, dural tears, cribriform plate and fovea

ethmoidalis fractures, as well as frontal lobe injury.[14]

CLASSIFICATION OF FRACTURES

Historically, there have been many classification systems based on clinical and radiologic examinations. Most have classified injuries based on the anatomic location, fracture pattern, displacement of the fracture, presence or absence of comminution, the walls of the sinus involved, and associated injuries to the nasoorbitoethmoidal complex (NOE) and the anterior cranial fossa and its contents.[16–19] With improvement in available imaging modalities, there have been modifications in the classification of fractures to include injury to the NFOT.[12] Elaborate classification schemes with multiple subdivisions do not add significantly to the management of frontal sinus injuries, hence simplicity should be the rule in whatever system that is used.[20]

Classification

1. Type 1: anterior wall fracture with minimal comminution, no associated NOE or orbital rim fractures[14]
2. Type 2: anterior wall comminuted fractures with possible extension to NOE and/or orbital rim[14]
3. Type 3: anterior and posterior wall fractures, posterior wall fractures without significant displacement or dural injury[14]
4. Type 4: anterior and posterior wall fractures with dural injury and cerebrospinal fluid leak[14]
5. Type 5: anterior and posterior wall fractures with dural injury, cerebrospinal fluid leak, and soft tissue or bone loss and/or severe disruption of the anterior cranial fossa.[14]

This classification system takes into account the principles widely accepted as determinants of surgery.

Of importance is the ability of the classification system to properly segmentalize injuries in a way that aids diagnosis and points the way to the appropriate treatment choices.

DIAGNOSIS

The frontal sinus region requires a significant amount of force to disrupt its skeletal framework. Therefore, a presumption must be made that other associated craniofacial injuries are present. Intracranial and cervical spine injuries must be assessed as soon as the patient is stabilized. A thorough but timely clinical examination must be performed, with the priority being proper radiographic examination. Multidetector computed tomographic (MDCT) scan is the standard of care for assessing frontal sinus injuries. MDCT scans allow evaluation of the fractures in different planes, with very thin slices, and 3-dimensional reconstruction that can be obtained to guide reconstruction (**Fig. 2**). A significant percentage of frontal sinus fractures have other associated facial fractures at the time of presentation; some may affect the patency of the airway. As such, definitive measures to secure the airway must be in place.

The primary clinical signs pointing to a frontal sinus fracture range from the sublime to more obvious features. Discoloration, swelling and bruising over the glabellar region are more subtle signs. Lacerations, loss of soft tissue in the frontal region, obvious depression or other contour deformities in the forehead, and orbital and NOE fractures are more definitive indications of skeletal disruption. Concomitant injuries to the specialized structures in the face, such as the globe, nose, or ears, are not infrequent, so early attention to these structures, especially the globe, is important.

SURGICAL MANAGEMENT

At the authors' institution, the treatment paradigm of these patients has shifted in recent years to a more measured and tailored approach. Some of this improvement has been influenced by the greater use of endoscopic techniques in sinus surgery. Patients are also demanding more cosmetically sensitive approaches to the sinus rather than the traditional bicoronal approach. Whatever the treatment method that is used, the goal is to preserve function, provide separation between the sinonasal tract and the brain, create a safe sinus environment, prevent infection, and restore cosmesis. Even if all these goals have been met, longterm follow-up is critical. Complications, some of which can be devastating, may develop several years after injury,[11,14,16] we therefore concur with some investigators, who advocate lifelong followup for these patients.[16] Fractures should ideally be repaired within the first 24–48 hours provided the patient's condition is stable. This is especially important for patients with CSF leaks, as the incidence of intracranial infection increases significantly after a week.

Incisional approaches to the frontal sinus comprise the bicoronal approach, brow incision, hairline endoscopic brow incision, transnasal endoscopic approach, butterfly incision, Lynch incision, or incision through an existing laceration.[15,21] The bicoronal incision is considered the workhorse of approaches, especially when extensive reconstruction is being performed. It allows a clear view of the area provided for cosmesis and facilitates the harvesting of a wide swath of pericranium and cranial bone to assist in the repair (**Figs. 3** and **4**).

The transnasal endoscopic approach and the hairline endoscopic brow approach have limited applicability. They are mainly used for small isolated anterior table fractures that require minimum fixation.

There are probably 5 categories that should be used to guide the management of frontal sinus fractures. It is important that these categories be simple and readily reproducible for developing standard management techniques.

1. Isolated anterior table fractures with or without displacement
2. Combined anterior-posterior table fractures with or without displacement
3. Isolated posterior fractures with displacement
4. Any fracture that disrupts the NFOT
5. Any fracture that results in dural disruption with or without underlying brain injury.

A

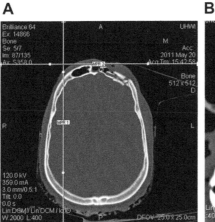

B

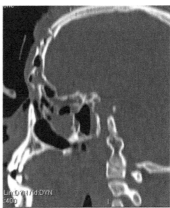

Fig. 2. (*A*) Axial view of comminuted fractures of both anterior and posterior tables. (*B*) Sagittal view of comminuted anterior and posterior table fractures.

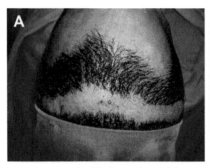 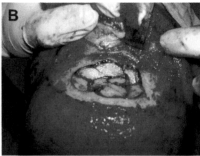

Fig. 3. (*A*) Bicoronal approach. (*B*) Comminuted fracture of the anterior table.

There is broad agreement in the treatment of isolated anterior table fractures. Nondisplaced or minimally displaced anterior table fractures are treated nonsurgically with antibiotics and decongestants.[15,16,21,22] These patients should have extended follow-up, which may include MDCT scans if the clinical examination dictates.

Displaced isolated anterior table fractures with no disruption of the NFOT should have reduction and fixation of the fragments with titanium or resorbable plates. It is important to thoroughly cleanse the wound of debris and remove entrapped devitalized sinus mucosa. In situations in which the comminution is extensive or fragments have been lost, harvesting cranial or iliac bone graft should be considered to recreate the contour of the anterior table (see **Fig. 4**).

The remaining categories of fractures pose a dilemma. Combined anterior-posterior table fractures with displacement require definitive separation from the brain (**Fig. 5**). These fractures are best approached by a bicoronal incision in which wide access and ability to procure a pericranial graft and cranial bone are assured. The bicoronal incision also facilitates neurosurgical repair of the dura and other neurosurgical injuries.[15,16] The main decision is whether to obliterate the

sinus or to cranialize it. If there is significant comminution of the posterior table, dural tears, injury to intracranial structures, or wide displacement, then cranialization is a better option. As has been said by numerous investigators, meticulous debridement of the sinus mucosa using rotary instruments is imperative for a good outcome (**Figs. 6** and **7**).[13,15,23,24] The authors prefer temporalis fascia to plug the NFOT followed by fibrin glue and a pedicled pericranial flap to further assure separation. However, muscle, bone, pericranium, and other sources of fascia can be used to seal the NFOT.[16,25] The anterior table is then reduced and fixated with titanium or resorbable plates.

When the posterior table is minimally displaced and not comminuted and there is no disruption of the dura, sinus obliteration can be considered. Debridement of all sinus mucosa and occlusion of the NFOT followed by placement of autogenous abdominal fat is appropriate. Several other materials can be used, namely, autogenous cancellous bone which we frequently prefer as it obviates the liquefaction necrosis that is sometimes noted with fat grafts, cadaveric cartilage, hydroxyapatite cement, and bioactive glass.[25] Despite the use of a second surgical site, the authors believe autogenous tissue sources produce better long-term results.

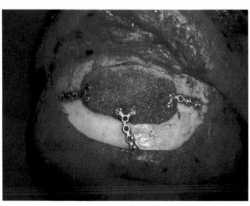 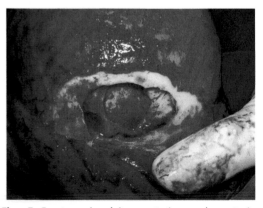

Fig. 4. Reconstruction with iliac graft.

Fig. 5. Fracture involving anterior and posterior tables with exposed dura.

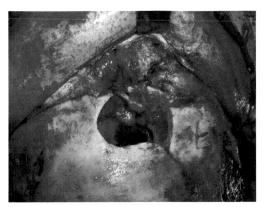

Fig. 6. Meticulous debridement of the sinus mucosa using rotary instruments is imperative for a good outcome.

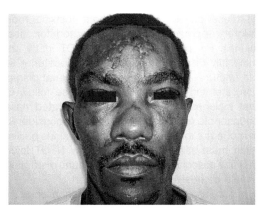

Fig. 8. Male patient 4 years after injury with undisplaced anterior and posterior table fractures conservatively managed with no functional sequelae.

When there is no displacement of both anterior and posterior table fractures, conservative management with close follow-up is done. This management should include MDCT scans to assess for intrasinus pathological conditions and NFOT obstruction (**Fig. 8**).

Isolated posterior table fractures are rare. These fractures require a bicoronal approach to facilitate craniotomy for neurosurgical repair of intracranial injuries and dural tears. After this has been accomplished, cranialization is performed as previously outlined.

Fractures that disrupt the NFOT are especially challenging. The recent historical thinking in the United States[16,25–27] has been to obliterate or cranialize these injuries because of the consensus that it inevitably leads to closure of the tract and attendant development of intrasinus and intracranial pathologic conditions. Sealing of the NFOT, as previously stated, can be performed with a variety of materials such as autogenous bone, temporalis muscle flaps, and pericranial and galeal flaps.[16,25]

As was discussed earlier, the sinus cavity can be filled with autogenous materials such as abdominal fat, iliac cancellous bone, muscle, pericranial flaps, or banked cadaveric tissue.[25,28,29] Synthetic materials that have been used include polytetrafluoroethylene, methylmethacrylate, bioactive glass, and calcium phosphate cements.[25] The largest series to date on the use of autologous fat had 250 patients with a median follow-up of 8 years. The overall complication rate was 18%, including a 5.2% incidence of abdominal wound complications (hematoma, seroma, or abscess), a 3% incidence of acute postoperative infection with necrosis of implanted fat, and a 3% incidence of recurrent chronic sinus infection.[25]

The main issue with synthetic material is the theoretical potential for infection of this avascular medium and possible foreign body reaction and material failure.[13] Overall, autogenous tissue is considered the gold standard.

Another viable option is stenting of the nasofrontal duct performed with tubes of various materials (rubber, gold, silicone). Such tubes are left in place for several weeks. Some studies report that about 30% of patients fail to maintain a patent duct after the catheter is removed. Postoperative scarring is the likely cause of this reocclusion.[15,25,30] In addition, surgeons may attempt to re-establish NFOT anatomy with a mucoperiosteal flap (Sewall-Boyden reconstruction), which, however, has been associated with restenosis and failure.[31]

With the prevalence of MDCT scans and the increased availability of endoscopic sinus procedures, some clinicians especially in Europe and the developing world are rethinking this blanket approach. Because of their greater ability to delineate small details, MDCT scans preoperatively identify more NFOT injuries. Does this mean that physicians should continue to aggressively treat

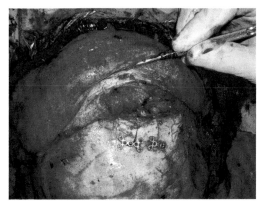

Fig. 7. Demonstrating open reduction internal fixation anterior table.

all these patients? The authors think a more tailored approach should be adopted for these injuries. For patients with mild NFOT injury and minimally displaced anterior and/or posterior table fractures with no intracranial or dural disruption, stenting of the NFOT with close follow-up that includes MDCT scans and indicated nasal endoscopic examinations, should be considered. In moderate to severe NFOT injuries, sinus obliteration must still be considered. Any NFOT injury that has associated intracranial or dural disruption, should be treated with cranialization.

In recent years, more reports that challenge the prevailing thinking are emerging. One such study was done by Smith and colleagues[31] in which a select group of patients with anterior table frontal sinus fractures involving the NFOT was treated with open reduction of the fracture without obliteration of the frontal sinus. Serial CT scans were obtained starting at 8 weeks after injury. Patients with persistent frontal sinus obstruction after medical treatment underwent an extended endoscopic frontal sinusotomy or a modified endoscopic Lothrop procedure. Mucociliary flow and clearance was re-established with conservative methods in most of the patients. This study involved a small cohort of patients, and management was patient dependent in terms of compliance and reliability. Hueman and Eller[32] described using balloon sinuplasty in managing a patient with nasofrontal duct injury and anterior table fracture. Seven months postoperatively, the patient demonstrated satisfactory NFOT function and facial contour clinically and radiographically. However, long-term studies are needed to verify the efficacy of these modified approaches. In **Figs. 9–11**, the authors describe a patient who had comminuted anterior table fracture with mild NFOT injury and was treated with stenting of the NFOT and plating of the anterior table. One year postoperatively, the patient

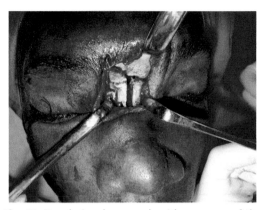

Fig. 10. Translesional approach with exposure of the fracture site.

demonstrated satisfactory facial aesthetics and a patent NFOT.

Fractures with dural and/or intracranial injury require a broad-based bicoronal approach to allow for neurosurgical repair. In most instances, this approach is followed by frontal sinus cranialization.

ENDOSCOPY

The bicoronal approach has been associated with instances of alopecia, scarring, and facial paresthesia, and, thus in recent years, there has been several small series that have described minimally invasive approaches to anterior table fractures[33–38] in an attempt to obviate these morbidities. The endoscopically assisted method was first described by Graham and Spring[39] in a 1996 study in which these investigators performed fracture reduction without internal fixation. Strong and colleagues[34] reported on a cadaver study describing the feasibility of performing endoscopic reduction and fixation. The investigators found

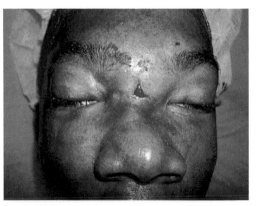

Fig. 9. Patient with open fracture anterior table frontal sinus with NFOT injury.

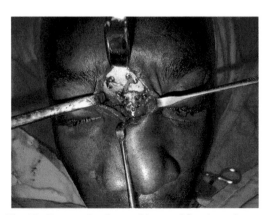

Fig. 11. Open reduction and internal fixation of anterior table after NFOT stenting.

that the fractures could be visualized, but they encountered difficulty with complete reduction and were unable to perform rigid fixation in a noninvasive manner. As an alternative, the investigators recommended camouflaging the anterior wall depression by endoscopically applying hydroxyapatite bone cement.[40]

Endoscopic approaches to frontal sinus fractures[37] have been suggested for acute fracture repair usually within 1 to 10 days of injury with or without fixation, delayed fracture repair, or fracture camouflage, which involves an observation period to allow for resolution of facial edema and then reconstruction with an alloplastic implant. The endoscopic approach can be performed via a transnasal route or a coronal incision. The transnasal approach allows intranasal drainage through the NFOT and provides cosmetic advantages because of the avoidance of an external incision.[41] However, endoscopic accessibility to the superior and lateral aspects of the frontal sinus is limited, and fracture reduction can prove to be difficult.

Kim and colleagues[42] reported on the feasibility of endoscopic reduction of anterior table fractures with Medpor implant, 0.85-mm sheets (Porex Surgical Inc, Newnan, GA, USA) in 10 cadavers and reported satisfactory postoperative results clinically and radiographically. This technique has been explored and has demonstrated efficacy in other studies.[34,37,40]

Steiger and colleagues[35] in their series stated that after 2 years of follow-up, all patients clinically showed good cosmetic results and were free of sinus complaints and radiographically had patent sinuses and reduced fractures. The methods used in this study were transnasal endoscopic approach and external endoscopically assisted trephination approach. One of the drawbacks is that this was a small series of 5 patients, and further studies are needed to validate this approach. Yoo and colleagues[43] reported another case report of transnasal endoscopic approach with modified balloon sinuplasty technique to splint the fracture segments in a 14-year-old man with good cosmetic outcome. In addition, this technique was recommended to be performed only in a subset of patients as described below.

1. Posteriorly displaced anterior table fractures[35]
2. Wide anterior-posterior diameter of the frontal sinus and recess[35]
3. Intact posterior frontal sinus table[35]
4. Recent history of trauma (loosely fixed)[35]
5. Fractures at or above the supraorbital rim.[37]

The reported benefits of these minimally invasive approaches compared with bicoronal approaches are better cosmesis, less scarring with subsequently reduced risks of infections, and mucocele formation.[33,35,37] Other advantages of endoscopic surgery include limited incisions, reduced soft tissue dissection, reduced risk of alopecia, minimal risk of postoperative paresthesia, reduced hospital stay, and improved patient selection. Disadvantages include a narrow field of view, lack of depth perception, and inability of the surgeon to operate bimanually without an assistant.[37] These results should be validated in a randomized clinical trial to make useful conclusions and comparisons.

Several other studies[33,42,44,45] have given credence and support to minimally invasive approaches to anterior table frontal sinus fractures, which are an alternative option in select patients. Kim and colleagues[41] described a transcutaneous transfrontal approach through a small eyebrow incision in 17 patients with closed anterior table fractures. All their patients reportedly achieved satisfactory aesthetic results and minimal complications. However, this method has inherent disadvantages such as the inability to perform concomitant rigid internal fixation and potential associated morbidities of facial paresthesia, bleeding, posterior table damage, and infection. However, these disadvantages were not reported in the investigators' series.

OUTCOME AND ASSESSMENT

The complications for all frontal sinus fractures can be separated into early and late complications. Early complications are usually wound infections, bleeding, cerebrospinal fluid leaks, NFOT obstruction with sinus congestions, and iatrogenic globe or brain injury.[22] Late complications present a more formidable challenge to the clinician and patient and may consist of mucoceles, mucopyoceles, osteomyelitis of the frontal bone, meningitis, and intracerebral abscess. The overall complication rate varies from 4% to 18%.[22,23,38]

However, the question arises, are these "complications" that are present in patients with a history of frontal sinus trauma, truly a result of the specific treatment or nontreatment of the fracture. This is the most vexing and, to date, unanswered question. To solve this issue, prospective controlled studies comparing patients with frontal sinus trauma with complications with other nontrauma groups followed over an extended period have to be designed.

The desired outcome for these patients is a cosmetically acceptable repair that recreates a safe functioning nasofrontal apparatus that is separated from the brain and remains disease

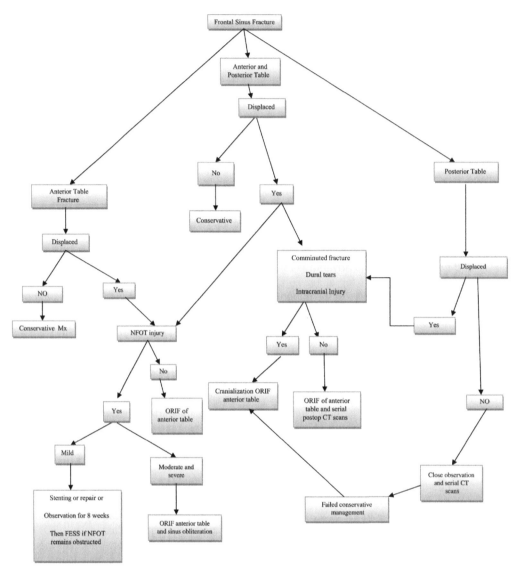

Fig. 12. Algorithm for the management of frontal sinus fractures. FESS, functional endoscopic sinus surgery; ORIF, open reduction internal fixation.

free over a long time. Recent studies report that investigators are succeeding in attaining this goal. The authors highlight their own approach in this regard in the algorithm listed (**Fig. 12**).

SUMMARY

More clinicians are reassessing the historical approach of obliteration or cranialization for more complex sinus fractures. The greater use of MDCT scans results in increased detection of fractures involving the NFOT. Does this mean that minimally displaced NFOT injuries should be operated on? This question is becoming more of

a dilemma for present-day surgeons. Bell and colleagues[22] talk about shifting toward sinus preservation in the management of several patients at a major trauma center. In a small series of patients, Gabrielli and colleagues[46] reported using stents to recreate drainage for patients who had injuries to the NFOT while maintaining the sinus.

Cone beam CT scans are available in several outpatient centers and doctors offices, thus allowing better postsurgical surveillance of the sinonasal complex. With the increased use of endoscopic procedures and their availability in most major and community hospitals, it is time to be more selective in the prevailing tendency to obliterate the sinus once damage has occurred to the floor of the sinus. Patient selection is important in this shift, along with strict postinjury long-term surveillance. As more centers that treat craniofacial trauma develop a more tailored treatment plan, more studies will be published to corroborate or dispute the efficacy of this type of treatment approach.

REFERENCES

1. Gray H, Williams PL, Bannister LH. Gray's anatomy: the anatomical basis of medicine and surgery. 38th edition. New York: Churchill Livingstone; 1995.
2. Cummings CW. Cummings otolaryngology—head and neck surgery. 4th edition. Philadelphia: Elsevier Mosby; 2005.
3. Anon JB, Rontal M, Zinreich SJ. Anatomy of the paranasal sinuses. New York, Stuttgart (Germany): Thieme, G. Thieme Verlag; 1996.
4. Blitzer A, Lawson W, Friedman WH. Surgery of the paranasal sinuses. Philadelphia, London: Saunders; 1985.
5. Bailey BJ. Head and neck surgery—otolaryngology. 2nd edition. Philadelphia: Lippincott-Raven; 1998.
6. McLaughlin RB Jr, Rehl RM, Lanza DC. Clinically relevant frontal sinus anatomy and physiology. Otolaryngol Clin North Am 2001;34(1):1–22.
7. Nahum AM. The biomechanics of maxillofacial trauma. Clin Plast Surg 1975;2(1):59–64.
8. Lee MK, Sakai O, Spiegel JH. CT measurement of the frontal sinus—gender differences and implications for frontal cranioplasty. J Craniomaxillofac Surg 2010;38(7):494–500.
9. Stammberger H. F.E.S.S: endoscopic diagnosis and surgery of the paranasal sinuses and anterior skull base: the Messerklinger technique and advanced applications from the Graz School. Tuttlingen (Germany): Endo; 2005.
10. Larrabee WF Jr, Travis LW, Tabb HG. Frontal sinus fractures—their suppurative complications and surgical management. Laryngoscope 1980;90(11 Pt 1): 1810–3.
11. Wolfe SA, Johnson P. Frontal sinus injuries: primary care and management of late complications. Plast Reconstr Surg 1988;82(5):781–91.
12. Stanwix MG, Nam AJ, Manson PN, et al. Critical computed tomographic diagnostic criteria for frontal sinus fractures. J Oral Maxillofac Surg 2010;68(11): 2714–22.
13. Bell RB. Management of frontal sinus fractures. Oral Maxillofac Surg Clin North Am 2009;21(2):227–42.
14. Manolidis S. Frontal sinus injuries: associated injuries and surgical management of 93 patients. J Oral Maxillofac Surg 2004;62(7):882–91.
15. Gerbino G, Roccia F, Benech A, et al. Analysis of 158 frontal sinus fractures: current surgical

16. management and complications. J Craniomaxillofac Surg 2000;28(3):133–9.
16. Gonty AA, Marciani RD, Adornato DC. Management of frontal sinus fractures: a review of 33 cases. J Oral Maxillofac Surg 1999;57(4):372–9 [discussion: 380–1].
17. Stanley RB Jr. Fractures of the frontal sinus. Clin Plast Surg 1989;16(1):115–23.
18. Newman MH, Travis LW. Frontal sinus fractures. Laryngoscope 1973;83(8):1281–92.
19. Donald PJ, Bernstein L. Compound frontal sinus injuries with intracranial penetration. Laryngoscope 1978;88(2 Pt 1):225–32.
20. Ioannides C, Freihofer HP. Fractures of the frontal sinus: classification and its implications for surgical treatment. Am J Otolaryngol 1999;20(5):273–80.
21. Chen KT, Chen CT, Mardini S, et al. Frontal sinus fractures: a treatment algorithm and assessment of outcomes based on 78 clinical cases. Plast Reconstr Surg 2006;118(2):457–68.
22. Bell RB, Dierks EJ, Brar P, et al. A protocol for the management of frontal sinus fractures emphasizing sinus preservation. J Oral Maxillofac Surg 2007; 65(5):825–39.
23. Strong EB, Pahlavan N, Saito D. Frontal sinus fractures: a 28-year retrospective review. Otolaryngol Head Neck Surg 2006;135(5):774–9.
24. Carboni A, Perugini M, Palla L, et al. Frontal sinus fractures: a review of 132 cases. Eur Rev Med Pharmacol Sci 2009;13(1):57–61.
25. Tiwari P, Higuera S, Thornton J, et al. The management of frontal sinus fractures. J Oral Maxillofac Surg 2005;63(9):1354–60.
26. Tedaldi M, Ramieri V, Foresta E, et al. Experience in the management of frontal sinus fractures. J Craniofac Surg Jan 2010;21(1):208–10.
27. Xie C, Mehendale N, Barrett D, et al. 30-year retrospective review of frontal sinus fractures: the charity hospital experience. J Craniomaxillofac Trauma 2000;6(1):7–15 [discussion: 16–8].
28. Kalavrezos ND, Gratz KW, Oechslin CK, et al. Obliteration of the frontal sinus with lyophilized cartilage in frontal fractures. Mund Kiefer Gesichtschir 1998; 2(Suppl 1):S66–9 [in German].
29. Thaller SR, Donald P. The use of pericranial flaps in frontal sinus fractures. Ann Plast Surg 1994;32(3): 284–7.
30. Wallis A, Donald PJ. Frontal sinus fractures: a review of 72 cases. Laryngoscope 1988;98(6 Pt 1):593–8.
31. Smith TL, Han JK, Loehrl TA, et al. Endoscopic management of the frontal recess in frontal sinus fractures: a shift in the paradigm? Laryngoscope 2002;112(5):784–90.
32. Hueman K, Eller R. Reduction of anterior frontal sinus fracture involving the frontal outflow tract using balloon sinuplasty. Otolaryngol Head Neck Surg 2008;139(1):170–1.

33. Chen DJ, Chen CT, Chen YR, et al. Endoscopically assisted repair of frontal sinus fracture. J Trauma 2003;55(2):378–82.

34. Strong EB, Buchalter GM, Moulthrop TH. Endoscopic repair of isolated anterior table frontal sinus fractures. Arch Facial Plast Surg 2003;5(6):514–21.

35. Steiger JD, Chiu AG, Francis DO, et al. Endoscopic-assisted reduction of anterior table frontal sinus fractures. Laryngoscope 2006;116(11):1978–81.

36. Strong EB, Kellman RM. Endoscopic repair of anterior table—frontal sinus fractures. Facial Plast Surg Clin North Am 2006;14(1):25–9.

37. Strong EB. Endoscopic repair of anterior table frontal sinus fractures. Facial Plast Surg 2009;25(1):43–8.

38. Gossman DG, Archer SM, Arosarena O. Management of frontal sinus fractures: a review of 96 cases. Laryngoscope 2006;116(8):1357–62.

39. Graham HD 3rd, Spring P. Endoscopic repair of frontal sinus fracture: case report. J Craniomaxillofac Trauma 1996;2(4):52–5.

40. Shumrick KA. Endoscopic management of frontal sinus fractures. Facial Plast Surg Clin North Am 2006;14(1):31–5.

41. Kim KS, Kim ES, Hwang JH, et al. Transcutaneous transfrontal approach through a small peri-eyebrow incision for the reduction of closed anterior table frontal sinus fractures. J Plast Reconstr Aesthet Surg 2010;63(5):763–8.

42. Kim KK, Mueller R, Huang F, et al. Endoscopic repair of anterior table: frontal sinus fractures with a Medpor implant. Otolaryngol Head Neck Surg 2007;136(4):568–72.

43. Yoo MH, Kim JS, Song HM, et al. Endoscopic transnasal reduction of an anterior table frontal sinus fracture: technical note. Int J Oral Maxillofac Surg 2008;37(6):573–5.

44. Mensink G, Zweers A, van Merkesteyn JP. Endoscopically assisted reduction of anterior table frontal sinus fractures. J Craniomaxillofac Surg 2009;37(4):225–8.

45. Forrest CR. Application of endoscope-assisted minimal-access techniques in orbitozygomatic complex, orbital floor, and frontal sinus fractures. J Craniomaxillofac Trauma 1999;5(4):7–12 [discussion: 13–4].

46. Gabrielli MF, Gabrielli MA, Hochuli-Vieira E, et al. Immediate reconstruction of frontal sinus fractures: review of 26 cases. J Oral Maxillofac Surg 2004;62(5):582–6.

Endoscopic Surgery of the Nose and Paranasal Sinus

Orville Palmer, MD, MPH, FRCSC[a],*, Jason A. Moche, MD[b],
Stanley Matthews, DDS[c]

KEYWORDS

- Endoscopic nasal surgery • Parasinuses
- Dacryocystorhinostomy
- Endoscopic cerebrospinal fluid repair
- Endoscopic pituitary surgery

ENDOSCOPIC SINUS SURGERY

Malte Erik Wigand and Wolfgang Draf were 2 highly accomplished surgeons who reported on endoscopic sinus surgery in the 1970s. It was Walter Messerklinger, however, who researched and reported on mucociliary clearance patterns of the nose and paranasal sinus. He managed to accomplish this with the use of the endoscope and computed tomography (CT) imaging.

Before the advent of endoscopic sinus surgery, most sinus surgeries were performed both externally and with the use of a headlight transnasally. Sinus surgery was aimed predominantly at the maxillary and the frontal sinuses. During the 1970s, the endoscopic examination of the nose using a microscope was advocated in Europe; however, this practice was not prevalent worldwide. Although the operating microscope was ideal for magnification, it did not facilitate the dexterity necessity for sinus surgery. Subsequently, the need for visualization of different areas of the nasal cavity in an angulated fashion became imperative.

The endoscope revolutionized the practice of endoscopic nasal surgery. As a result, external sinus surgery is performed less frequently today, and more emphasis is placed on functional endoscopy and preservation of normal anatomy. The main drawback of the endoscope is that the image obtained is two-dimensional. However, it has the advantage of providing good magnification and angulations for examination of the nasal cavity. It is a valuable and convenient office tool because of its portability. The combination of endoscopy and CT imaging has enhanced the understanding of inflammatory disease of the sinus and has helped us to better understand the pathophysiologic processes that exist in the sinonasal tract. Mucosal preservation techniques in endoscopy have led to a decreased risk of significant scarring, and new bone formation previously unseen in traditionally more aggressive procedures. Today, mucosal preservation is of paramount importance in the diagnosis and surgical management of the sinonasal tract.

The osteomeatal complex is recognized as the final pathway for sinus drainage, and could possibly be a major contributing factor in the pathologic processes existing in the sinuses.

Technical advancements have led to significant improvement in the instrumentation used in endoscopic sinus surgery. The increased resolution of the screens used in this type of surgery has enhanced the ease and safety of these procedures.

The authors have nothing to disclose.

[a] Otolaryngology-Facial Plastics and Reconstruction, Harlem Hospital Center, Columbia University, 506 Lenox Avenue, New York, NY 10037, USA
[b] Division of Otolaryngology, Department of Surgery, Harlem Hospital Center, Columbia University, 506 Lenox Avenue, New York, NY 10037, USA
[c] Oral and Maxillofacial Surgery, Department of Dentistry, Woodhull Medical and Mental Health Center, 760 Broadway, Room 2C-320, Brooklyn, NY 11206, USA
* Corresponding author.
E-mail address: odp3@columbia.edu

Oral Maxillofacial Surg Clin N Am 24 (2012) 275–283
doi:10.1016/j.coms.2012.01.006
1042-3699/12/$ – see front matter © 2012 Elsevier Inc. All rights reserved.

Expansion of the endoscope is possible when removing skull-base tumors and closing skull-base defects. In addition, it helps in the extension of surgical procedures beyond the limits of the paranasal sinus. With the advent of CT-assisted navigation systems, the accuracy and safety of paranasal sinus surgery has vastly improved.

The development of the Hopkins rod in endoscopic surgery is of vital importance. Before the Hopkins rod was available, the use of traditional instrumentation was associated with significant scarring and osteogenesis caused by damage to and denuding of bone, and was associated with chronic inflammation and significant pain.

Tru-Cut instruments enable clean removal of the diseased mucosa in sinus surgery. These instruments are significantly less traumatic in skull-base and sinonasal surgery, as they allow cleaner openings of the sinus ostium and accurate removal of aspects of the middle and superior turbinate, which facilitates more precise surgery.

The microdebrider, a descendant of Tru-Cut instruments, was first developed by orthopedic surgeons for arthroscopic procedures. The advantage of the microdebrider is that it is connected to a suction device used to remove tissue, bony particles, and nasal polyp during the procedure.

Nasal endoscopes are available in 0°, 30°, 45°, and 70° angulations. Although the 0° is the preferred choice for most endoscopic sinus surgery, the other angulated endoscopes help to facilitate a more accurate diagnosis and assist in certain technical aspects of the surgery.

CT imaging in endoscopic surgery is of paramount importance for the diagnosis, intraoperative management, and navigation guidance system. In recent years, there has been a significant increase in the resolution of CT imaging. Anatomic detail can be assessed preoperatively and reviewed intraoperatively. Anatomic details of the osteomeatal complex can be seen. The relationship of the cribriform plate to the superior wall of the ethmoidal sinus and attachments of the uncinate process are also of surgical importance.

The use of magnetic resonance imaging (MRI) scans has been increasing in the diagnosis and treatment of sinus and skull-base disease. MRI is helpful in differentiating inflammatory disease from neoplasm. MRI clearly defines the extent of soft tissue disease, especially disease adjacent to the skull base, as well as neoplastic processes involving the lamina papyracea. An MRI scan also helps in the characterization of gliomas and other soft tissue processes involving the skull base.

Interactive computer imaging helps intraoperatively in endoscopic surgery of the previously operated sinus. It is also useful in disease of the frontal recess, sphenoid, and skull base. Computer imaging has its limitations, however. The accuracy of interactive imaging is about 2 mm. As a result, its use does not reduce the importance of good endoscopic visualization and careful use of instruments.

Anatomy of the Nose and the Lateral Nasal Wall

The anatomy of the lateral nasal wall is highly variable, and a thorough understanding of the anatomy is necessary before proceeding with any nasal endoscopic procedure.

In general, the nasal cavity is divided into 2 nasal cavities by the nasal septum. The medial wall of each cavity is smooth and flat, whereas the lateral wall is irregular. The lateral wall is made irregular by projections known as turbinates or conchae.

These projections are the most prominent feature of the lateral nasal wall. Turbinates are usually 3 to 4 in number. Turbinates appear as cylindrical coils of bone, delicately covered by ciliated columnar epithelium. A turbinate normally contains an air cell, in which case it is termed a concha.[1,2]

The superior and middle conchae are processes of the ethmoidal bone, whereas the inferior concha is an independent bone of the skull. The conchae subdivide each nasal cavity into meati.

Humidification and temperature regulation of inspired air is provided by the conchae, which is highly glandular and vascular mucosal tissue. It is common for a prominence to be seen at the anterior attachment of the middle turbinate. This prominence, known as the agger nasi cell, varies in size. The agger nasi cells overlie the lacrimal sac, separated from it by a thin layer of bone. These cells are considered a remnant of the nasoturbinate bones seen in animals.[1]

Meati are named according to the conchae above them. For example, the superior meatus is inferior to the superior concha. The sphenoethmoidal recess lies above the superior conchae and drains the sphenoid sinus. The superior meatus drains the posterior ethmoidal air cells. The middle meatus is inferior to the middle concha. The anterior group of sinuses (the frontal, maxillary, and anterior ethmoidal) drains into the middle meatus. The inferior meatus is inferior to the inferior concha. The nasolacrimal duct opens in its anterior third. This opening is covered by a mucosal valve known as the Hassner valve. The course of the nasolacrimal duct lies just deep to the agger nasi cell.

The uncinate (hook-like) process forms the first layer, or lamella, of the middle meatus. The uncinate process is a wing-shaped or boomerang-shaped piece of bone that attaches anteriorly to the posterior edge of the lacrimal bone, and inferiorly to the superior edge of the inferior turbinate. The superior attachment of the uncinate process is highly variable. It may be attached to the lamina papyracea, the roof of the ethmoidal sinus, or the middle turbinate. The configuration of the ethmoidal infundibulum and its relationship to the frontal recess depends largely on the behavior of the uncinate process. The uncinate process can be classified into 3 types depending on its superior attachment. The anterior insertion of the uncinate process cannot be identified clearly because it is covered with mucosa, which is continuous with that of the lateral nasal wall.[3]

In type I, the uncinate process bends laterally in its uppermost portion and inserts into the lamina papyracea. Here the ethmoidal infundibulum is closed superiorly by a blind pouch called the recessus terminalis (terminal recess).

In type II, the uncinate process extends superiorly to the roof of the ethmoidal bone. The frontal sinus opens directly into the ethmoidal infundibulum. In these cases a disease in the frontal recess may spread to involve the ethmoidal infundibulum and the maxillary sinus secondarily. Sometimes the superior end of the uncinate process may divide into 3 branches: 1 is attached to the roof of the ethmoid, 1 is attached to the lamina papyracea, and the third is attached to the middle turbinate.[3]

In type III, the superior end of the uncinate process turns medially to become attached to the middle turbinate. Here also, the frontal sinus drains directly into the ethmoidal infundibulum.[3]

The hiatus semilunaris is a two-dimensional space that lies between the anterior wall of the bulla and the free posterior margin of the uncinate process. Through this hiatus there is a cleftlike space known as the ethmoidal infundibulum. The ethmoidal infundibulum is bound medially along its entire length by the uncinate process and its lining mucosa. The anterior groups of sinuses drain into this area.[2]

The paranasal sinuses

The paranasal sinuses are pneumatic areas in the frontal, ethmoid, sphenoid, and maxillary bones, lined by mucous membrane (respiratory epithelium), which is continuous with that of the nasal cavity.

The frontal sinuses are paired and located in the frontal bone (superciliary arch). The ethmoid air cells are located in the ethmoid bones bilaterally, in the upper part of the nasal cavity between the frontal and sphenoid sinuses.

The sphenoid sinus relationships are: superiorly, pituitary gland and the optic nerves and chiasm; laterally, the cavernous sinus with its contents

(ophthalmic and maxillary division of cranial nerve V, cranial nerves III, IV, VI, and the internal carotid artery); the nasopharynx is located below the sinus.[2]

The maxillary sinus is located in the maxillae bilaterally. Medially, it is related to the nasal cavity; superiorly, to the orbit (infraorbital nerve); and inferiorly, to the teeth of the upper jaw. Drainage is poor because the opening is located high on the medial wall of the sinus. The rate of infection is also higher because of the intimate association between maxillary molars.[2]

The osteomeatal complex is an anatomic unit into which the frontal, ethmoid, and maxillary sinuses drain. This complex consists of the maxillary ostium, infundibulum, hiatus semilunaris, uncinate process, bulla ethmoidalis, and anterior portion of the middle meatus.

Pathophysiology

During the 1950s and 1960s Messerklinger did extensive research and reported on the mucociliary action of the nose and paranasal sinus in fresh cadavers. He discovered that the drainage of sinuses to their respective natural ostia was not random but followed a sequence of patterns that appeared to be genetically determined. In cases where the natural pathways were blocked by inflammatory processes and/or tumors, the direction of mucous flow through the natural ostium was unaffected. This understanding provides a template for the complete physiologic process behind functional endoscopic sinus surgery. The transportation of mucous secretion in the maxillary sinus starts at its floor. It is then transported along the medial, anterior, posterior, and lateral walls to converge at the natural ostium of the maxillary sinus.[4]

The natural maxillary atrium opens in the posterior third of the ethmoidal infundibulum. The ethmoidal infundibulum opens into the middle meatus by way of the hiatus semilunaris. The mucus is then taken from the semilunaris along the medial surface of the inferior turbinate, usually under the Eustachian tube, into the nasopharynx. Drainage of mucus from the frontal sinus region is unique. It starts along the interfrontal septum, then moves superiorly, then laterally over the roof, then inferiorly to the floor, then toward the natural ostium.

Because of various shallow depressions in the frontal sinus, it is not uncommon to have some degree of recycling of mucus in the frontal sinus before it actually reaches the natural ostium. After passing through the frontal ostium, mucus drains into the frontal recess. The secretion then empties into the ethmoidal infundibulum, where there is a wide variation in anatomy. The secretion subsequently merges with the maxillary sinus and empties into the nasopharynx under the Eustachian tube.

The ethmoidal air cells anterior and inferior to the ground lamella tend to drain along a similar pathway to the maxillary sinuses. However, the posterior ethmoidal cells located posterosuperior to the ground lamella drains into the sphenoethmoidal recess. From here they drain into the nasopharynx, usually above the Eustachian tube. Sphenoidal sinus mucus drains into the sphenoethmoidal recess and joins that of the posterior ethmoidal cells to drain into the nasal pharynx. From the foregoing discussion there are 2 major routes of drainage of the paranasal sinuses along the lateral nasal wall. Mucus from the frontal anterior ethmoidal cells and maxillary sinuses drains below the Eustachian tube. Mucus from the posterior ethmoidal and sphenoidal sinus drains into the nasal pharynx, usually above the Eustachian tube.

ENDOSCOPIC PITUITARY SURGERY

Under general anesthesia and endotracheal intubation, the patient is put in a supine position with head elevated at 20° to 30°. A Mayfield headrest is commonly used with the arch of the navigation system. A 4-mm 0° endoscope is inserted in the nasal cavity that has the most space between the lateral nasal wall and the nasal septum. The endoscope is carried to the middle and superior turbinate, and the posterior aspect of the superior turbinate is removed if indicated.[5]

An inferior sphenoidotomy is then performed and the sphenoid is widened in a rostrocaudal direction. The rostral end of the sphenoid is resected. The sphenoidal rostrum is then removed using a high-speed drill. The rostrum is usually left intact because this material can be used in the subsequent reconstruction of the floor of the sella turcica. A bony window that is created by the removal of the sphenoidal rostrum is widened again using a micro drill.

Continuing the procedure under image guidance, the floor of the sella is then removed using the micro drill. The dura is exposed rostrally to the tuberculum sellae, caudally to the clival indentation, and anteriorly to the cavernous sinus bilaterally. The site of the abnormality will determine the site of incision into the dura. Most of these procedures are undertaken by the 0° scope, although the 70° or 30° scope may facilitate excision of pituitary lesions depending on the size and extent.[6]

After successful removal of the pituitary tumor, it is important that an angled endoscope be placed in the cavity for confirmation of complete removal. If necessary, curved instruments can facilitate resection of the diseased tissue. After resection, the cavity is irrigated thoroughly to prevent clot buildup. Packing the sella region with gelfoam and fibrin glue decreases dead space. The floor of the sella is then reconstructed with the rostral sphenoid bone removed. If this is inadequate, the mucosal flap of the nasal septum may be used. Gelfoam may be substituted by abdominal fat.

Endoscopic Repair of Septal Perforation/ Septoplasty

Septal perforation is most commonly caused by previous septal surgery. However, other causes can include trauma, septal hematoma, abscess, chronic nose picking, button-battery insertion, and collagen vascular diseases. Most septal perforations are asymptomatic, but when symptoms do occur, complaints may include bleeding, dryness, nasal whistling, and nasal obstruction. Asymptomatic septal perforation requires no treatment. Patients experiencing mild symptoms usually benefit from frequent nasal irrigation and the application of antibiotic ointment. For patients with more severe symptoms, septal buttons may be useful. Symptomatic patients who are not responding to medical treatment are usually offered corrective septal surgery.

Most septal perforation occurs in the cartilaginous area. Reconstructing a septal perforation greater than 2 cm in its widest diameter can be undertaken with ease with the open or endoscopic approach. Larger perforation tends to be more difficult to repair with either technique. Although the septal perforation can be done under local anesthetic, general anesthesia remains the preferred method. Temporalis fascia or ear cartilage is usually harvested to assist in the septal closure. The septum is infiltrated with 1% lidocaine with epinephrine. A unilateral hemitransfixion incision is then made. The hemitransfixion incision is taken to the floor of the nose toward the lateral nasal wall under the inferior turbinate. This procedure facilitates extensive harvesting of mucosa onto the lateral wall to create ease of closure of the septal perforation. An extensive elevation of the mucoperichondrium and mucoperiostium is undertaken unilaterally. A 2- to 3-cm longitudinal incision is made on the side of the elevated flap on the dorsal aspect of the septum, allowing for an upper as well as a lower transposition flap.[7]

The flaps are then advanced to cover the perforation, and sutured with interrupted 4-0 Vicryl or chromic catgut suture. The upper naked septum is left uncovered. Occasionally a relief incision is made longitudinally at the junction of the floor and lateral wall of the nasal cavity, but this can cause stenosis of the nasal aperture. At this stage the temporalis fascia or harvested cartilage is shaped to be slightly smaller than the bony or cartilaginous defect. The graft is placed in position through the hemitransfixion incision. Silastic splints are then placed in both nostrils bilaterally to keep the graft and flap intact, and the nasal cavity is packed. The nasal pack is removed after 2 to 3 days and the silastic sheets removed after 2 to 4 weeks.[8]

Septoplasty is another procedure with better short-term and long-term outcomes when done endoscopically. The indication for this procedure is the same as for the traditional open approach. The procedure is done predominantly with a 0° endoscope. Endoscopy provides superior visualization while performing this procedure, with consequent more precise placement of the mucosal incision, more conservative cartilage removal, and more accurate reconstruction. Endoscopy is a valuable tool for teaching residents (**Fig. 1**).

Endoscopic Closure of Cerebrospinal Fluid Rhinorrhea

The diagnosis, localization, and treatment of cerebrospinal fluid (CSF) rhinorrhea have always been a controversial subject. The diagnosis of CSF leak is usually not difficult; however, localization and surgical closure can be somewhat challenging. The challenge usually surrounds the cause and the size of the defect. Craniofacial trauma accounts for about 75% of CSF rhinorrhea. Another 15% to 20% is caused by surgical injury. A small percentage is caused by spontaneous leak or is associated with some other pathologic condition.

Traditionally these CSF rhinorrhea were treated intracranially. The intracranial approach is not free from complications such as anosmia and all the neurologic changes associated with brain retraction. In addition, there is a high rate of recurrence with this approach. The endoscopic

approach offers superior visualization of the site of the leak. In addition, the repair can be successful with fewer intracranial complications. Anosmia postoperatively tends to be rare. Endoscopy in combination with the navigation system increases the accuracy and ease of repair of CSF rhinorrhea.

Initially fluorescein dye was the gold standard. The use of intrathecal dye injection has been associated with transient neurologic complications, so its use is not advocated. Thin-slice CT cisternography is also of historical significance; however, its use is no longer indicated in the management of CSF rhinorrhea. High-resolution fine-slice CT scan, usually done coronally and axially, is the investigation of choice for locating a defect in CSF rhinorrhea. It can also indirectly indicate other soft tissue anomalies associated with CSF rhinorrhea.

CT scan is also superior to MRI for identification of bony defects and bony erosion. It is also highly sensitive in the identification of arachnoidal granulation, which is usually associated with spontaneous CSF rhinorrhea. In addition, posttraumatic CSF leak associated with skull-base trauma can be easily picked up on high-resolution CT, making it undoubtedly the investigation of choice.

MRI can be used in association with high-resolution CT in those cases for which the localization of the leak is challenging. MR cisternography with a long retention time is the method of choice when MRI is being used, but is definitely the investigation of second choice in localization of CSF rhinorrhea. It is used in combination with plain high-resolution CT in cases where the leak is inactive.

β_2-Transferrin is a specific type of transferrin found in CSF rhinorrhea. The transferrin test is 97% to 99% sensitive and is also extremely specific. It is reassuring for the surgeon if β_2-transferrin is found in nasal secretion. One drop of CSF fluid is usually adequate for analysis. Even when contaminated, this test offers a very high degree of sensitivity and specificity. The fluid is collected in a plain glass blood tube as it drips from the nasal cavity when the patient is instructed to lean forward.

Surgical Management of CSF Rhinorrhea

Various methods and materials have been used for the closure of CSF rhinorrhea. Materials include local flaps (mucoperichondrial, pericranial, dural), free fascia (tensor fasciae latae and temporalis fasciae), muscle grafts, synthetic dura, septal cartilage, and adhesives. In the authors' experience abdominal fat has become the standard material of practice, and can be administered by

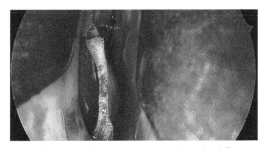

Fig. 1. Elevated bilateral mucoperichrondrial flaps.

itself or in combination with other materials. The procedure is usually done under general anesthesia. After identifying the sight of the leak by radiologic means, the nose is injected with 1% lidocaine with epinephrine and a topical decongestant is applied with neurosurgical cottonoid. Using a 0° endoscope the area of leak is identified.

For leak of the sphenoid sinus associated with postoperative leak from pituitary surgery, interactive navigation is indicated. The leaking site is identified; fine biopsies are done if other abnormalities are suspected. The dura is elevated for a few millimeters, and the fat graft isolated from the abdominal wall or the thigh is then impregnated with the fibrin glue. It is then placed at the site of the leak, usually anchored under the elevated dura. The graft can be further supported by septal cartilage or a mucosal flap.[9] A nasal pack is inserted. A lumbar drain is placed at this point or just before the start of the endoscopic procedure. The patient is put on bed rest and stool softeners, and told to avoid straining. For very small posttraumatic defects of less than 2 cm^2, lumber drainage may not be used. Lumbar drainage is almost always used in spontaneous CSF rhinorrhea regardless of size.[9]

Endoscopic Sinus Surgery

Chronic inflammatory disease is the most common indication for endoscopic sinus surgery. There are a host of procedures that can be undertaken in the sinonasal cavity, unilaterally, bilaterally, in various combinations, or in association with septal or turbinate surgery. Coronal CT scan of the nose and paranasal sinus is the investigation of choice in the management and treatment of inflammatory disease of the sinonasal tract (**Fig. 2**).

Specific procedures sometimes require additional views, such as sagittal views to accurately

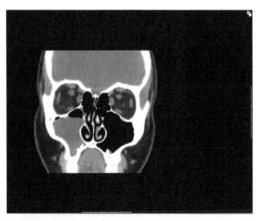

Fig. 2. Coronal CT of nose and paranasal sinus with right-side antrochoanal polyp.

determine insertion of the uncinate process in frontal sinoplasty. Axial views are required for the complex anatomy of the skull base, especially when neoplastic lesions are suspected. Endoscopic surgical procedures of the paranasal sinuses comprise limited anterior ethmoidectomy, total ethmoidectomy, exploration of the frontal sinus recess and the frontal ostium with or without frontal balloon sinoplasty, sphenoidotomy and sphenoid sinus exploration, middle meatal antrostomy with or without balloon maxillary antral sinoplasty medial maxillectomy, and dacrocystorhinostomy.

These procedures can be done under general or local anesthesia depending on the comfort level of the patient, the extent of the surgery undertaken, and the comfort level of the surgeon involved. The authors tend to do most procedures with the patient under general anesthesia.

Preoperatively the CT scan is scrutinized to determine the anatomy of the lateral nasal wall, the insertion of the uncinate process in relation to the skull base, detailed anatomy of the osteomeatal complex, height of the cribriform plate relative to the ethmoidal roof, and the extent and nature of the sinonasal inflammatory process.

Endoscopic Nasal Examination

This procedure is conducted before every endoscopic nasal procedure. The patient is placed in the supine position, the head elevated 15° to 20°, and the nose decongested with topical decongestant–soaked neurosurgical cottonoids: one placed along the length of the medial edge of the inferior turbinate, one in the middle meatus, and one placed along the medial aspect of the extent of the middle turbinate. A 30° scope is next used to examine the nasal cavity. The first pass is made along the floor of the nasal cavity just medial to the inferior turbinate, examining the inferior aspect of the nasal cavity thoroughly, followed by the nasopharynx, posterior pharyngeal wall, and Eustachian tube. The endoscope is then redirected in the area of the middle meatus, looking along the skull base and sphenoid ostium. The middle meatus, middle turbinate, osteomeatal complex, and anterior nasal cavity in the area of the nasal lacrimal pathway are then examined. A second pass is used to view the superior turbinate, superior meatus, sphenoethmoidal recess, and anterior skull base.

Ethmoidectomy

A 0° endoscope is used for most of this procedure. An osteotome is used to remove the middle portion of the uncinate process to facilitate access and visualization of the bulla ethmoidalis. Using small endoscopic forceps or a microdebrider, the anterior ethmoidal air cells are removed, avoiding injury to adjacent mucosa. It is not uncommon to find a perforation in the basal lamella. If it is not present, the ground lamella can be punctured and the posterior ethmoidal cells entered. Diseased mucosa is selectively removed under direct vision, taking advantage of the Tru-Cut nature of the endoscopic instruments used.

Dissection is taken back to the posterior wall of the ethmoidal sinus, which is located approximately 7 cm from the nasal aperture. Loose bone, mucosal fragments, and diseased tissue are removed. The sinus is then irrigated; a 30° endoscope is introduced to examine the cavity to ensure removal of all diseased mucosa. The sinus is packed with the standard Medtronic absorbable pack. The anterior end of the middle turbinate is frequently shaved with a microdebrider or resected to create better osteomeatal ventilation (**Fig. 3**).

Sphenoid Surgery

Sphenoid sinusotomy is done either in isolation or in combination with ethmoidectomy. Chronic inflammatory isolated sphenoidal disease is commonly associated with the immunocompromised patient. It is not uncommon to see sphenoidal inflammatory disease in association with chronic ethmoidal disease. Preparation similar to that for ethmoidectomy is undertaken. A 0° endoscope is usually passed medial to the middle turbinate. The superior turbinate is identified .For proper exposure, the posterior aspect of the superior

turbinate is removed using Tru-Cut endoscopic forceps. At this stage the sphenoidal ostium is identified; when visibility is not possible, identification of the anterior safe entry of the sphenoidal sinus should be facilitated by navigational guidance. The sphenoidal sinus is entered and the polyp, cyst, or diseased mucosa is removed leaving intact normal mucosa. The ostium is widened rostrocaudally. No packs are needed for isolated sphenoid exploration (**Fig. 4**).[10]

Frontal Sinus Exploration

This procedure is normally done in combination with ethmoidectomy. Navigation guidance is needed when there is extensive disease or complex anatomy. Again a 0° scope is used to examine the osteomeatal complex. After ethmoidectomy is completed, the superior aspect of the uncinate process is used as a guide to the frontal recess. Visualization can be optimized at this stage using the 70° endoscope. The frontal recess is cleared of its inflammatory disease, polyps, and any abnormal mucosa. Occasionally the anterior aspect of the middle turbinate is removed to facilitate exposure. The frontal sinus ostium is identified and removal of the abnormal mucosa undertaken. Enlargement of the ostium is then done by forceps and an osteotome.

Some mention should be made at this point about balloon sinoplasty of the frontal sinus. Balloon sinoplasty was prompted by the success of balloons in other disciplines such as gastroenterology, cardiology, and vascular surgery. It is not uncommon to have postoperative frontal sinus ostium stenosis after the type of surgery described in previous paragraphs. Balloon sinoplasty offers an atraumatic means of dilating the frontal sinus ostium and frontal recess with minimal injury to the surrounding tissue.[11]

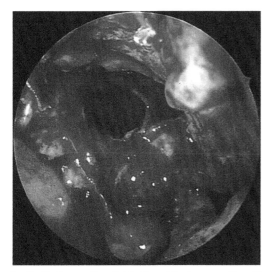

Fig. 3. Postoperative right ethmoidectomy cavity with resected anterior middle turbinate.

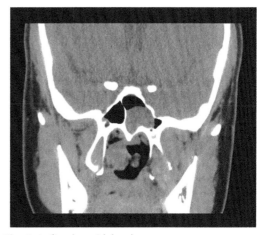

Fig. 4. Left sphenoidal polyp.

After removal of the diseased mucosa of the frontal recess, a guide is placed in the frontal recess. A balloon catheter with an illuminated tip is then introduced through the placed guide. Accurate placement is facilitated by accurate marking and calibration on the length of the catheter. In addition, information on the placement is ascertained by the pinpoint elimination of the anterior aspects of the frontal sinus by the illuminated catheter tip. The natural ostium is dilated, then the catheter is slightly retracted and the frontal recess dilated. Short-term and long-term outcomes of frontal sinoplasty seem to be encouraging; however, data are still forthcoming and its impact on sinus surgery is still evolving.

Middle Meatal Antrostomy

By far the most common surgery of the maxillary antrum is middle meatal antrostomy. This procedure can be done by backbiting osteotome, balloon dilation similar to that undertaken for frontal sinoplasty, or a combination of both. Surgery of the maxillary ostium is normally undertaken in combination with ethmoidectomy. The uncinate process is usually a guide to the natural ostium of the maxillary sinus, which is usually found inferior to the inferior aspect of the uncinate process. Its visualization is sometimes enhanced by the removal of the inferior aspect of the uncinate process. Under direct vision, the antrum is entered using a curved forceps with atraumatic tip. The natural ostium is usually widened anteroposteriorly to about 8 mm. Loose mucosa is removed immediately. The sinus is then irrigated. A 30° and a 70° scope can be passed through the ostium to examine the extent of the mucosal disease of the maxillary sinus, and removal of maxillary polyps and cysts can be facilitated.

Surgery of the anterior wall of the maxillary sinus can be somewhat limited using this approach.[12] The endoscopic Caldwell-Luc technique can assist in the complete examination of the maxillary sinus (**Fig. 5**).[13]

Endoscopic Medial Maxillectomy

Endoscopic medial maxillectomy is now the procedure of choice for the removal of benign and malignant disease processes isolated to the lateral nasal wall, the most common of which is an inverted papilloma. The origin of inverted papilloma is most commonly the maxillary sinus, lamina papyracea, or ethmoidal sinus.

There is a range of procedures for this disease, including endoscopically assisted resection, endoscopic maxillectomy, medial maxillectomy using a lateral rhinotomy, or endoscopically assisted

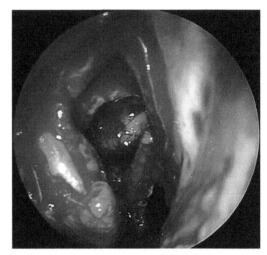

Fig. 5. Left ethmoidectomy is seen on the left. Middle meatal antrostomy is depicted on the lower right.

maxillectomy in combination with a lateral rhinotomy. Patients who undergo a lateral rhinotomy and medial maxillectomy have recurrent disease on the order of 25% to 30%, whereas the endoscopic approach by itself or in combination with an open procedure leads to recurrence on the order of 7% to 9%.

For the endoscopic approach, the nasal cavity is first examined. Tumor extent is endoscopically evaluated. Under endoscopic vision, an incision is made in the mucosa just anterior to the tumor. Tumors usually appear on the lateral nasal wall in the vicinity of the inferior turbinate. An osteotome is then used to enter the bony lateral wall. The maxillary antrum is entered through this osteotomy. The tumor is removed using a combination of direct-removal suction and a microdebrider. For tumors involving the inferior turbinate, the total removal of the inferior turbinate along with varying amounts of the lateral nasal wall is removed, depending on the extent of the tumor.[14] Tumors involving the ethmoidal sinus can be removed by endoscopic total ethmoidectomy as already described. The sphenoid cavity can be explored as described earlier. Tumor can be removed in its entirety under direct vision.

The maxillary sinus is then packed using ribbon gauze. The pack is removed within 48 hours under sedation. Subsequent follow-up and surveillance for recurrence is done endoscopically. Complications, namely epistaxis, double vision, and frontal sinus obstructive disease, are uncommon with both the open and the endoscopic approach. The hospital stay for endoscopic medial maxillectomy is 1 day, compared with 6 days for procedures involving an open approach. Endoscopic medial maxillectomy is not associated with a facial scar, although facial deformity as a result of scarring in the middle third of the face is rare with the open approach.

Dacryocystorhinostomy

Endoscopic dacryocystorhinostomy (DCR) is one of many techniques used to either unblock or create a new opening in the nasolacrimal system. The traditional approach to DCR typically involves an open surgical procedure. Endoscopic DCR is a minimally invasive procedure, used to bypass the nasolacrimal duct, and can be laser assisted.

Endoscopic DCR is indicated for patients diagnosed with lacrimal sac or nasolacrimal duct obstruction (NLDO). NLDO can be caused by several congenital or acquired factors, and is a common but not life-threatening condition. Presenting symptoms include excessive epiphora and dacryocystitis. Conventional treatment of NLDO includes warm compresses, massage, and probing the nasal passage. If NLDO is left untreated, these symptoms persist and may cause embarrassment for the patient. There is a greater prevalence of NLDO in elderly women than in their male counterparts. Sprekelsen and colleagues[15] hypothesized that long-term use of cosmetics may be an important factor.

Endoscopic DCR has many advantages over the standard external DCR approach. One of the key advantages is the avoidance of cosmetic scarring by entering the nasal cavity. Using endoscopy, surgical damage to the angular vein is avoided and the canthal ligaments are preserved. Bilateral surgery can be performed simultaneously in one setting. Decreased operating time and reduced intraoperative bleeding allows for the procedure to be performed on a day-surgery basis.[15]

Endoscopic surgery of the nose and paranasal sinus has revolutionized sinus surgery in a profound way. Open sinus surgery is now rarely performed. The endoscopic approach has not only provided improved surgical outcomes, it has also shortened the length of stay in hospital and has become a valuable teaching tool.

REFERENCES

1. Nayak SR, Kirtane MV, Ingle MV. Functional endoscopic sinus surgery—I (anatomy, diagnosis, evaluation and technique). J Postgrad Med 1991; 37(1):26B, 26–30.

2. Hiatt JL, 1934, Gartner LP, 1943. Textbook of head and neck anatomy. Original illustrations by Jerry L. Gadd 2002(3):209–17.

3. Balasubramanian T. Drtbalu's otolaryngology—uncinate process 2011; online rhinology textbook. Available at: http://sites.google.com/site/drtbalusotolaryngology/rhinology/uncinate-process. Accessed August 20, 2011.

4. Stammberger H, Hawke M. Essentials of endoscopic sinus surgery. St Louis (MO): Mosby; 1993.

5. Nyquist GG, Anand VK, Brown S, et al. Middle turbinate preservation in endoscopic transsphenoidal surgery of the anterior skull base. Skull Base 2010; 20(5):343–7.

6. Nakao N, Itakura T. Surgical outcome of the endoscopic endonasal approach for non-functioning giant pituitary adenoma. J Clin Neurosci 2011; 18(1):71–5.

7. Lee HR, Ahn DB, Park JH, et al. Endoscopic repairment of septal perforation with using a unilateral nasal mucosal flap. Clin Exp Otorhinolaryngol 2008;1(3): 154–7.

8. Paradis J, Rotenberg BW. Open versus endoscopic septoplasty: a single-blinded, randomized, controlled trial. J Otolaryngol Head Neck Surg 2011;40(Suppl 1): S28–33.

9. Schmerber S, Righini C, Lavielle JP, et al. Endonasal endoscopic closure of cerebrospinal fluid rhinorrhea. Skull Base 2001;11(1):47–58.

10. Wang Q, Lan Q, Lu XJ. Extended endoscopic endonasal transsphenoidal approach to the suprasellar region: anatomic study and clinical considerations. J Clin Neurosci 2010;17(3):342–6.

11. Govindaraj S, Adappa ND, Kennedy DW. Endoscopic sinus surgery: evolution and technical innovations. J Laryngol Otol 2010;124(3):242–50.

12. Robey A, O'Brien EK, Leopold DA. Assessing current technical limitations in the small-hole endoscopic approach to the maxillary sinus. Am J Rhinol Allergy 2010;24(5):396–401.

13. Masterson L, Al Gargaz W, Bath AP. Endoscopic Caldwell-Luc technique. J Laryngol Otol 2010; 124(6):663–5.

14. Durucu C, Baglam T, Karatas E, et al. Surgical treatment of inverted papilloma. J Craniofac Surg 2009; 20(6):1985–8.

15. Sprekelsen MB, Barberan MT. Endoscopic dacryocystorhinostomy: surgical technique and results. Laryngoscope 1996;106(2 Pt 1):187–9.

Revision Sinus Surgery

Satish Govindaraj, MD[a], Abib Agbetoba, MD[a],
Samuel Becker, MD[b],*

KEYWORDS

- Sinus • Rhinosinusitis • Revision surgery • Inflammation

Chronic rhinosinusitis (CRS) is a common illness affecting approximately 18 to 22 million Americans per year, placing a significant burden on patient quality of life and the health care system. Direct treatment costs have been estimated to range from $3.5 to $5 billion annually.[1,2] When symptoms persist despite optimal medical management, surgical intervention represents the preferred treatment. Functional endoscopic sinus surgery (FESS) is currently the gold standard in management of CRS refractory to medical management, and has a success rate for symptom improvement of more than 90%. However, symptom improvement correlates poorly with disease resolution, and up to approximately 20% of patients go on to require surgical revision. Those patients requiring revision endoscopic sinus surgery (RESS) are therefore in a minority but represent a therapeutic challenge for the otolaryngologist.[3] Before embarking on revision sinus surgery, a thorough reassessment of the patient's underlying disorder should be conducted. A key concept is that chronic sinusitis is a multifactorial disease with surgery serving as an adjunct to medical management and control of environmental factors. In addition, continued medical therapy plays a pivotal role in disease maintenance following revision surgery. Major contributing factors leading to RESS can be general host, environmental, and local host factors.[4] In those patients who have failed an initial attempt at endoscopic sinus surgery, a checklist should be completed evaluating each of these categories before an attempt at surgical revision (**Table 1**). The categories most amenable to revision sinus surgery are inadequate surgery extirpation or postoperative scarring either caused by poor operative technique or inadequate postoperative care. Lazar and colleagues[5] found that fibrous bands, adhesion formations, and recurrence of nasal polyposis are among the most common postsurgical findings in patients undergoing revision sinus surgery. Other factors contributing to failures in primary sinus cases include lateralization of the middle turbinate, scarring and stenosis of sinonasal ostia, retained anterior and posterior ethmoidal cells, residual uncinate, and the presence of initial frontal sinus disease. In addition, patients who have developed significant neosteogenesis as a result of mucosal stripping from prior surgical intervention also pose a significant challenge in revision cases. This problem can be difficult or impossible to resolve with revision surgical intervention and seems to be associated with a poorer long-term prognosis as well as persistent sinonasal pain.

This article examines revision surgical treatment of persistent inflammatory sinus disease. Advancements in endoscopic sinus surgery have enabled most revision sinus surgery to be conducted using this technique. The addition of stereotactic image guidance has been a useful adjunct in surgically managing these patients. Open surgical approaches may have a role in revision sinus surgery cases, although these are more commonly confined to the occasional trephination or osteoplastic flap procedure in patients who fail revision surgery with an extended frontal sinus approach.

PREOPERATIVE EVALUATION
History

Patients who are candidates for revision sinus surgery should undergo a complete medical reassessment as if they were being evaluated for the

[a] Department of Otolaryngology, The Mount Sinai Medical Center, 1 Gustave L. Levy Place, New York, NY 10029, USA
[b] Becker Nose and Sinus Center, LLC, 800 Bunn Drive, Suite 202, Princeton, NJ 08540, USA
* Corresponding author.
E-mail address: Sam.s.becker@gmail.com

Oral Maxillofacial Surg Clin N Am 24 (2012) 285–293
doi:10.1016/j.coms.2012.01.010
1042-3699/12/$ – see front matter © 2012 Elsevier Inc. All rights reserved.

oralmaxsurgery.theclinics.com

Table 1
Checklist prior to surgical revision

Environmental	General Host	Local Host
Cigarette smoke	Reactive airway	Iatrogenic
Chemical irritants	Immunodeficiency Genetic factors:	Neosteogenesis Nasal polyps
Inhalant allergy	Cystic fibrosis	
Emotional stress	Kartagener Samter triad	

first time. Documentation of the patient's initial complaints and the operative records are also important items to secure. It is critical to understand whether the patient's complaints before the first surgical procedure were of sinus origin, as well as reviewing and evaluating the patient before medical therapy. Common symptoms such as nasal obstruction, hyposomia, and headaches are all amenable to RESS in primary failures.[6] In addition, understanding the extent of the initial procedure, as well as identifying any orbital or intracranial violation, allows for critical preoperative planning to help decrease surgical complications and postoperative morbidity.

Some of the key areas to evaluate are potential genetic predisposition (cystic fibrosis, cilia dysmotility, immunodeficiency, autoimmune state), allergy assessment if clinical suspicion exists, and environmental exposure to dust, mold, chemicals, and smoke inhalation. Smoking cessation is critical in smokers with CRS undergoing elective endoscopic sinus surgery. Failure to maintain abstinence can lead to quick relapse and poor postoperative wound healing.

Any patients who had their first operations for chronic sinusitis or polyposis before the age of 18 years should be evaluated for a cystic fibrosis variant. However, the possibility of cystic fibrosis should also be considered in patients who present even later in life if they have had multiple disease recurrences. Among the most difficult cohort of patients to treat are those with the Samter triad and asthma-associated nasal polyposis. It is important that they understand that their disease process is chronic and requires ongoing medical care. Asthma has been extensively cited in the literature as being a prognosticator for poor surgical outcomes in endoscopic sinus surgery.[7–9] Mendelsohn and colleagues[9] reported a 5-year polyp recurrence rate of 45% in asthmatic patients, and this rate was as high as 90% in patients with Samter triad, with associated revision rates of 25% and 37% respectively,

compared with 10% for controls. If both the physician and the patient are not vigilant with regard to ongoing medical therapy and regular routine endoscopic follow-up, the likelihood of further revision sinus surgery is high. In any patient undergoing revision sinus surgery, evaluation of both active and passive immunocompetence is a consideration, in addition to allergy evaluation.

Physical Examination

A complete head and neck examination should be performed in the initial visit. The presence of lymphadenopathy may suggest sarcoidosis, chronic serous otitis media could be associated with Wegener granulomatosis, or laryngeal findings of posterior glottic erythema and edema may reveal underlying gastroesophageal reflux.

Diagnostic nasal endoscopy is an essential component of the preoperative physical examination, particularly in patients who have undergone prior surgical procedures. This endoscopy can often provide more information regarding the anatomy and the presence of active disease than routine imaging. When identified on endoscopy, reactive nasal mucosa should be controlled with topical and oral steroids before surgical intervention. Typically a course of 20 to 30 mg of prednisone daily for 3 to 7 days before surgery is sufficient. The steroids also help stabilize lower airway reactivity as well as reduce sinonasal inflammation. In addition, any purulence within the sinonasal cavity should be cultured and treated with the appropriate antibiotic. The cavity should be assessed for evidence of iatrogenic factors contributing to recurrent or recalcitrant disease (**Table 2**).

Radiographic Evaluation

The radiologic assessment should include review of films taken before the first surgical procedure whenever possible, and then compared with the present studies. Khalil and colleagues[10]

Table 2
Iatrogenic factors

Physiological Problem	Common Anatomic Source
Lateralization of middle turbinate	Absence of middle turbinate
Mucus recirculation	Residual uncinate process
Scarring of bulla to middle turbinate	Residual ethmoid bony partitions
Scarring of frontal recess	Scarring of sphenoid sinus ostia

retrospectively reviewed computed tomography (CT) scans of 63 patients undergoing revision sinus surgery and found lateralized middle turbinates in 11.1% of the reviewed imaging slides, residual uncinate process in 57.1%, and persistent anterior and posterior ethmoid cells in 92.1% and 96% respectively. Stereotactic computer-assisted navigation systems are commonly used for revision sinus surgery cases. The key areas for review in the preoperative CT evaluation are shown in **Table 3**.

ENDOSCOPIC REVISION SINUS SURGERY
General Concepts

Normal anatomic relationships have been altered in a revision sinus surgery case, thus the identification of constant landmarks at the outset of the surgery is vital. The key landmarks to identify are the maxillary sinus roof, medial orbital wall, and the skull base either within the posterior ethmoid or sphenoid sinus. The roof of the maxillary sinus serves as a landmark in 2 ways: correlation with the level of the sphenoid ostium and a safe height for posterior dissection through the ethmoids to the sphenoid sinus. In addition, initial identification of the medial orbital wall as it joins the roof of the maxillary sinus is critical because maintaining a lateral dissection plane along the orbit avoids working medially where the skull base is thin and more at risk. Once in the sphenoid sinus, the lowest point of the skull base can be identified. Dissection can now proceed in a posterior to anterior direction along the skull base and medial orbit. Because the dissection is brought anteriorly, the location of the anterior ethmoid artery is important to avoid inadvertent injury to this structure. Dissection is therefore only performed in this area after the anatomy of the skull base has become evident.

Instrumentation

The revision sinus surgery case requires both manual and powered instrumentation. Through cutting instruments are essential for the removal of bony partitions without stripping mucosa. Non–through cutting instruments such as the Blakesley forceps are helpful in fracturing thickened osteitic bone along the skull base or medial orbital wall. When thickened bone is fractured with non–through cutting forceps, it is not typically removed in the jaws of these forceps because of the possibility of stripping mucosa. Instead, it is teased out from the mucosa and then removed.

Powered instrumentation includes angled microdebriders and diamond burr drills. Microdebriders allow the expeditious removal of bony partitions and loose mucosa without stripping mucoperiosteum. In addition, angled debriders of 60° and 90° are an efficient way of removing polyps from the frontal recess and from the maxillary sinus. Powered drills play a role in the removal of osteitic bone that is not amenable to manual instrumentation. The 15° and 70° angled diamond burr drills are used in areas where the osteitic bone is too thick or cannot be fractured with forceps. However, when the diamond burrs are used, it is with the understanding that mucosal sacrifice is inevitable and adjacent mucosa needs to resurface the area, thus they should be used selectively.

Maxillary Sinus

The most common problem related to the maxillary sinus is the presence of residual uncinate process, which can result in either blunting or scarring at the anterior aspect of the antrostomy or failure to communicate the true and iatrogenic ostia with resultant mucus recirculation. Residual infraorbital ethmoid (Haller) cells are also identified frequently and may result in persistent

---

Table 3
Preoperative CT evaluation

Site	Evaluation
Skull base	Slope, height, erosions, asymmetry, neosteogenesis
Medial orbital wall	Integrity, residual uncinate position, erosion
Ethmoid vessels	Anterior/posterior ethmoid vessels relative to skull base
Posterior ethmoid	Vertical height, presence of Onodi cell, neosteogenesis
Maxillary sinus	Infraorbital ethmoid cells, accessory ostia
Sphenoid sinus	Position of intersinus septum, location of carotid artery and optic nerve and whether dehiscent
Frontal recess/sinus	Presence of agger nasi and supraorbital pneumatization, frontal sinus drainage, anterior-posterior diameter of frontal sinus

inflammation. In addition, if the maxillary sinus extends medially into the nasal cavity, entrapment of airflow occurs with mucosal drying and secondary impairment of mucociliary clearance.

With respect to residual uncinate process, the most useful instruments are a ball tip seeker, backbiter forceps, and an angled (30° or 45°) endoscope. The residual uncinate process is located anteriorly and can hide the natural ostium when examined with a 0° scope. A 30° or 45° angled endoscope is required to obtain a better view of the area. A ball tip seeker is then used to medialize this segment of uncinate and the curved 60° microdebrider for tissue removal. Another option is to use the backbiter for both dissection and removal of residual uncinate in this area (**Fig. 1**). At times, there is failure to communicate the true ostium with the surgically created opening. This situation is easily managed, even in the office setting, through the use of a backbiter to remove the intervening tissue and communicate both openings (**Fig. 2**). An angled (60°) microdebrider can be used to obtain the same result.

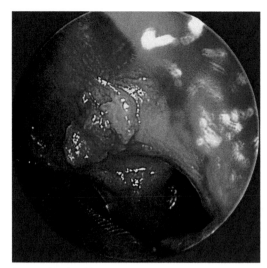

Fig. 2. The backbiter is used to remove the intervening tissue between the natural ostium and surgical ostium of the maxillary sinus.

Ethmoid Sinus

The ethmoid region is a common area for residual bony partitions along the skull base and medial orbital wall. These areas may be sources of persistent inflammation and cellular obstruction with secondary neosteogenesis. In addition, if prior surgery has removed or perforated the middle turbinate, clearing the skull base of bony partitions or polyps becomes dangerous. There is a potential risk of cerebrospinal fluid (CSF) leaks secondary to

possible absence of the middle turbinate, the medical boundary of the dissection, and failure to identify dural invaginations at the superior attachment of the middle turbinate. The use of stereotactic navigation can be helpful in these cases. The location of the anterior ethmoid artery should be evaluated on preoperative CT scan because, at times, the artery may be passing through an area of neosteogenic bone, or may be hanging freely from the ethmoid roof.

The surgical technique requires initial identification of the medial orbital wall to establish the lateral extent of the dissection, which is best achieved by using a through cutting forceps to remove these bony partitions while preserving mucosa. The medial wall of the maxillary sinus can be used as a reference point for the plane of the lamina papyracea. An angled Blakesley can be used to palpate the medial orbital wall for residual bony partitions. Once the medial orbital wall is cleared, the skull base can then be identified in the sphenoid sinus or posterior ethmoid region. In all surgical procedures, a 0° telescope should be used until the medial orbital wall and skull base have been identified. If the skull base is not readily identified in the posterior ethmoid sinus, it is important to identify the sphenoid sinus ostium and widen the ostium to determine the location of the skull base roof within the sphenoid sinus. As mentioned, this is the lowest point of the skull base, thus moving from posterior to anterior, staying adjacent to the medial orbital wall, is the safest way to avoid intracranial entry. The key to safely clearing the skull base is palpating behind each bony partition before removal (**Fig. 3**). If space can be felt behind

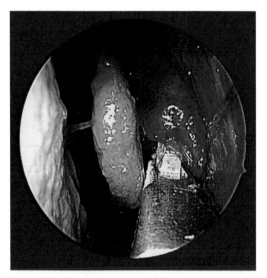

Fig. 1. The backbiter is used here to resect the residual uncinate process after reflecting it medially.

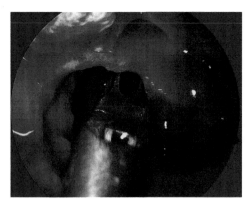

Fig. 3. An angled instrument is used to palpate behind a bony partition in the ethmoid cavity before removal.

a bony partition it should be safe for removal. In addition, the instrument should be angled laterally to decrease the risk of intracranial penetration medially where the skull base at times slopes. If the bone is too thick to remove with a through cutting forceps, it may be gently fractured with a Blakesley forceps, teased away from the surrounding mucosa with a curette or ball-tipped seeker and then removed. In certain circumstances, a wide area of bony neosteogenesis may be present and an angled drill will be necessary. Mucosal sacrifice is inevitable in this situation, and a reliance on healthy adjacent mucosa, postoperative debridement, and antibiotic coverage is necessary until the area is resurfaced. In the posterior ethmoid region, a 15° drill is adequate; however, because the dissection progresses anteriorly, it is necessary to transition to an angled endoscope and 70° drill.

Sphenoid Sinus

The sphenoid sinus serves as a critical structure to identify in the revision sinus surgery case. It anatomically defines the lowest point of the skull base, marks the posterior extent of the dissection, and serves as a posterior landmark for the medial orbital wall. The most common iatrogenic sequela of the sphenoid sinus is scarring of the ostium. At times, the ostium may be densely osteitic, requiring a drill for entry. Adhesion and scarring of the superior turbinate to the face of the sphenoid are also causes for recurrent sphenoid sinus disease. In each of these cases, stereotactic navigation is helpful. The last posterior ethmoid cell typically has a pyramidal shape with the apex pointing superolaterally toward the anterior clinoid process. Once this has been identified, attention is directed medially and the superior meatus is identified by palpation. The posterior boundary of

the superior meatus is the superior turbinate and the inferior portion of the superior turbinate is then resected with a through cutting forceps. This resection leads the surgeon directly back to the natural ostium, which lies medial to the superior turbinate, and the ostium can then be palpated and widened. Once entry has been established, widening of the ostium can be accomplished using either a mushroom punch or rotating sphenoid punch (**Fig. 4**). The wall is then resected until it is flush with skull base. A drill may be required when the bone is thick. After opening the sinus, irrigation can be performed to evacuate any retained secretions or crusts.

Frontal Sinus

Revision endoscopic frontal sinus surgery is an area of significant recent advancement. With the appropriate anatomy, frontal sinus inflammatory disease can be treated endoscopically with only select cases requiring open approaches such as trephination or an osteoplastic flap. The main iatrogenic sequelae causing frontal sinus obstruction are residual cells obstructing the frontal recess region and neosteogenesis from prior mucosal stripping. The key concepts to remember are to remove all bony partitions within the frontal recess while leaving a fully mucosalized ostium of at least 4 to 5 mm diameter. This task can be challenging in the setting of neosteogenesis.

Endoscopic management of the frontal sinus often requires angled endoscopes and proper instrumentation. The Draf classification describes 3 levels of frontal sinus dissection (**Table 4**).[11] In the revision sinus surgery case, the minimum of a Draf IIa procedure is usually recommended. In cases that have failed a prior Draf II procedure,

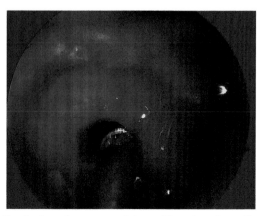

Fig. 4. A mushroom punch is used here to enlarge the ostium of the sphenoid sinus. Because of its round head, the instrument is able to cut in all directions.

Table 4
Classification of Draf frontal sinusotomy

Type	Description
Draf I	Anterior ethmoidectomy, frontal recess drainage pathway confirmed
Draf IIa	Create an opening between lamina papyracea and middle turbinate insertion
Draf IIb	Removal of frontal sinus floor between lamina papyracea and nasal septum
Draf III	Bilateral IIb with removal of upper nasal septum and lower frontal sinus septum

a transseptal frontal sinusotomy (Draf III) can be performed if the anatomy is amenable.

Draf IIa

This procedure was described by Stammberger[12] as "uncapping the egg" and involves expanding the frontal sinus recess from lamina papyracea to middle turbinate by removing residual bony partitions and air cells. Triplanar CT reconstructions are used to identify the frontal sinus drainage pathway and conceptualize the anatomy as it will be seen endoscopically. The first step is confirmation of the frontal sinus drainage pathway. This step can be done gently with a malleable probe. The ostium often lies between the uncinate process and middle turbinate in a medial location. Once identification of the ostium is done with a probe, the area below the sinus can then be expanded. In a Draf IIa, the ostium is not enlarged, and the patient's ostium dimensions are preserved. Anterior expansion with a frontal sinus curette fractures any residual agger nasi cells. This expansion should be done in an anterolateral direction. Once fracture of the bony partitions is complete, a curved microdebrider may be used to remove bony fragments and mucosal tags. Alternatively, larger bony fragments can be teased out with a curved probe and removed with a giraffe forceps. This anterior exposure facilitates working in the frontal recess and is termed uncapping the egg.[4,13] Lateral extension of the ostium is performed with a curved mushroom punch to the medial orbital wall. An alternative is to down fracture fragments with a curved hook. Medial dissection is expanded to the middle turbinate insertion and posterior dissection is conducted to the posterior table of the frontal sinus. In most cases, there is a supraorbital ethmoid air cell posteriorly

of variable size. When this is identified, the bony partition between the supraorbital ethmoid cell and the frontal sinus should be removed. Once completed, a wide fully mucosalized frontal sinus ostium will be present (**Fig. 5**).

Draf IIb

The Draf IIb removes the frontal sinus floor on 1 side from the lamina papyracea to nasal septum. In this procedure, the frontal ostium is enlarged beyond its normal anatomic dimensions. The indications are failure of a prior Draf IIa procedure. The same steps for the Draf IIa procedure are performed with the addition of resecting the anterior one-third of the middle turbinate where it borders the frontal sinus and expanding the ostium medially to the nasal septum. The anterior one-third of the middle turbinate can be resected using straight-through cutting forceps (**Fig. 6**A). In the revision case, a prior partial middle turbinate resection may have been performed. If this is the case, the anterior resection should be carried superiorly to the level of the skull base, taking care more posteriorly not to resect the region where the dura invaginates into the turbinate attachment. The floor of the sinus is removed from lamina papyracea to the nasal septum (see **Fig. 6**B).

Draf III (transseptal frontal sinusotomy)

The Draf III procedure is a bilateral Draf IIb procedure with resection of the intervening segment of superior nasal septum and the adjacent frontal intersinus septum. There is up to a 10% risk of

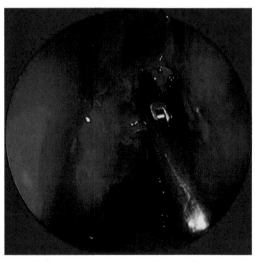

Fig. 5. A frontal sinus instrument is used to resect the bony septation between the supraorbital ethmoid air cell and the frontal sinus ostium, resulting in a larger frontal sinus drainage pathway.

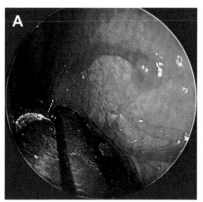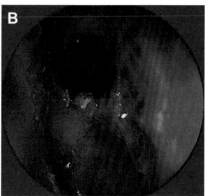

Fig. 6. (*A*) A straight-through cutting instrument is used to resect the middle turbinate at its skull base attachment. (*B*) Left frontal sinus ostium enlarged from nasal septum on left to medial orbital wall on right. In this revision case, the anterior wall of the frontal sinus was also enlarged with a drill because of stenosis of the frontal ostium from prior surgery.

a CSF leak and not all patients have anatomy suitable for this procedure. The distance between the anterior and posterior table of the frontal sinus (anteroposterior [AP] diameter) should be at least 5 mm. Evaluation of the preoperative CT scan is required with careful attention to the AP diameter of the frontal sinus, the width of the ethmoid cavity, and the thickness of the nasofrontal beak (the bone at the anterior aspect of the ostium). A thick nasofrontal beak translates into additional drilling time and an increased incidence of postoperative scarring.

The procedure is begun by identification of the more patent frontal sinus; however, when both sinuses are involved, it may be initiated with resection of the midline superior septum and entering the frontal sinus in the midline. The skull base is always identified posteriorly with this procedure to avoid the risk of CSF leak. More commonly, bilateral Draf IIb procedures are first performed. Once the ostia have been enlarged to the nasal septum, the superior septum is resected after injecting it with 1% lidocaine with 1:100,000 epinephrine. A sickle knife or beaver blade is used to make a superiorly based U-shaped flap on the nasal septum. This mucosa is removed with a 60° microdebrider. The segment of bony septum at the floor of the frontal sinus is removed as well as the frontal intersinus septum, which brings both frontal sinuses into continuity. Further enlargement may be performed anteriorly by thinning the anterior nasofrontal beak with a curette or 70° drill. Care is taken to preserve mucosa along lateral and posterior walls of the sinus and to preserve mucociliary clearance.

Complications of Endoscopic Sinus Surgery

The major complications of endoscopic sinus surgery are in 2 main categories: intracranial and intraorbital injuries (**Table 5**). In most series, these potential complications occur in approximately 1:200 cases. Preoperative discussion and detailed explanation before obtaining informed consent are essential. Although the complications were previously thought to occur at increasing frequency in patients undergoing revision procedures, recent review of the literature has suggested that the rates of major and minor complications do not increase in patients undergoing RESS, with major complications occurring at a rate of 0.3% to more than 1.3%.[14] The risk of CSF leak should be adjusted accordingly in those patients having multiple revision procedures, those with dense osteitic bone or neosteogenesis along the skull base, and those undergoing transseptal frontal sinusotomy. Although major complications are rare, minor complications such as scarring, disease persistence, synechiae formation, and mucoceles are more common.

Postoperative Care and Debridement

The long-term success of revision sinus surgery depends on diligent postoperative medical

Table 5
Complications of endoscopic sinus surgery

Major	Minor
Orbital	Scarring
Hemorrhage	Bleeding
Muscle injury	Infection
Optic nerve injury	Epiphora
Internal carotid injury	
Central nervous system	
CSF leak	
Encephalocele	
Brain abscess	

management and office debridement. The office should have a complete set of instruments available for removal of residual bony partitions and lysis of synechiae. Endoscopically directed cultures should be performed as needed. The mucosal appearance is the critical sign of whether a postoperative cavity has healed completely and is likely to remain stable. Residual areas of edema along the skull base or medial orbital wall suggest residual bony partitions. Palpation and removal of these areas with curettes or through cutting instruments can be performed after topical anesthesia. In addition, intralesional steroids can be administered in select cases, especially in the frontal recess.

Medical management involves the use of antibiotics, nasal steroids, nasal saline irrigations, and antibiotic irrigations. The duration of oral steroids and other medical management depends on the endoscopic appearance of the postoperative cavity. To alleviate the risk of introducing infection, aggressive irrigations are not initiated until 2 weeks after surgery. Nasal saline preparations are easily available over the counter to keep the cavity moist between debridements. Patients are seen in the office for 4 to 6 weeks of weekly debridement. Topical nasal steroids are usually continued long-term, especially in the revision patient who may need indefinite treatment.

OPEN REVISION SINUS SURGERY
Caldwell-Luc

The Caldwell-Luc approach to the maxillary sinus is not commonly performed for the management of standard inflammatory sinus disease, although some clinicians have shown good results in revision patients. In patients with neoplastic processes, including inverted papilloma, the Caldwell-Luc is an ideal adjunct to the endoscopic approach, especially in those tumors with anterior or lateral attachment. For this reason, a brief description of the procedure is presented because it has already been well described.[15,16] An incision is made in the upper gingivobuccal sulcus leaving a cuff of mucosa for reapproximation on the dental side of the incision. Unipolar cautery can be used to take the dissection to the face of the maxilla. An incision is made through the periosteum, and a periosteal elevator is used to elevate superiorly. Medial elevation to the piriform aperture and lateral extension to the lateral wall of the maxilla is performed. As the periosteum is elevated superiorly the infraorbital nerve bundle is identified. Entry into the maxillary sinus is performed with a 2-mm osteotome and mallet in the canine fossa. A small square is created to accommodate

a Kerrison rongeur. The bony opening is enlarged to the size needed for disease clearance. Closure of the incision is performed with a 3-0 chromic suture in a running horizontal mattress fashion. The horizontal mattress everts the mucosal edges well and prevents retraction of mucosa and food trapping in the wound.

Frontal Sinus Trephination and Frontal Intersinus Septectomy

The frontal sinus trephination creates a medial window in the medial floor or anterior wall of the frontal sinus and is used in inflammatory cases in which frontal sinus cells are inaccessible via an endoscopic approach. The technique requires either an infrabrow or intrabrow incision that is taken down to the underlying periosteum and bone. Transillumination or image guidance can then be used to confirm location of the frontal sinus. A 5-mm cutting burr is used to enter the frontal sinus. Care is taken to avoid the area of the supraorbital nerve. Once the sinus has been entered, expansion of the entry site is performed with a Kerrison rongeur. Once widened, dissection can be performed via the trephination site or a combined above and below approach may be used. In the case of a unilateral obstructed frontal sinus that is not amenable to an endoscopic approach, trephination with endoscopic frontal intersinus septectomy can be used. This technique allows for a passive drainage pathway from the obstructed frontal sinus to the contralateral unaffected sinus. A trephination is performed on the diseased frontal sinus and then resection of the intersinus septum is done with a diamond burr drill and Kerrison rongeur. It is vital that careful attention is paid to removing the inferior aspect of the intersinus septum to allow for optimal drainage of the diseased sinus into the patent contralateral sinus. Initial studies evaluating this technique have shown promising results in both subjective and objective postoperative clinical and radiographic outcomes.[17]

Osteoplastic Flap

The osteoplastic flap with or without obliteration is a procedure reserved for intractable frontal sinus inflammatory disease not amenable to a transseptal frontal sinusotomy, failure of Draf III frontal sinusotomy, and for resection of select frontal sinus tumors. A standard bicoronal incision is typically performed extending from each helical crus. A subgaleal plane is identified and elevated to 2 cm above the supraorbital rims. At this point, blunt dissection is used to further elevate the flap and identify the supraorbital neurovascular bundles. A safe dissection area is the midline. A radiographic template is cut to the dimensions of the frontal sinus or, preferably, computer-assisted imaging is used to identify the outline of the frontal sinus. The periosteum is incised a few millimeters outside the template and elevated 2 mm on either side. Low-profile miniplates are drilled and then removed. An oscillating saw is used to make a 2-mm vertical trough and then the saw is beveled toward the sinus until entry into the frontal sinus is achieved. The vertical cuts at the supraorbital rim can be completed with an osteotome if desired and a horizontal saw cut can be made in the midline above the root of the nose to make it easier to fracture the sinus in this region. If obliteration is planned, all mucosa is removed by both Freer elevation and drilling the entire bony surface under magnification with the operating microscope to ensure complete mucosal removal. If possible, obliteration is avoided and a wide opening is made into the nasal cavity. This combined above and below approach involves combining a classic Draf III procedure from below with the osteoplastic flap. Typically, the transnasal endoscopic procedure is performed initially and, if it is clear that all the disease cannot be removed, the external approach is performed. For reconstruction at the end of the procedure, the bone flap is then replaced and miniplates reapplied. The wound is closed with the use of 2-0 Vicryl sutures in an interrupted fashion. This layer must incorporate the galea aponeurosis. The skin is closed with staples. Suction drains are placed for 24 hours. Staple removal is done at 10 days.

SUMMARY

Revision sinus surgery for the treatment of inflammatory disease has been revolutionized with the advent of endoscopic sinus surgery. Clinical trials have shown statistically significant positive outcome data for both patient symptoms and quality of life, as well as improvements in objective findings on postoperative nasal endoscopy and CT imaging for patients undergoing RESS.[18] Overall success rates have ranged from 50% to 90.9% as reported in literature, with many studies showing comparable results with that of primary FESS.[5,14] In only select cases is open surgery required. The keys to successful revision surgery are adjunctive medical management, aggressive postoperative debridement, mucosal preservation, and removal of osteitic bone. It is also important for both the physician and patient to understand the underlying disease process and comorbid factors so that anticipated postoperative outcomes can be met with realistic expectations.

REFERENCES

1. Pleis JR, Lucas JW. Summary health statistics for U.S. adults: National Health Interview Survey, 2007. Vital Health Stat 10 2009;(240):1–159.
2. Ahmed J, Pal S, Hopkins C, et al. Functional endoscopic balloon dilation of sinus ostia for chronic rhinosinusitis. Cochrane Database Syst Rev 2011;7:CD008515.
3. Senior BA, Kennedy DW, Tanabodee J, et al. Long-term results of functional endoscopic sinus surgery. Laryngoscope 1998;108(2):151–7.
4. Palmer JN, Kennedy DW. Revision endoscopic sinus surgery. Philadelphia: Elsevier Mosby; 2005.
5. Lazar RH, Younis RT, Long TE, et al. Revision functional endonasal sinus surgery. Ear Nose Throat J 1992;71(3):131–3.
6. Bhattacharyya N. Clinical outcomes after revision endoscopic sinus surgery. Arch Otolaryngol Head Neck Surg 2004;130(8):975–8.
7. Lawson W. The intranasal ethmoidectomy - an experience with 1,077 procedures. Laryngoscope 1991; 101(4):367–71.
8. Kennedy DW. Prognostic factors, outcomes and staging in ethmoid sinus surgery. Laryngoscope 1992;102(12 Pt 2 Suppl 57):1–18.
9. Mendelsohn D, Jeremic G, Wright ED, et al. Revision rates after endoscopic sinus surgery: a recurrence analysis. Ann Otol Rhinol Laryngol 2011;120(3):162–6.
10. Khalil HS, Eweiss AZ, Clifton N. Radiological findings in patients undergoing revision endoscopic sinus surgery: a retrospective case series study. BMC Ear Nose Throat Disord 2011;11:4.
11. Weber R, Draf W, Kratzsch B, et al. Modern concepts of frontal sinus surgery. Laryngoscope 2001;111(1):137–46.
12. Stammberger H. "Uncapping the Egg" the endoscopic approach to frontal recess and sinuses. Tuttlingen (Germany): Karl Storz; 2004. p. 15–7.
13. Kuhn FA, Bolger WE, Tisdahl RG. The agger nasi cell in frontal recess obstruction: an anatomic, radiologic and clinical correlation. Operat Tech Otolaryngol Head Neck Surg 1991;2:226–31.
14. Moses RL, Cornetta A, Atkins JP Jr, et al. Revision endoscopic sinus surgery: the Thomas Jefferson University experience. Ear Nose Throat J 1998; 77(3):190, 193–195, 199–202.
15. Bailey BJ, Calhoun KH, Friedman NR, et al. Atlas of head and neck surgery-otolaryngology. 2nd edition. Philadelphia: Lippincott Williams & Wilkins; 2001. p. 918–20.
16. Kennedy DW. Diseases of the sinuses diagnosis and management. Hamilton (Ontario): BC Decker; 2001.
17. Reh DD, Melvin TA, Bolger WE, et al. The frontal intersinus septum takedown procedure: revisiting a technique for surgically refractory unilateral frontal sinus disease. Laryngoscope 2011;121(8):1805–9.
18. McMains KC, Kountakis SE. Revision functional endoscopic sinus surgery: objective and subjective surgical outcomes. Am J Rhinol 2005;19(4):344–7.

Removal of Parotid, Submandibular, and Sublingual Glands

Mohammed Nadershah, BDS*, Andrew Salama, MD, DDS

KEYWORDS

- Parotidectomy • Submandibular gland • Sublingual gland
- Facial nerve

PAROTID GLAND
Surgical Anatomy

The parotid gland is the largest of the paired major salivary glands. The anatomy and localization of the facial nerve is the most critical step in surgery of the parotid gland. The facial nerve is a mixed nerve carrying motor, sensory, and parasympathetic fibers; it has 5 intracranial segments and 1 extracranial segment. The motor fibers originate from the facial nucleus of the pons. The nerve enters the temporal bone through the internal acoustic meatus after being joined by the nervus intermedius. The nerve takes a labyrinthine course traveling anteriorly toward the geniculate ganglion. It travels posteriorly along the medial wall of the tympanic cavity toward the second genu at the oval window. Just before exiting the skull, the nerve divides to give rise to the posterior auricular nerve and motor branches to the posterior belly of the digastric and stylohyoid muscles. The last segment of the nerve exits the skull through the stylomastoid foramen and provides motor innervations for the muscles of facial expression.[1] The facial nerve divides the parotid gland into a larger superficial lobe and a smaller deep lobe. It then turns anterolaterally into the parotid gland and splits into 2 major branches. This division is an important surgical and anatomic landmark that is termed pes anserinus (Latin for goose's foot). It further branches into temporal, zygomatic, buccal, marginal mandibular, and cervical branches (**Fig. 1**). Davis and colleagues[2] studied 350

cervicofacial halves and described 6 different branching patterns without a common pattern. However, in all of the cadavers, the upper temporal and zygomatic branches were noted to be branches of the upper division of the facial nerves, whereas the marginal mandibular and the cervical branches were of the lower division. The buccal branch demonstrated the most anatomic variability and cross-innervation, with the highest number of cross-innervations occurring between the zygomatic and buccal branches.[3] All muscles of facial expression receive motor innervations from the facial nerve on their deep surface except for the mentalis, buccinator, and levator anguli oris.

The parotid duct, also known as the Stensen duct, runs 13 mm inferior and parallel to the zygomatic arch. The parotid duct is 4 to 6 cm in length and 5 mm in diameter. It exits the gland from its anteromedial surface and travels superficial to the masseter muscle. The duct turns medially at the anterior border of the muscle through the buccinator muscle to empty into the oral cavity. The orifice into the oral cavity, the parotid papilla, is typically buccal to the upper second molar. Accessory parotid glands are found overlying the masseter muscle in nearly 20% of patients. This finding is clinically significant, as a tumor may arise in the accessory gland and present as a mass anterior to the main parotid gland.[4]

The secretory parasympathetic innervation originates from the inferior salivatory nucleus, and the efferent fibers travel through the glossopharyngeal nerve. The superior cervical ganglion supplies

The authors have nothing to disclose.

Department of Oral and Maxillofacial Surgery, Boston Medical Center, Boston University, 850 Harrison Avenue, 5th Floor, Boston, MA 02118, USA

* Corresponding author.

E-mail address: mnadershah@gmail.com

Oral Maxillofacial Surg Clin N Am 24 (2012) 295–305

doi:10.1016/j.coms.2012.01.005

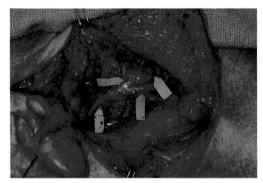

Fig. 1. Facial nerve branches during a superficial parotidectomy procedure (*blue arrows*).

the sympathetic innervation. A terminal branch of the external carotid artery, namely the transverse facial artery, provides the gland's arterial blood supply. The venous return is through the retromandibular vein, which drains into both the external and internal jugular veins. The lymphatic drainage of the parotid glands is rich and complex. Intraparenchymal lymph nodes receive drainage from the ears, soft palate, and posterior nasopharynx. Periparotid lymph nodes, superficial to the gland's capsule, serve as lymphatic basins for the scalp, the auricle, and the temporal region. Both of these systems drain into the superficial and deep cervical lymphatic chains.[4]

MANAGEMENT OF A PAROTID SWELLING

A parotid swelling or mass warrants a thorough history and physical examination to help elucidate the cause. Diagnostic tools include fine-needle aspiration, ultrasonography, computed tomography (CT), magnetic resonance imaging (MRI) (**Fig. 2**), and sialography (**Fig. 3**). Parotid swellings can be categorized into inflammatory, obstructive, autoimmune, or pathologic origin.

Inflammatory or infectious disorders, including viral or bacterial sialadenitis, are typically associated with fever, tenderness, and a rapid clinical course. Chronic or recurrent infectious sialadenitis is characterized by multiple bouts of acute exacerbations with clinically quiescent phases. Management of acute bacterial sialadenitis involves adequate hydration, antibiotics, and medical supportive treatment. Chronic refractory sialadenitis may be managed with a superficial parotidectomy (SP).

Obstructive sialadenitis is typically associated with postprandial pain and swelling. It is most commonly caused by sialoliths (66%).[5] Sialoliths, however, are more common in submandibular glands (80%–90%); the parotid gland is involved

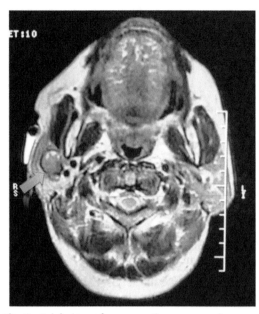

Fig. 2. Axial view of a magnetic resonance image at the midparotid level. The arrow points to a deep-lobe lesion of the right parotid gland.

in only 5% to 10% of cases. Sublingual sialoliths are uncommon (0%–5%).[6] Initial conservative treatment includes adequate hydration, sialogogues, and anti-inflammatory medications. If conservative measures fail, surgical options are considered, including intraoral sialolithectomy if the stone is located distally in the duct, sialadenectomy and, introduced more recently, sialoendoscopy.[7] Transparotid stone retrieval is a surgical option but requires dissection of the nerve and isolation of the duct, which may be complicated in the setting of recalcitrant obstruction and infection.

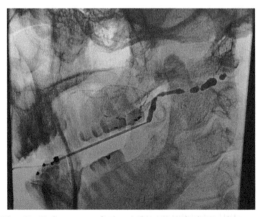

Fig. 3. Sialogram of the left parotid duct, demonstrating a sausage-like appearance caused by multiple strictures resulting from chronic sialadenitis.

Autoimmune diseases should be included in the differential diagnosis of a parotid swelling. Primary Sjögren syndrome is a chronic autoimmune disease affecting the salivary and lacrimal glands, which often presents with bilateral parotid swelling associated with dry mouth and dry eyes. Secondary Sjögren syndrome is associated with other systemic autoimmune disorders such as lupus erythematosus and scleroderma,[8] and is more common in women in the fourth or fifth decades of life.[9] Objective diagnostic criteria as established by the European Study Group include ocular symptoms, oral symptoms, evidence of keratoconjunctivitis sicca, focal sialadenitis identified by biopsy of minor salivary glands, instrumental evidence of involvement of salivary glands, and the presence of autoantibodies. The application of this system showed high specificity (97.5%) and sensitivity (94.2%) for diagnosing primary Sjögren syndrome.[10]

Eighty percent of major tumors of the salivary glands arise in the parotid glands, 80% of which are benign and approximately 80% of which are located in the superficial lobe.[11] Clinical signs suggestive of malignancy include weakness of the facial nerve, rapid tumor doubling time/growth rate, pain, and cervical lymphadenopathy. Complete or partial weakness of the facial nerve is always associated with an infiltrating malignancy.[12,13] A slow-growing tumor pattern does not necessarily exclude a malignant tumor. Fine-needle aspiration cytology (FNAC) is a useful minimally invasive technique for evaluation of a parotid or neck mass. FNAC has high sensitivity (73%–86.6%) and high specificity (97% for benign vs 85% for malignant). However, it is operator sensitive, with the most frequent error being false-negative results caused by inadequate sampling technique.[14]

An open parotid biopsy is generally not advocated because of the risk of tumor seeding. SP has served as the conventional therapeutic and diagnostic modality. SP is also indicated for a suspected metastasis to parotid lymph nodes, which may arise regionally from a cancer of the nose, sinus, regional skin, and oropharynx, or rarely from a distant site. Although intraparotid lymph nodes are generally confined to the superficial lobe, a total parotidectomy should be considered for grossly metastatic disease to the parotid bed. More recently, extracapsular dissection (ECD) has proved to be a viable alternative to SP in the treatment of benign tumors of the parotid gland. ECD entails leaving about 2 to 3 mm of loose areolar tissues around the tumor's capsule (without exposure of the facial nerve) in contrast to enucleation, which has a high recurrence rate

(20%–45%).[15] McGurk and colleagues[16] reviewed 821 patients with parotid tumors and divided them, based on clinical examination only, into simple (discrete, smaller than 4 cm, mobile, n = 662) and complex (deep, fixed, facial palsy, larger than 4 cm, n = 159). Patients in the simple group were treated using extracapsular dissection (n = 503) or SP (n = 159). Only 32 patients (5%) of the simple group were found to have a malignancy (SP = 20, ECD = 12). However, the 5-year and 10-year cancer-specific survival rates were not statistically different (SP = 98%, ECD = 100%). Moreover, the ECD group showed significantly lower morbidity (transient palsy of facial nerve, Frey syndrome, and amputation neuroma).[16] Another alternative to SP is partial superficial parotidectomy (PSP) or function-preserving parotidectomy, in which only the tumor-bearing area of the parotid parenchyma is removed after the dissection and preservation of the main trunk and adjacent branches of the facial nerve. Roh and colleagues[17] conducted a randomized clinical trial to compare conventional SP or total parotidectomy with PSP for benign parotid tumors. The investigators concluded that PSP results in improved cosmetic, sensory, and salivary functions without compromising local disease control.

Surgical Technique

Parotid surgery presents special challenges to the surgeon, because most of the tumors removed are benign and patients commonly expect complete function of the facial nerve after surgery. The surgery may be further complicated by other factors including previous irradiation, infection, and previous surgery. Tumor size and the special relationship of the tumor to the facial nerve may also increase the complexity of parotid surgery. The importance of understanding the surgical anatomy of the facial nerve cannot be overemphasized.[18]

Beahrs[19] described the surgical technique that is still most commonly used today. The aim of surgery is to safely remove the tumor with normal adjacent parotid tissue margins while preserving the function of the facial nerve provided there is no direct nerve involvement. Guntinas-Lichius and colleagues[20] found that temporary weakness of the facial nerve was associated with older age (>70 years), larger tumors (>70 cm^3), and longer surgeries (>260 minutes), whereas permanent injury of the facial nerve was associated with revision parotid surgery. The incidence of temporary injury of the facial nerve ranges from 18% to 40%, whereas the incidence of permanent injury ranges from 2% to 4%.[20–22] The value of continuous operative monitoring of the facial nerve using a nerve integrity monitor (NIM) has been questioned. Deneuve and colleagues[23] found no significant difference in the occurrence of disorders of the facial nerve with or without the use of the NIM. Although prednisone was shown to be effective for treating Bell palsy,[24,25] postoperative prednisone did not improve the rate of recovery from injury to the facial nerve.[26]

The surgery is typically performed under general anesthesia with oral intubation. The endotracheal tube should be secured to the opposite side with the patient's head rotated laterally toward the contralateral shoulder. The skin should be prepared and draped to expose the ears, the corner of the mouth, the lateral canthus, and the neck to allow for observation of facial twitching during the dissection. A reverse Trendelenburg position aids in minimizing blood loss.

The modified Blair incision is commonly used for routine parotid surgery. The incision should follow the crease just anterior to tragus and curve gently below the ear lobule before it becomes almost horizontal in the upper neck about 2 cm below the mandibular angle, preferably along a skin crease. The incision in the preauricular region may be modified to endaural design to conceal scarring. Cross-hatching the incision with a blade or using intradermal dye markings may aid in alignment of the incision during closure. The dissection is carried through the subcutaneous tissues to the parotid fascia while avoiding entering the gland or the tumor mass. The assistant should exert a constant upward and anterior traction of the skin flap while the surgeon maintains countertraction in a posterior direction. The flap may be raised to the anterior border of the parotid gland by creating tunnels parallel to the course of the branches of the facial nerve. At this point, only blunt dissection should be done and the masseter muscle fascia should be identified. Failure to dissect beyond the gland anteriorly will make it difficult to remove the gland later on. The tail of the parotid and the key inferior landmarks are then exposed by identifying the sternocleidomastoid muscle (SCM). The fascia overlying the muscle provides a safe plane to elevate the tail of the gland. The greater auricular nerve (GAN) and the external jugular vein (EJV) will be encountered. Some surgeons advise against ligating the EJV early in the dissection to avoid edema and venous congestion in the gland.

The GAN is a sensory nerve that provides sensation to the skin overlying the parotid gland, the mastoid area, and the pinna of the ear. The GAN travels deep to the SCM, then turns and runs along its superficial surface before entering the inferior surface of the parotid. This nerve is divided as close to the gland as possible in an attempt to save sensory branches if possible, and to serve as a potential nerve graft if needed. Preserving the posterior branch of the GAN may result in less sensory loss.[27] Next, the posterior border is dissected off the cartilaginous ear canal down to the level of the cartilaginous pointer. The posterior belly of the digastric muscle must be dissected and identified.

In 1940, Janes was the first surgeon to describe the identification of the facial nerve trunk (FNT).[28,29] Multiple anatomic landmarks have been described for identifying the location of the FNT. The posterior digastric muscle was studied as a potential landmark and the FNT and was found, on average, to be 4.5 mm anterocranial to its superior border.[29,30] In a cadaveric study, Holt[31] found that the mean distance from the stylomastoid foramen to the digastric muscle was 9 mm. Because of its great variability, the posterior digastric muscle is not always a reliable landmark, which can be explained by the effect of retraction during surgery, change in neck positioning, or tissue contracture in cadaveric studies.

The tragal pointer is another landmark that has been studied. The FNT is 1 to 2 cm deeper than the tragal pointer.[29,30] In a radiographic study using CT and MRI, The FNT was found to be 1 to 1.5 cm caudal to the pointer.[32] However, it has the disadvantages of being blunt, difficult to localize, asymmetric, and sometimes irregular.[33]

Bony landmarks are generally considered to be more reliable because they are not affected by retraction. The tympanomastoid fissure has been considered one of the best anatomic landmarks because of its invariable relation to the FNT.[29,33–35] De Ru and colleagues[29] found the average distance from tympanomastoid fissure to the FNT to be 2.7 mm. The styloid bone is a deeper bony landmark, and exposure of this landmark may result in injury to the FNT.[19,36] In addition, it may be absent in about one-third of the population.[2] Careful identification of the FNT is indicated by twitching in facial muscles and is confirmed by the division into temporofacial and cervicofacial main trunks, also known as the pes anserinus. The posterior auricular artery or one of its branches runs in close proximity to the main FNT, and should not be ligated until identification of the facial nerve is confirmed.

The retrograde approach to identify the facial nerve by tracing its distal branches proximally has been advocated.[37] A disadvantage of this method is increased surgical time, especially if the tumor is large enough to distort the position of the branches of the facial nerve.[33] However, other studies have shown no significant difference in the surgical time and effectiveness of tumor excision, in addition to the potential advantage of removing less normal parotid tissue with this technique.[38,39]

Dissection of the tumor-bearing portion of the gland follows identification of the FNT, which should be confirmed with a nerve stimulator. For superficial tumors the gland is elevated anteriorly with gentle traction of the tumor. A fine-tipped instrument such as a McCabe dissector may be used for fine dissection of the parotid tissues. Meticulous hemostasis can be achieved with bipolar cautery or a Harmonic scalpel. Several submillimeter arteries that follow the FNT can be a source of great frustration. Following the linear path of the nerve with particular attention to the branches and branch points will ensure a complete and safe plane for tumor extirpation. Deep-lobe tumors pose a surgical dilemma, as one must weigh the balance of adequate retraction and tumor margins. Deep-lobe tumors may often not be appreciated until surgery, whereupon the nerve is identified with the tumor lying beneath the trunk (**Fig. 4**). Distal dissection of the nerve will facilitate elevation and mobilization of the branches. Delicate circumferential dissection is then performed, with careful attention to the deep structures including the terminal branches of the external carotid artery. Identification of larger deep-lobe tumors with parapharyngeal infiltration can be revealed by MRI. Often, deep-lobe or dumbbell tumors can be manually dissected by light finger dissection. Malignant tumors of the deep lobe may require a mandibulotomy or mandibular splitting technique for safe oncologic margins. Additional access may be afforded by dividing the digastric muscle and/or dislocating the mandible anteriorly.

FREY SYNDROME

One of the most common late complications following parotidectomy is Frey syndrome, also known as the auriculotemporal nerve syndrome or gustatory sweating. Baillarger[40] first described the condition in 1853 after draining a parotid abscess in 2 patients. In 1923, Lucja Frey[41] was able to relate the gustatory sweating to the auriculotemporal nerve. However, the pathophysiology of the condition was explained by Thomas[42] in 1927. He postulated that the postganglionic parasympathetic fibers originating from the otic ganglion undergo aberrant regeneration and supply the sweat glands in the skin, resulting in production of sweat and erythema of the skin during eating.

The latent time required for the development of this condition has been reported to vary between 2 weeks and 2 years in most cases, although there is a case report of development of this syndrome after more than 8 years postoperatively.[43] The self-reported subjective incidence of Frey syndrome after parotidectomy is about 10%. However, when patients are asked about the symptoms this figure increases to about 40%.[44] Objective evaluation is inconsistent in the literature. Minor[45] described an iodine-starch test to facilitate clinical diagnosis. Unfortunately, there is no universally accepted classification for the severity of this syndrome. However, there have been some attempts at classification through subjective questionnaires (eg, social embarrassment, frequency of wiping, intensity, smell of sweat).[46–49]

Probably the best way to prevent or mitigate Frey syndrome is to minimize exposure of the parotid wound bed, by performing a partial parotidectomy when appropriate.[50] There is an increased incidence of gustatory sweating with thinner skin flaps.[51] Moreover, postoperative radiation decreased the incidence of this syndrome.[52] The placement of different barriers to prevent aberrant regeneration has been described, including temporoparietal fascia flap,[47] superficial musculoaponeurotic system (SMAS),[53] SCM flap,[52,54] lyophilized dura, polyglactin, expanded polytetraflouroethylene,[55] and acellular dermis.[56]

Medical and surgical options are available for the treatment of Frey syndrome. Medical treatment includes topical anticholinergic medications[57] and injection of botulinum toxin A.[48] Surgical options include reelevation of the skin flap with placement of a barrier[58] and tympanic neurectomy.[59]

SIALOCELE

Sialocele is a discrete subcutaneous salivary collection that accumulates after parotidectomy or trauma of the parotid gland. Sialocele typically

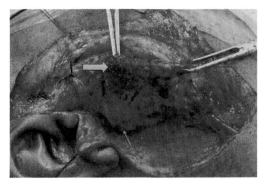

Fig. 4. Parotid deep-lobe tumor (*large arrow*) is dissected from underneath the facial nerve (*small arrow*).

starts within the first week of the surgery and often resolves within a month. Clinically it presents as a nontender fluctuance at the angle of the mandible. The incidence after parotidectomy varies from 6% to 40%.[60–62] Treatment options include observation, needle aspiration, and pressure dressing. Botulinum toxin A may also used to treat sialoceles. The incidence may be lower if the drain is left for a longer period of time, especially with a PSP, for which there is more normal saliva-producing tissue than in the case of a total SP.[62]

SUBMANDIBULAR GLAND
Surgical Anatomy

The submandibular gland (SMG) occupies the triangle formed by the mandible and the anterior and posterior bellies of the digastric muscle. The mylohyoid muscle divides the gland into a smaller anterior part and a larger posterior part connected at the posterior free edge of the muscle. The SMG duct, also known as the Wharton duct, originates from the anterior surface of the gland and travels 5 cm anteriorly before it drains into the oral cavity just lateral to the lingual frenum (**Fig. 5**). The lingual nerve carries sensory innervations to the anterior

two-thirds of the tongue and parasympathetic fibers to the SMG. It courses in a lateral to medial direction, double-crossing the Wharton duct first by passing below the nerve then by crossing it medially (**Fig. 6**). The motor function of the tongue is controlled by the hypoglossal nerve, which is inferior and medial to the posterior third of the SMG just below the posterior belly of the digastric muscle.[63] Another vital surgical landmark is the marginal branch of the facial nerve. This nerve runs in a subplatysmal plane within the superficial layer of the deep cervical fascia, which is continuous with the SMG capsule. Subfascial dissection allows for a safe plane of dissection. The vascular supply to the gland is provided by the facial artery and vein. It is critical to remember that the facial nerve is always superficial to the facial vein.

Surgical Technique

There are many surgical approaches described in the literature for the surgical excision of the SMG. Open approaches include lateral transcervical, transoral, submental, and retroauricular approaches. The endoscopic approach is classified as either an endoscopic-assisted technique or a completely endoscopic robot-assisted technique. Each one of these approaches has advantages and disadvantages. However, the lateral transcervical approach remains the most popular technique.[64]

The lateral transcervical approach is a familiar technique to most surgeons and allows for removal of larger masses via direct and easy access. However, its disadvantages include

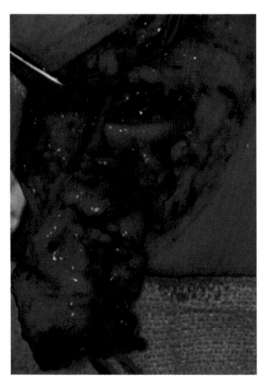

Fig. 5. The submandibular duct is still attached just before completion of the excision of the submandibular gland.

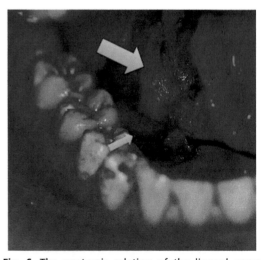

Fig. 6. The anatomic relation of the lingual nerve (*large arrow*) to the submandibular duct (*small arrow*) is demonstrated after the excision of a simple ranula and the sublingual gland involved.

a visible scar and a risk of injury to the facial, lingual, and hypoglossal nerves. The incision is placed 1.5 to 2 cm below the inferior border of the mandible in a skin crease. The dissection extends deep to the platysma. The platysma should be divided and the superficial layer of the deep cervical fascia identified. Large or extra-glandular tumors may require leaving a segment of platysma over the gland to avoid tumor spillage. The marginal mandibular nerve is identified and protected. To decrease the chance of nerve injury, the facial vein at the inferior border of the gland should be ligated and retracted superiorly with fascia covering the gland (Hayes-Martin maneuver). The facial artery or its branches to the gland must be ligated. Several approaches to the gland may then used, however, the authors favor the inferior approach. The lower aspect of the gland is raised in a cephalad direction and the digastric tendon is identified. The dissection is carried in a superior and medial direction, and the mylohyoid muscle must be retracted to allow exposure of the small anterior part of the SMG. At this point, the lingual nerve is identified with the attached submandibular ganglion. The fibers extending from the ganglion to the gland are released. The hypoglossal nerve may be identified and protected. The SMG duct is ligated as close as possible to its opening into the oral cavity. A drain may be placed and the incision is closed in layers. Complications of SMG excision using this approach include hematoma formation (2%–10%), infection (2%–9%), formation of a fistula (1%–3%), marginal mandibular nerve injury (7.7%–36%), hypoglossal nerve injury (0%–7%), and lingual nerve injury (0%–22.5%).[64–70]

The submental approach is carried through a horizontal incision in the midline at the level of the hyoid bone in a skin crease, thus allowing direct access to the SMG from its anterior aspect. Roh[71] compared this technique with the traditional lateral transcervical approach and found no difference in nerve injury, operative time, incision length, and hospital stay. However, patients had higher satisfaction with the submental approach because the scar is concealed. Chen and colleagues[72] described an endoscopic-assisted submental approach that allows for a smaller incision.

Roh[73] also described the use of a retroauricular hairline incision (RAHI) for removal of an upper neck mass and compared this approach with the traditional lateral transcervical approach.[74] He concluded that the RAHI had comparable rates of complications but higher patient satisfaction because of the hidden scar. However, care must be taken with this approach to avoid injuring hair follicles and the GAN.

The transoral excision of the SMG was first described by Downton and Qvist[75] in 1960, and was reintroduced by Hong and Kim.[76] It has the advantage of avoiding skin scars and has a lower chance of injuring the marginal mandibular nerve. Hong and Yang[77] reported a temporary change in tongue sensation in 74% and temporary limitation in tongue movement in 70.1%, which resolved spontaneously in all patients. Weber and colleagues[78] reported their experience with this technique. The investigators found a temporary change in tongue sensation in 43% of the patients, which resolved in 2 months. None of the patients experienced any restriction of tongue movement. Endoscopic-assisted transoral surgery may provide better visualization and illumination of the surgical landmarks, but has the disadvantages of increased cost, increased surgical time, and a steep learning curve.[63,64]

More recently, Monfared and colleagues[79] used a porcine model to report endoscopic excision of the SMG using CO_2 insufflation. An operative pocket was created using balloon dissection and was maintained using low-pressure (maximum 4 mm Hg) CO_2 insufflation. Terris and colleagues[80] used a cadaveric model to compare the endoscopic technique with the robot-assisted endoscopic technique, and concluded that the latter offers three-dimensional visualization and better surgical instrumentation in areas difficult to access. The time needed for setup of the robot was offset by the shorter operative time. Further clinical studies are needed to validate the efficiency of this technique.

SUBLINGUAL GLAND
Surgical Anatomy

The sublingual glands (SLG) are the smallest pair of the major salivary glands. The almond-shaped SLG is located above the mylohyoid muscle in the space between the mandible and the genioglossus muscles, just below the oral mucosa. Unlike the other major salivary glands, it lacks a true fascial capsule. It drains into the oral cavity through approximately 10 ducts, known as the ducts of Rivinus. Occasionally some of the anterior ducts may collect into a larger common duct, known as the Bartholin duct, which empties into the Wharton duct.

The sympathetic innervation to the SLG is derived from paravascular nerves along the facial artery; the parasympathetic supply comes from the submandibular ganglion via the lingual nerve. The arterial supply comes from the sublingual artery (branch of the lingual artery) and the submental artery (branch of the facial artery), with the venous drainage reflecting the arterial supply.

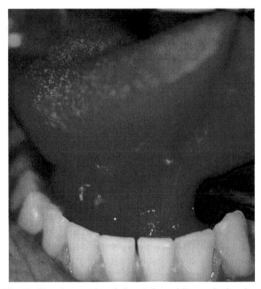

Fig. 7. Simple ranula of the right sublingual gland.

The lymphatics of the SLG drain into the submandibular lymph nodes.

ORAL RANULA

One of the most common indications for the removal of the SLG is for the treatment of a ranula. A ranula is a result of the phenomena known as mucus retention and mucus extravasation. A ranula is classified as simple (**Fig. 7**), which is limited to the oral cavity, or plunging, which extends through the mylohyoid muscles into the neck (**Fig. 8**). The treatment options include observation,[81,82] sclerotherapy (OK-432),[83] marsupialization,[84] and resection of the ipsilateral SLG along with the ranula.[85,86] The best treatment approach remains controversial. However, the high recurrence rate after marsupialization (about 67%) makes it a less appealing option compared with resection of the SLG along with the ranula (1.2%).[86] There have been some reports considering the ranula as an oral manifestation of human immunodeficiency virus infection and sometimes as the only presentation of the disease.[87–89] The procedure may be performed under local anesthesia but our preference is to use general anesthesia. A shoulder roll is placed and a nasal endotracheal tube is used. Ranulas may present at various stages, but are more easily manipulated when they are decompressed. A linear incision is made 1 cm medial to and parallel to the ipsilateral mandible. The mucosa is incised and bipolar cautery is used obtain hemostasis. Blunt dissection with peanut gauze dissectors is used to identify the superior aspect of the gland. Cannulation of the Wharton duct may help to identify critical landmarks including the lingual nerve. The medial aspect gland is dissected and the lingual nerve identified. Gentle lateral retraction of the gland will expose the relationship of the lingual nerve and the Wharton duct. The gland is dissected from the floor of the mouth anteriorly using blunt dissection. The posterior lateral dissection is completed last, and although a true capsule does not exist, a clean plane of dissection is achievable. Meticulous hemostasis should be achieved to prevent a floor-of-mouth hematoma, which may cause airway obstruction in severe cases.

SUMMARY

Removal of the major salivary glands is the treatment of choice for many pathologic conditions. Understanding the regional surgical anatomy is

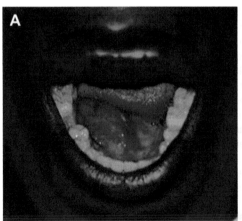
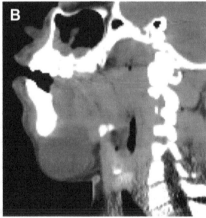

Fig. 8. (A) Intraoral view of a right plunging ranula. (B) Sagittal view of the patient's CT scan showing the extension of the ranula below the mylohyoid muscle.

of utmost importance for the surgeon involved in treating these conditions. Parotidectomy requires a high level of attention to detail. Treatment-planning decisions should be made based on the underlying nature of the abnormality. The surgical approach centers on safe identification of the facial nerve. Removal of the submandibular and sublingual glands is straightforward, and requires an in-depth understanding of the anatomy of the floor of the mouth and level Ib of the neck.

REFERENCES

1. Greywoode JD, Ho HH, Artz GJ, et al. Management of traumatic facial nerve injuries. Facial Plast Surg 2010;26(6):511–8.
2. Davis RA, Anson BJ, Budinger JM, et al. Surgical anatomy of the facial nerve and parotid gland based upon a study of 350 cervicofacial halves. Surg Gynecol Obstet 1956;102(4):385–412.
3. Gosain AK. Surgical anatomy of the facial nerve. Clin Plast Surg 1995;22(2):241–51.
4. Hsu AK, Kutler DI. Indications, techniques, and complications of major salivary gland extirpation. Oral Maxillofac Surg Clin North Am 2009;21(3): 313–21.
5. Marchal F, Dulguerov P, Becker M, et al. Specificity of parotid sialoendoscopy. Laryngoscope 2001; 111(2):264–71.
6. Bodner L. Salivary gland calculi: diagnostic imaging and surgical management. Compendium 1993; 14(5):572, 574–6, 578 passim; quiz: 586.
7. Maresh A, Kutler DI, Kacker A. Sialoendoscopy in the diagnosis and management of obstructive sialadenitis. Laryngoscope 2011;121(3):495–500.
8. Moutsopoulos HM, Zerva LV. Anti-Ro (SSA)/La (SSB) antibodies and Sjögren's syndrome. Clin Rheumatol 1990;9(1 Suppl 1):123–30.
9. Mandel L, Surattanont F. Bilateral parotid swelling: a review. Oral Surg Oral Med Oral Pathol Oral Radiol Endod 2002;93(3):221–37.
10. Vitali C, Bombardieri S, Moutsopoulos HM, et al. Assessment of the European classification criteria for Sjögren's syndrome in a series of clinically defined cases: results of a prospective multicentre study. The European Study Group on Diagnostic Criteria for Sjögren's Syndrome. Ann Rheum Dis 1996;55(2):116–21.
11. Guzzo M, Locati LD, Prott FJ, et al. Major and minor salivary gland tumors. Crit Rev Oncol Hematol 2010; 74(2):134–48.
12. Hocwald E, Korkmaz H, Yoo GH, et al. Prognostic factors in major salivary gland cancer. Laryngoscope 2001;111(8):1434–9.
13. Lima RA, Tavares MR, Dias FL, et al. Clinical prognostic factors in malignant parotid gland tumors. Otolaryngol Head Neck Surg 2005;133(5):702–8.
14. Riley N, Allison R, Stevenson S. Fine-needle aspiration cytology in parotid masses: our experience in Canterbury, New Zealand. ANZ J Surg 2005;75(3): 144–6.
15. Leverstein H, van der Wal JE, Tiwari RM, et al. Surgical management of 246 previously untreated pleomorphic adenomas of the parotid gland. Br J Surg 1997;84(3):399–403.
16. McGurk M, Thomas BL, Renehan AG. Extracapsular dissection for clinically benign parotid lumps: reduced morbidity without oncological compromise. Br J Cancer 2003;89(9):1610–3.
17. Roh JL, Kim HS, Park CI. Randomized clinical trial comparing partial parotidectomy versus superficial or total parotidectomy. Br J Surg 2007;94(9):1081–7.
18. Beahrs OH, Adson MA. The surgical anatomy and technic of parotidectomy. Am J Surg 1958;95(6): 885–96.
19. Beahrs OH. The surgical anatomy and technique of parotidectomy. Surg Clin North Am 1977;57(3): 477–93.
20. Guntinas-Lichius O, Gabriel B, Klussmann JP. Risk of facial palsy and severe Frey's syndrome after conservative parotidectomy for benign disease: analysis of 610 operations. Acta Otolaryngol 2006; 126(10):1104–9.
21. Yuan X, Gao Z, Jiang H, et al. Predictors of facial palsy after surgery for benign parotid disease: multivariate analysis of 626 operations. Head Neck 2009; 31(12):1588–92.
22. Koch M, Zenk J, Iro H. Long-term results of morbidity after parotid gland surgery in benign disease. Laryngoscope 2010;120(4):724–30.
23. Deneuve S, Quesnel S, Depondt J, et al. Management of parotid gland surgery in a university teaching hospital. Eur Arch Otorhinolaryngol 2010; 267(4):601–5.
24. Sullivan FM, Swan IR, Donnan PT, et al. Early treatment with prednisolone or acyclovir in Bell's palsy. N Engl J Med 2007;357(16):1598–607.
25. Hato N, Yamada H, Kohno H, et al. Valacyclovir and prednisolone treatment for Bell's palsy: a multicenter, randomized, placebo-controlled study. Otol Neurotol 2007;28(3):408–13.
26. Roh JL, Park CI. A prospective, randomized trial for use of prednisolone in patients with facial nerve paralysis after parotidectomy. Am J Surg 2008; 196(5):746–50.
27. Brown JS, Ord RA. Preserving the great auricular nerve in parotid surgery. Br J Oral Maxillofac Surg 1989;27(6):459–66.
28. Heeneman H. Identification of the facial nerve in parotid surgery. Can J Otolaryngol 1975;4(1): 145–51.
29. de Ru JA, van Benthem PP, Bleys RL, et al. Landmarks for parotid gland surgery. J Laryngol Otol 2001;115(2):122–5.

30. Reid AP. Surgical approach to the parotid gland. Ear Nose Throat J 1989;68(2):151–4.

31. Holt JJ. The stylomastoid area: anatomic-histologic study and surgical approach. Laryngoscope 1996; 106(4):396–400.

32. Casselman JW, Mancuso AA. Major salivary gland masses: comparison of MR imaging and CT. Radiology 1987;165(1):183–9.

33. Robertson MS, Blake P. A method of using the tympanomastoid fissure to find the facial nerve at parotidectomy. Aust N Z J Surg 1984;54(4):369–73.

34. Nishida M, Matsuura H. A landmark for facial nerve identification during parotid surgery. J Oral Maxillofac Surg 1993;51(4):451–3.

35. Lawson HH. Value of the tympanomastoid fissure in the exposure of the facial nerve. Br J Surg 1988; 75(4):309.

36. Hogg SP, Kratz RC. Surgical exposure of the facial nerve. AMA Arch Otolaryngol 1958;67(5):560–1.

37. Conley J. Search for and identification of the facial nerve. Laryngoscope 1978;88(1 Pt 1):172–5.

38. Scarpini M, Bonapasta SA, Ruperto M, et al. Retrograde parotidectomy for pleomorphic adenoma of the parotid gland: a conservative and effective approach. J Craniofac Surg 2009;20(3):967–9.

39. Emodi O, El-Naaj IA, Gordin A, et al. Superficial parotidectomy versus retrograde partial superficial parotidectomy in treating benign salivary gland tumor (pleomorphic adenoma). J Oral Maxillofac Surg 2010;68(9):2092–8.

40. Baillarger M. Mémoire sur l'oblitération du canal Sténon. Gazette Médicale de Paris 1853;23:194–7 [in French].

41. Frey L. Le syndrome du nerf auriculo-temporal. Rev Neurol 1923;2:97–104 [in French].

42. Thomas A. Le double réflexe vaso-dilatateur et sudoral de la face consecutive aux blessures de la loge parotidienne. Rev Neurol (Paris) 1927;1:447–60 [in French].

43. Malatskey S, Rabinovich I, Fradis M, et al. Frey syndrome—delayed clinical onset: a case report. Oral Surg Oral Med Oral Pathol Oral Radiol Endod 2002;94(3):338–40.

44. de Bree R, van der Waal I, Leemans CR. Management of Frey syndrome. Head Neck 2007;29(8): 773–8.

45. Minor V. Eines neues verfahren zu der klinisichen untersugung der schweissabsonderung. Dtsch Z Nervenheilkd 1928;101:258–61 [in German].

46. Hays LL. The Frey syndrome: a review and double blind evaluation of the topical use of a new anticholinergic agent. Laryngoscope 1978;88(11): 1796–824.

47. Ahmed OA, Kolhe PS. Prevention of Frey's syndrome and volume deficit after parotidectomy using the superficial temporal artery fascial flap. Br J Plast Surg 1999;52(4):256–60.

48. Beerens AJ, Snow GB. Botulinum toxin A in the treatment of patients with Frey syndrome. Br J Surg 2002;89(1):116–9.

49. Luna-Ortiz K, Sanson-RioFrio JA, Mosqueda-Taylor A. Frey syndrome. A proposal for evaluating severity. Oral Oncol 2004;40(5):501–5.

50. Witt RL. The significance of the margin in parotid surgery for pleomorphic adenoma. Laryngoscope 2002;112(12):2141–54.

51. Singleton GT, Cassisi NJ. Frey's syndrome: incidence related to skin flap thickness in parotidectomy. Laryngoscope 1980;90(10 Pt 1):1636–9.

52. Casler JD, Conley J. Sternocleidomastoid muscle transfer and superficial musculoaponeurotic system plication in the prevention of Frey's syndrome. Laryngoscope 1991;101(1 Pt 1):95–100.

53. Allison GR, Rappaport I. Prevention of Frey's syndrome with superficial musculoaponeurotic system interposition. Am J Surg 1993;166(4):407–10.

54. Filho WQ, Dedivitis RA, Rapoport A, et al. Sternocleidomastoid muscle flap preventing Frey syndrome following parotidectomy. World J Surg 2004;28(4): 361–4.

55. Dulguerov P, Quinodoz D, Cosendai G, et al. Prevention of Frey syndrome during parotidectomy. Arch Otolaryngol Head Neck Surg 1999;125(8):833–9.

56. Sinha UK, Saadat D, Doherty CM, et al. Use of AlloDerm implant to prevent Frey syndrome after parotidectomy. Arch Facial Plast Surg 2003;5(1): 109–12.

57. Bremerich A, Eufinger H, Rustemeyer J, et al. Frey syndrome. Mund Kiefer Gesichtschir 2001;5(1): 33–6 [in German].

58. MacKinnon C, Lovie M. An alternative treatment for Frey syndrome. Plast Reconstr Surg 1999;103(2): 745–6.

59. Hays LL, Novack AJ, Worsham JC. The Frey syndrome: a simple, effective treatment. Otolaryngol Head Neck Surg 1982;90(4):419–25.

60. Upton DC, McNamar JP, Connor NP, et al. Parotidectomy: ten-year review of 237 cases at a single institution. Otolaryngol Head Neck Surg 2007;136(5): 788–92.

61. Wax M, Tarshis L. Post-parotidectomy fistula. J Otolaryngol 1991;20(1):10–3.

62. Witt RL. The incidence and management of siaolocele after parotidectomy. Otolaryngol Head Neck Surg 2009;140(6):871–4.

63. Guerrissi JO, Taborda G. Endoscopic excision of the submandibular gland by an intraoral approach. J Craniofac Surg 2001;12(3):299–303.

64. Beahm DD, Peleaz L, Nuss DW, et al. Surgical approaches to the submandibular gland: a review of literature. Int J Surg 2009;7(6):503–9.

65. Preuss SF, Klussmann JP, Wittekindt C, et al. Submandibular gland excision: 15 years of experience. J Oral Maxillofac Surg 2007;65(5):953–7.

66. Torroni AA, Mustazza MC, Bartoli DD, et al. Transcervical submandibular sialoadenectomy. J Craniofac Surg 2007;18(3):613–21.

67. Milton CM, Thomas BM, Bickerton RC. Morbidity study of submandibular gland excision. Ann R Coll Surg Engl 1986;68(3):148–50.

68. Smith WP, Peters WJ, Markus AF. Submandibular gland surgery: an audit of clinical findings, pathology and postoperative morbidity. Ann R Coll Surg Engl 1993;75(3):164–7.

69. Berini-Aytes L, Gay-Escoda C. Morbidity associated with removal of the submandibular gland. J Craniomaxillofac Surg 1992;20(5):216–9.

70. Smith AD, Elahi MM, Kawamoto HK Jr, et al. Excision of the submandibular gland by an intraoral approach. Plast Reconstr Surg 2000;105(6):2092–5.

71. Roh JL. Removal of the submandibular gland by a submental approach: a prospective, randomized, controlled study. Oral Oncol 2008;44(3):295–300.

72. Chen MK, Su CC, Tsai YL, et al. Minimally invasive endoscopic resection of the submandibular gland: a new approach. Head Neck 2006;28(11):1014–7.

73. Roh JL. Retroauricular hairline incision for removal of upper neck masses. Laryngoscope 2005;115(12): 2161–6.

74. Roh JL. Removal of the submandibular gland by a retroauricular approach. Arch Otolaryngol Head Neck Surg 2006;132(7):783–7.

75. Downton D, Qvist G. Intra-oral excision of the submandibular gland. Proc R Soc Med 1960;53: 543–4.

76. Hong KH, Kim YK. Intraoral removal of the submandibular gland: a new surgical approach. Otolaryngol Head Neck Surg 2000;122(6):798–802.

77. Hong KH, Yang YS. Surgical results of the intraoral removal of the submandibular gland. Otolaryngol Head Neck Surg 2008;139(4):530–4.

78. Weber SM, Wax MK, Kim JH. Transoral excision of the submandibular gland. Otolaryngol Head Neck Surg 2007;137(2):343–5.

79. Monfared A, Saenz Y, Terris DJ. Endoscopic resection of the submandibular gland in a porcine model. Laryngoscope 2002;112(6):1089–93.

80. Terris DJ, Haus BM, Gourin CG, et al. Endo-robotic resection of the submandibular gland in a cadaver model. Head Neck 2005;27(11):946–51.

81. Mortellaro C, Dall'Oca S, Lucchina AG, et al. Sublingual ranula: a closer look to its surgical management. J Craniofac Surg 2008;19(1):286–90.

82. Pandit RT, Park AH. Management of pediatric ranula. Otolaryngol Head Neck Surg 2002;127(1):115–8.

83. Roh JL. Primary treatment of ranula with intracystic injection of OK-432. Laryngoscope 2006;116(2): 169–72.

84. Baurmash HD. Marsupialization for treatment of oral ranula: a second look at the procedure. J Oral Maxillofac Surg 1992;50(12):1274–9.

85. Seo JH, Park JJ, Kim HY, et al. Surgical management of intraoral ranulas in children: an analysis of 17 pediatric cases. Int J Pediatr Otorhinolaryngol 2010;74(2):202–5.

86. Zhao YF, Jia Y, Chen XM, et al. Clinical review of 580 ranulas. Oral Surg Oral Med Oral Pathol Oral Radiol Endod 2004;98(3):281–7.

87. Butt F, Chindia M, Kenyanya T, et al. An audit of ranulae occurring with the human immunodeficiency virus infection. J Oral Maxillofac Pathol 2010;14(1): 33–5.

88. Chokunonga E, Levy LM, Bassett MT, et al. Aids and cancer in Africa: the evolving epidemic in Zimbabwe. AIDS 1999;13(18):2583–8.

89. Syebele K, Butow KW. Oral mucoceles and ranulas may be part of initial manifestations of HIV infection. AIDS Res Hum Retroviruses 2010;26(10):1075–8.

An Update on Squamous Carcinoma of the Oral Cavity, Oropharynx, and Maxillary Sinus

Joshua E. Lubek, DDS, MD[a],*, Lewis Clayman, DMD, MD[b,c]

KEYWORDS

- Squamous carcinoma • Oral cavity • Oropharynx
- Maxillary sinus

There are more than 45,000 new cancer cases involving the head and neck diagnosed each year within the United States. Squamous cell carcinoma (SCC) accounts for the majority of cases, often occurring within the oral cavity and oropharynx. Overall 5-year survival rates (60%) have not changed dramatically over the past few decades.[1] New demographic patterns are also emerging with younger patients (less than age 45 years) and those patients without tobacco or alcohol abuse developing these cancers.[2,3]

The anatomic sites composing the oral cavity are the alveolar ridge/gingiva, retromolar pad, buccal mucosa, floor of mouth, hard palate, and anterior two-thirds of the tongue. Recent literature suggests that cancers of the buccal mucosa and the gingiva are more aggressive than previously thought.

The oropharynx is composed of the tongue base, soft palate, tonsils, and posterior pharyngeal wall. Cancers of the oropharynx typically present with advanced-stage disease due to its rich lymphatic system that facilitates early nodal spread, resulting in a high incidence of early nodal metastases. Current literature suggests a strong link between human papillomavirus (HPV) and oropharyngeal cancers leading to much debate

regarding treatment strategies involving these aggressive tumors.[2]

Improvements in technology have resulted in better imaging pretherapy and post-therapy, minimally invasive surgery, improved radiotherapy techniques, and reconstructive options. These advancements are leading to improvements in cancer treatment and quality of life.

This article reviews current literature and various controversial topics involving the diagnosis and treatment strategies for patients with oral cavity/oropharyngeal cancers. Although not considered cancer within the oral cavity, maxillary sinus SCC is discussed. The proximity to the oral cavity and late presentation often make it difficult for clinicians to establish primary origin (maxillary gingiva vs maxillary sinus).

HUMAN PAPILLOMAVIRUS

High-risk oncogenic HPV types (HPV-16 and HPV-18) have a significant role in the pathogenesis of oropharyngeal SCC. Various studies have demonstrated that 35% to 65% of oropharyngeal tumors contain high-risk HPV. This strong association is thought to result from the relationship

The authors have no financial interests to disclose.

[a] Maxillofacial Oncology/Microvascular Surgery, Department of Oral & Maxillofacial Surgery, University of Maryland, 650 West Baltimore Street, Baltimore, MD 21201, USA
[b] Oral & Maxillofacial Surgery, 2150 Appian Way, Suite 201, Pinole, CA 94564, USA
[c] Department of Otolaryngology–Head & Neck Surgery Wayne State University 5E UHC 4201 St Antoine, Detroit, MI 48201, USA
* Corresponding author.
E-mail address: jlubek@umaryland.edu

between the oropharyngeal mucosa and the mucosal-associated lymphoid tissue of the pharyngeal and lingual tonsils. The crypt-like tissue harbors persistent HPV infection leading to stable oncoprotein expression and carcinomatous transformation. This correlation has important implications because patients with HPV-associated oropharyngeal SCC have a better prognosis than do those with non–HPV-related tumors. The most recent National Comprehensive Cancer Network guidelines include HPV testing for oropharyngeal SCC. The difference in overall survival in patients with HPV-positive and HPV-negative carcinomas at nonoropharyngeal SCC sites has not been demonstrated. Prevention of HPV-positive oropharyngeal SCC with the HPV vaccination has not yet been demonstrated.[2,4]

The link between oral SCC and high-risk HPV is not as clearly defined. HPV identified within oral carcinomas is variable ranging from 4–80%. The majority of these studies used nonquantitative polymerase chain reaction (PCR) methods to detect HPV DNA, which lacks specificity for oncogenic infection. In a large multicenter trial of 766 oral cancers, HPV DNA was identified in only 4% of tumors.[5] Lopes and colleagues[6] screened 142 consecutive cases of oral SCC using both conventional PCR with consensus primers and type-specific quantitative PCR. The investigators demonstrated a low prevalence of high-risk HPV (2%) and concluded that there is little evidence to suggest that oral cavity SCC is associated with high-risk HPV and that routine testing of oral cancers for HPV could not be justified. One criticism of this article was the lack of stratification between young and old patients with oral SCC who had HPV isolated from the tumors. The prevalence of oral SCC in younger patients is increasing and HPV may be implicated as a causative factor.

PANENDOSCOPY

According to the literature, head and neck synchronous and metachronous second primary cancers have been reported to occur with a frequency varying from 3% to 21%. This risk has been hypothesized due to the field cancerization change thought to occur within the mucosa of the entire aerodigestive tract after exposure to exogenous carcinogens, such as tobacco and alcohol.[7] In the past, many clinicians advocated panendoscopy, involving laryngoscopy, bronchoscopy, and esophogoscopy, in all patients diagnosed with a head and neck malignancy. Arguments against this rationale include increased iatrogenic risk (ie, esophageal perforation), increased cost, and low yield in diagnosis. This

controversy is further complicated by improvements in diagnostic imaging (ie, positron emission tomography [PET], MRI, CT, and ultrasound) and office-based flexible endoscopy and by the increased incidence of newly diagnosed patients who have never abused tobacco or alcohol. A recent study comparing diagnostic panendoscopy in patients with a past history of tobacco abuse with nontobacco users identified a synchronous primary rate of 12% in the tobacco user group whereas no second primary carcinomas were found in the nontobacco user cohort. The investigators concluded that panendoscopy is unlikely to result in the identification of a synchronous carcinoma in patients who have never used tobacco.[8] Haerle and colleagues[9] evaluated the accuracy of PET/CT scan versus panendoscopy for detection of second primary tumors in 311 patients. The prevalence of second primary tumors was 6.1% with PET/CT scan compared with 4.5% with panendoscopy. An additional 5 cancers were detected with PET/CT scan that were missed within the field of the panendoscopy. Recent evidence suggests that symptom-directed panendoscopy performed after PET/CT imaging provides better identification of synchronous and unknown primary tumors. Routine panendoscopy should still be considered for patients with significant risk factors, such as tobacco abuse, and in situations requiring better tumor visualization to aid in assessing stage and in planning surgical resection.[10,11]

CANCER OF THE ORAL CAVITY AND OROPHARYNX—SURGERY AND RADIATION

Early-stage cancers of the oral cavity and oropharynx are generally treated with surgery or radiotherapy. Advanced-stage tumors (stage III/IV disease) require multimodality treatment. Most guidelines recommend that advanced resectable oral SCC be treated with surgery followed by radiotherapy or concurrent chemoradiotherapy (CCRT) depending on pathologic features identified postresection. Surgery as the first-line modality for tumors within the oral cavity has been considered for various reasons. The oral cavity is easily accessible surgically compared with other regions within the head and neck. Surgical removal of the tumor allows for pathologic assessment of tumor histology and margins. Pathologic staging of the tumor accurately determines the adequacy of resection and the need for adjuvant therapy if the tumor is "upstaged." Improvements in reconstructive surgery (computer-assisted/simulated design and microvascular surgery) have allowed for better functional outcomes than are customary after radiation therapy for bulky disease. This has helped shift away from the concept of chemoradiotherapy as an organ preservation technique.[12]

Advocates for using radiotherapy as a primary modality list technological improvements in technique for improved outcomes with less patient morbidity. Intensity-modulated radiation therapy (IMRT) can deliver high doses of radiation with precision while minimizing damage to surrounding tissues. IMRT can conform to the irregular shape of a tumor, delivering higher doses directly to the tumor cells and potentially destroying more radio-resistent tumor cells. The technique requires more precise planning due to the sharp dose falloff gradient between the gross tumor and the surrounding normal tissue. Numerous data suggest that IMRT provides locoregional control (90%) and is well tolerated by patients. Most studies only compare conventional radiotherapy with IMRT without having surgery as a separate study arm.[13]

The most recent National Comprehensive Cancer Network guidelines recommend that surgery or definitive radiotherapy can be used to treat early-stage T1/T2, N0/N1 oropharyngeal disease. More advanced-stage tumors require a combination of CCRT or surgery followed by adjuvant radiotherapy or CCRT.[2] Most clinicians still consider radiotherapy or CCRT as first-line therapy in oropharyngeal carcinoma due to the equivalent response rates compared with surgery. Arguments against using surgery as primary treatment include the high probability that cervical metastases are present (15%–75%) requiring adjuvant radiotherapy. Quality of life is an important factor in considering treatment options. Speech and swallowing function are diminished by all of the treatment modalities selected. *Organ preservation* is a term used liberally but a more important concept is that of *functional organ preservation*. The value of an anatomically preserved structure if it no longer functions correctly and destroys a patient's quality of life must be questioned. Surgical approaches to the oropharynx often involve highly invasive approaches (ie, mandibulotomy and pull-through techniques) that many consider too morbid, affecting speech and swallowing musculature. Improvements in oncologically safe access surgery, such as transoral robotic surgery and free flap oropharyngeal reconstruction, are making some clinicians reconsider surgery as a first-line therapy. Removal of gross tumor can allow for more narrowly focused adjuvant radiotherapy, minimizing side effects, such as mucositis, esophageal stricture, xerostomia, or swallowing dysfunction.[14–17] Kim and colleagues[18] compared treatment outcomes and quality of life in 133 patients with oropharyngeal cancer treated either with surgery or radiation-based therapy. The investigators concluded that disease-free and overall survival rates were equivalent at 3 years. Most quality-of-life parameters were equivalent; however, patients reported better outcomes in the categories of dry mouth, pain medication requirements, and weight gain in the surgery-based therapy cohort.

ADJUVANT CHEMORADIOTHERAPY AND INDUCTION CHEMOTHERAPY

Two large, clinical, randomized, prospective multicenter trials conducted in the United States (Radiation Therapy Oncology Group [RTOG] 95-01) and in Europe (European Organisation for Research and Treatment of Cancer [EORTC] 22931) identified high-risk features (extracapsular spread and close/positive margins), selecting patients who would benefit from the addition of chemotherapy to the adjuvant radiotherapy. The RTOG trial found statistical improvement in locoregional control and disease-free survival. The European study showed significant improvement in survival; however, more patients received a higher dose of radiotherapy in that trial.[19–21] Other adverse pathologic features, such as multiple nodes, perineural invasion, perivascular invasion, and advanced-stage tumors, might benefit from adjuvant CCRT.[21] Although CCRT improves locoregional control and disease-free survival, increased complications, both short-term (ie, mucositis) and long-term (ie, swallowing difficulties), are increased.[22–24]

Induction chemotherapy remains controversial in the management of oral cavity/oropharyngeal cancer. Some investigators think it downsizes the tumor before surgery or CCRT. Other investigators suggest that it helps decrease the rate of distant metastasis. Of concern is that often the induction chemotherapy outcome data are compared with historical data or trials in which a surgical arm has not been included. A randomized trial by Licitra and colleagues[24] evaluated 195 patients with resectable oral cavity tumors that were randomized to surgery or induction chemotherapy followed by surgery. Five-year survival rates were similar in both cohorts and no statistical difference was seen in locoregional control or distant metastasis. A randomized phase III multicenter study examined 5-year and 10-year follow-up data on 237 patients with stage III or stage IV disease. Significant differences were found in patients considered nonoperable with 21% and 16% survival rates compared with 8% and 6%.[25] The benefits of induction chemotherapy may yet be demonstrated in unresectable advanced cancers, especially using triple-drug therapies (cisplatin/5-fluorouracil/docetaxel).[26]

SURGICAL MARGINS

The goal of surgical resection of the primary site is to remove all malignant disease. Although controversy exists as to what is considered a negative surgical margin and its true implications on prognosis, a majority of the current literature suggests the most significant histopathologic predictor of recurrence at the primary site is the ability to achieve a negative surgical margin.[27,28] Most clinicians consider a surgical margin negative when the normal tissue beyond the margin is greater than 5 mm. The debate over what is considered a clear margin still remains. Kurita and colleagues[27] reported on a series of 148 oral SCC patients and concluded that a margin of less than 5 mm adversely affected local control. Binahmed and colleagues[29] reviewed a tumor registry of 425 oral cavity carcinomas. The investigators defined a negative margin as less than 2 mm and found that involved and close margins affected local recurrence only. In their series and contrary to other published series, positive margins were the only factor that increased the risk of regional and distant failure. A surgeon's ability to achieve clear margins is often difficult, with reported rates between 40% and 70%. Inherent problems with margin assessment include histologic and quantitative errors. Evidence suggests that severe dysplasia and carcinoma in situ have significant negative impact on local control and recurrence; however, many pathologists consider only invasive carcinoma a positive result. After resection and specimen fixation, margin shrinkage is highly variable and reported to range from 15% to 50%. To compensate for this, most surgeons resect with a clinical margin of 1 cm to 1.5 cm. Data suggesting that a larger clinical margin results in fewer positive pathologic margins are inconclusive.[28,30] Hanasono and colleagues[31] demonstrated a significant decrease in positive pathologic margins in patients treated for advanced-stage oral cavity squamous carcinoma reconstructed with microvascular free flaps compared with those reconstructed before the introduction of free flaps. Genetic changes within the histologic margins can also help explain failure at so-called negative margins. Brennan and colleagues[32] evaluated p53 mutations in DNA of 72 surgical margins reported as negative for microscopic carcinoma on final pathology. Neoplastic p53 mutations were found in at least one surgical margin in 52% of patients and this correlated positively with recurrence.

Vital dyes have also become an important cost-effective tool to assist surgeons with intraoperative margin assessment. Toluidene blue is reported to have a sensitivity ranging from 84% to 100%. Reports of high false-positive rates (30%–50%) are thought to occur due to retention of the stain in the tissues after biopsy, trauma, and inflammation.[33] Lugol iodine solution binds tissue glycogen. Tissue glycogen is inversely proportional to the amount of keratinization in the tissue. Dysplastic and malignant cells have increased glycolysis and, therefore, do not pick up the Lugol stain. Lugol stain is reported to have a sensitivity and specificity greater than 80% for delineation of dysplastic margins.[34]

MANAGEMENT OF THE N0 NECK

Neck metastasis is the single most important prognostic indicator in head and neck carcinoma. The incidence of occult cervical metastasis from carcinoma of the oral cavity is reported to vary from 10% to 40%.[35,36] This rate is reportedly even greater involving cancers of the oropharynx. Thin mucosal tissue and a rich submucosal lymphatic system are thought to be reasons for the risk of early neck metastases. Although tumor thickness is thought to be the single greatest risk factor for cervical lymph node spread, no universal tumor depth has been established as an absolute indication for neck dissection. A general consensus among clinicians is that if the occult risk of neck disease is greater than 20%, then elective neck dissection (END) should be performed. Various studies report this risk when a depth of invasion is greater than 3 mm (range 2–10 mm). This risk-benefit of elective neck treatment is difficult to analyze because clinicians and patients are torn between overtreatment, risking increased morbidity, and the benefit of removal of regional disease. Clinical examination combined with various imaging modalities have reported sensitivities and specificities ranging from 40% to 100%. In a study of 106 patients, Stuckensen and colleagues[37] found a sensitivity of 70%, 84%, and 66% and a specificity of 82%, 68%, and 74% for PET, ultrasound, and CT scan, respectively. The accuracy of preoperative PET/CT fusion imaging in the N0 neck is also debated. Problems include poor resolution, lack of noncontrast CT, and inability to detect metastasis smaller than 4 mm.[35,38]

Controversy regarding END results from lack of randomized prospective trials. To date there are only 4 randomized trials comparing END with observation of the N0 neck in oral cancers. Of those studies, 3 used surgery for treatment of the primary tumor. The study by Vandenbrouck and colleagues[39] used radiation to treat the primary cancer within the oral cavity. All 4 studies demonstrated a benefit with END on nodal metastasis and disease-specific survival. Only the study by Kligerman and colleagues[40] reached a statistically significant difference in disease-specific survival (14% in the observation group vs 42% END group). Despite this lack of prospective randomized data, many retrospective studies report that a watch-and-wait approach results in increased risk of more advanced neck disease (N2–N3) and decreased overall survival if END is not performed. Ebrahimi and colleagues[41] retrospectively evaluated 153 patients with thick T1 and T2 cancers. Patients who underwent END had a 22% regional failure compared with a 92% regional nodal failure rate in the observational group.[35,36,41,42]

To help overcome the problem of unnecessary lymph node dissection in the N0 neck, the technique of sentinel lymph node biopsy (SLNB) is being investigated. SLNB involves the injection of technetium Tc 99m sulfur colloid in several locations around the tumor. Using a probe to detect the radioactive tracer, the first echelon lymph nodes are evaluated. If they are positive, then a formal lymph node dissection is performed. The use of SLNB in the management of cutaneous melanoma and breast cancer is well established but its use for oral cavity squamous cell carcinoma (OSCC) is more controversial. Arguments against SLNB for OSCC include the highly variable lymphatic drainage patterns of the head and neck, resulting in multiple sentinel nodes needed for evaluation, and the difficulty in locating the actual sentinel nodes, especially in an irradiated field. In comparison, the morbidity associated with the standard supraomohyoid neck dissection is low and the node harvest is easily and accurately evaluated histopathologically. SLNB may have high false-negative rates due to operator inexperience and histologic sectioning/evaluation of the specimen. Advocates for the use of SLNB for head and neck cancers give the following reasons: decreased morbidity and avoidance of an unnecessary neck dissection, identification of positive nodes outside the normal lymphatic pattern, and as an alternative for patients who do not want an END but desire a more thorough evaluation than observational treatment. A large prospective multicenter trial in the United States using SLNB for evaluation of T1/T2 N0 oral SCC found a negative predictive value of 96%. It also reported that the false-negative rate for experienced surgeons was 0%.[43] Results from a European multicenter prospective trial showed an overall sensitivity of 93%. In that trial, 34% of patients were clinically upstaged. Sentinel node identification from the floor of mouth subsite was more difficult to ascertain and resulted in a site-specific sensitivity of 80%.[44]

TRANSORAL ROBOTIC SURGERY

New advances in technology facilitate minimal access surgery to areas within the head and neck that were not previously accessible without large transcervical or face-splitting incisions. Transoral robotic surgery allows access to tumors within the posterior oral cavity and oropharynx via multiple robotic arms and a high-definition/magnification camera. The operator sits at a separate console and via remote control can operate the various instruments. Electrocautery, laser, and standard dissection instruments can be used with the robot. Advantages include surgical access via minimal approaches that provide for tumor removal, resulting in definitive pathologic assessment while minimizing transection and resection of critical swallowing musculature. Recent trials with this new technique also suggest the need for lower postoperative radiation dosages, thus decreasing patient morbidity.[45,46] Successful free flap reconstruction is also performed with robotic assistance.[47,48] Weinstein and colleagues[49] reported on a case series of 47 patients who underwent transoral robotic surgery surgical resection for advanced oropharyngeal cancers. Two-year disease-specific survival was 90%. Only 1 patient required percutaneous endoscopic gastrostomy tube placement; 38% of patients avoided adjuvant chemotherapy and 11% of patients avoided chemoradiotherapy. Although this technology shows promise, long-term follow-up outcome data are needed. Other concerns include costs in regard to equipment and training.

TRANSORAL CARBON DIOXIDE LASER SURGERY

The carbon dioxide (CO_2) laser has been the standard laser used for oncologic surgery with an established safety record.[50–52] The earliest data demonstrated its efficacy and safety with endolaryngeal surgery using a laser coupled to an operating microscope.

Advantages of the laser include the following. (1) Lack of physical contact with the tissue permits a no-touch technique. The target tissue does not quaver and retract the way it does with electrocautery, decreasing the amount of heat-induced shrinkage of the surgical margin. This can allow for accurate analysis by a pathologist because the zone of thermal necrosis adjacent to the laser beam is usually less than 0.3 mm and is further reduced in a rapid superpulsed mode.[53] (2) Sealing of small blood vessels of less than 500 μm results in a relatively dry field, which can amount to shorter surgery and anesthesia times.[54] (3) There is reduced postoperative edema. Henstrom and colleagues[55] reported on a series of 20 patients with tongue base resection in which 10 patients avoided tracheostomy and the other 10 were decannulated an average of 16 days after surgery. (4) The dual capability to ablate and incise allows the laser to be used simultaneously to resect and to ablate well beyond a known dysplastic margin. This permits a wide mucosal margin to be established while preserving the substructure and allowing rapid re-epithelialization. This is useful for ablation of dysplastic margins while minimizing extensive mucosal resection.[56] A prospective study by Jerjes and colleagues[57] using transoral CO_2 laser resection of T1/T2 oral SCC in 90 patients demonstrated rates of locoregional control comparable to those with conventional surgical techniques.

Disadvantages of the laser include cost, bulky machinery with a delicate articulated arm that tends to get in the way, and the need for trained technical personnel. Protective eyewear, wet sponges/drapes, and laser-safe endotracheal tubes are required to protect against fire and burns to patient and staff. Although it is not difficult to gain proficiency, the lack of tactile feedback requires a period of surgical adjustment and familiarity. In regards to specific cancer site management, resection of floor of mouth OSCC can be performed safely in the region of the submandibular ducts, particularly if a pulsed mode is used, because the high-flow ductal system rarely becomes obstructed. The laser should be avoided in areas requiring alveolar osteotomies because it tends to melt the mineral content of the bone and delay healing.[52]

CANCER OF THE GINGIVA

Gingival cancers account for less than 10% of oral cavity cancers. They are seen more frequently in the elderly, female population and often without a history of tobacco or alcohol abuse.[58] Controversy exists about the relevance of bony invasion of these tumors and their management with respect to occult neck disease. According to the current staging guidelines by the American Joint Committee on Cancer superficial erosion of the bone or tooth socket by a gingival primary does not upstage a tumor to a T4 size.[59] A problem with this classification can be attributed to the minimal thickness of the attached gingiva (2–3 mm thickness), often resulting in early bone invasion. Bone invasion is associated with an increase in nodal metastasis and worse overall survival.[58,60] In a recent review of 72 patients with gingival cancers, 42% of patients with cervical metastatic disease had bony invasion compared with 17% of the N0 patients having bony involvement. The investigators also reported an occult nodal metastasis rate of 36% for T1 lesions and 55% for advanced-stage (T3/T4) tumors of the mandibular gingiva, respectively.[58] Debate exists as to the best imaging modality for evaluation of bone invasion. Recent literature suggests that MRI has the highest sensitivity and negative predictive value; however, the addition of PET/CT may further improve these outcomes.[61] Confusion exists as to the type of resection required after dental extraction. The theory of seeding the extraction socket with tumor, thereby allowing for deep bony involvement, has many investigators advocating for segmental mandibulectomy. Other reasons for selection of segmental mandibulectomy versus marginal resection are to achieve better access, allowing for a negative margin and improved survival outcomes.[58,62,63]

There are few data to guide the treatment of carcinomas of the maxillary gingiva, alveolus, and hard palate. Recent evidence suggests that this rare subsite is more aggressive than previously suspected and that regional failure in the previously undissected neck occurs far too often.[58,64,65] Simental and colleagues[66] reviewed 26 patients and found an incidence of 27% of occult nodal metastasis. Montes and colleagues[64] conducted a large retrospective multicenter review of 146 patients with maxillary SCC. The investigators found a regional metastatic rate of 31% with 7.5% of patients dying with distant disease. Within the clinically N0 necks, 14% developed nodal disease. There was a 28% regional metatstatic rate for maxillary tumors assessed at 4 cm or less in size (T1/T2). Regional salvage rates were approximately 50%. Based on their results, the investigators concluded that selective neck dissection (levels I–III) should be strongly considered for maxillary squamous carcinoma clinically staged T2 and greater.

CANCER OF THE BUCCAL MUCOSA

The incidence of buccal SCC in North America is approximately 10%. Worldwide, buccal cancers compose a large majority of the oral cancers (30%) largely due to the high prevalence of betel nut use. Locoregional failure rates are high, ranging from 30% to 80%.[67–69] Reasons suggested for these high failure rates include the intrinsic aggressive tumor behavior with early local lympho-vascular invasion into the surrounding buccal fat pad, lack of a good anatomic barrier, and the difficulty in achieving clear surgical margins without resecting the full thickness of the cheek. Lin and colleagues[67] reported on a series of 182 patients with buccal SCC and concluded that postoperative radiotherapy should be considered in early-stage (T1/T2 N0) disease because of high recurrence rates (40%) with surgery alone.

MAXILLARY SINUS SQUAMOUS CARCINOMA

Maxillary sinus SCC accounts for 3% of all head and neck cancers and 80% of all paranasal sinus cancers. These rare tumors are often asymptomatic until they present as advanced-stage cancers. Important predictors of locoregional control and survival include tumor size and the ability to achieve negative surgical margins. Although rates of lymph node metastasis are reported low (9%–14%), elective treatment of the neck with either surgery or radiation has been shown to improve regional control and survival.[70–72] Paulino and colleagues[73] recommended elective treatment of the neck based on an occult nodal rate of 28.9% in a series of 42 patients with maxillary sinus SCC.

The Ohngren line is an imaginary line extending from the medial canthus of the eye to the angle of the mandible passing through the maxillary sinus. It is a useful guide to help assist clinicians in treatment planning. Tumors below this line involve the maxillary infrastructure and those above this line involve the suprastructure. Often tumors below this line require a low or partial maxillectomy and have a better prognosis. Reconstruction of the low maxillectomy defect is often easier and amenable to either prosthetic obturator or free flap reconstruction without major cosmetic deformity or major speech and swallowing difficulties. Tumors above this line often present late with frequent invasion through the posterior sinus wall and involvement in the pterygoid space. Involvement of the orbital rim requires orbital floor resection and reconstruction. Tumors that have invaded the pterygoid space have a poor prognosis and are difficult to resect with any truly negative margin.[71]

SUMMARY

Squamous carcinomas of the oral cavity, oropharynx, and the maxillary sinus often present a difficult challenge in diagnosis and treatment. Many of these cancers present in advanced stages requiring multimodality treatment with surgery and chemoradiotherapy. Although tobacco and alcohol abuse remain the most common risk factors, new trends are emerging, including younger nonsmoker patient populations with links to HPV (oropharyngeal carcinoma). SCC of the gingiva, buccal mucosa, and maxillary sinus are more aggressive than previously suspected with higher rates of locoregional recurrence. Improvements in technology are allowing for better access surgery with robotic approaches, decreased treatment morbidity with IMRT, laser therapy, and computer-assisted microvascular reconstruction. Management of the N0 neck remains controversial with the future of sentinel lymph node biopsy showing promise.

REFERENCES

1. Woolgar JA, Rogers S, West CR, et al. Survival patterns oral SCCa. Oral Oncol 1999;35:257–65.
2. National Comprehensive Cancer Network Clinical Practice Guidelines in Oncology. Head and neck cancers V.1.2011. Available at: http://www.nccn.org. Accessed January 14, 2012.
3. Myers JN, Elkins T, Roberts D, et al. Squamous cell carcinoma of the tongue in young adults: increasing incidence and factors predicting treatment outcomes. Otolaryngol Head Neck Surg 2000;122:44–51.
4. Marur S, D'Souza G, Westra WH, et al. HPV-associated head and neck cancer: a virus-related cancer epidemic. Lancet Oncol 2010;11:781–9.
5. Herrero R, Castellsague X, Pawlita M, et al. Human papillomavirus and oral cancer; the International Agency for Research on Cancer multicenter study. J Natl Cancer Inst 2003;95:1772–83.
6. Lopes V, Murray P, Williams H, et al. Squamous cell carcinoma of the oral cavity rarely harbours oncogenic human papillomavirus. Oral Oncol 2011;47:698–701.
7. Slaughter DP, Southwick HW, Smejkal W. Field cancerization in oral stratified squamous epithelium clinical implications of multicentric origin. Cancer 1953;6:963–8.
8. Rodriguez-Bruno K, Ali MJ, Wang SJ. Role of panendoscopy to identify synchronous second primary malignancies in patients with oral cavity and oropharyngeal squamous cell carcinoma. Head Neck 2011;33(7):949–53.
9. Haerle SK, Strobel K, Hany TF, et al. FDG-PET/CT versus panendoscopy for the detection of synchronous second primary tumors in patients with head and neck squamous cell carcinoma. Head Neck 2010;32(3):319–25.
10. Rennemo E, Zatterstrom U, Boysen M. Synchronous second primary tumors in 2016 head and neck cancer patients: role of symptom-directed panendoscopy. Laryngoscope 2011;121:304–9.
11. Rudmik L, Lau HY, Matthews TW, et al. Clinical utility of PET/CT in the evaluation of head and neck squamous

cell carcinoma with an unkown primary: a prospective clinical trial. Head Neck 2011;33(7):935–40.

12. Vaughan ED. Functional outcomes of free tissue transfer in head and neck cancer reconstruction. Oral Oncol 2009;45:421–30.

13. Lee N, Puri DR, Blanco AI, et al. Intensity modulated radiation therapy in head and neck cancers: an update. Head Neck 2007;29:387–400.

14. Mowry SE, Ho A, Lotempio MM, et al. Quality of life in advanced oropharyngeal carcinoma after chemo-radiation versus surgery and radiation. Laryngoscope 2006;116(9):1589–93.

15. Tschudi D, Stoeckli S, Schmid S. Quality of life after different treatmentmodalities for carcinoma of the oropharynx. Laryngoscope 2003;113(11):1949–54.

16. Allal AS, Nicoucar K, Mach N, et al. Quality of life in patients with oropharynx carcinomas: assessment after accelerated radiotherapy with or without chemotherapy versus radical surgery and postoperative radiotherapy. Head Neck 2003;25(10):833–9.

17. Borggreven PA, Aaronson NK, Verdonck-de Leeuw IM, et al. Quality of life after surgical treatment for oral and oropharyngeal cancer: a prospective longitudinal assessmentof patients reconstructed by a microvascular flap. Oral Oncol 2007;43(10): 1034–42.

18. Kim TW, Youm HY, Byun H, et al. Treatment outcomes and quality of life in oropharyngeal cancer after surgery-based versus radiation-based treatment. Clin Exp Otorhinolaryngol 2010;3(3):153–60.

19. Bernier J, Domenge C, Ozsahin M, et al. Post-operative irradiation with or without concomitant chemotherapy for locally advanced head and neck cancer. N Engl J Med 2004;350:1945–52.

20. Cooper JS, Pajak TF, Forastiere AA, et al. Post-operative concurrent radiotherapy and chemotherapy for high-risk squamous cell carcinoma of the head and neck. N Engl J Med 2004;350:1937–44.

21. Bernier J, Cooper JS, Pajak TF, et al. Defining risk levels in locally advanced head and neck cancers: a comparative analysis of concurrent postoperative radiation plus chemotherapy trials of the EORTC(#22931) and RTOG(#9501). Head Neck 2005;27:843–50.

22. Machtay M, Moughan J, Trotti A, et al. Factors associated with severe late toxicity after concurrent chemoradiation for locally advanced head and neck cancer: an RTOG analysis. J Clin Oncol 2008;26:3582–9.

23. Langendijk JA, Doornaert P, Verdonck-de Leeuw IM, et al. Impact of late treatment related toxicity on quality of life among patients with head and neck cancer treated with radiotherapy. J Clin Oncol 2008;26:3770–6.

24. Licitra L, Guzzo M, Mariani L, et al. Primary chemotherapy in resectable oral cavity squamous cell cancer: a randomized controlled trial. J Clin Oncol 2003;21(2):327–33.

25. Zorat PL, Paccagnella A, Cavaniglia G, et al. Randomized phase III trial of neoadjuvant chemotherapy in head and neck cancer: 10-year follow-up. J Natl Cancer Inst 2004;96:1714–7.

26. Paccagnella A, Mastromauro C, D'amanzo P, et al. Induction chemotherapy before chemoradiotherapy in locally advanced head and neck cancer: the future? Oncologist 2010;15(Suppl 3):8–12.

27. Kurita H, Nakanishi Y, Nishizawa R, et al. Impact of different surgical margin conditions on local recurrence of oral squamous cell carcinoma. Oral Oncol 2010;46:814–7.

28. Upile T, Fisher C, Jerjes W, et al. The uncertainty of the surgical margin in the treatment of head and neck cancer. Oral Oncol 2007;43:321–6.

29. Binahmed A, Nason RW, Abdoh AA. The clinical significance of the positive surgical margin in oral cancer. Oral Oncol 2007;43:780–4.

30. Cheng A, Cox D, Schmidt BL. Oral squamous cell carcinoma margin discrepancy after resection and pathologic processing. J Oral Maxillofac Surg 2008;66:523–9.

31. Hanasono MM, Friel MT, Klem C, et al. Impact of reconstructive microsurgery in patients with advanced oral cavity cancers. Head Neck 2009;31: 1289–96.

32. Brennan JA, Mao L, Hruban RH, et al. Molecular assessment of histopathologic staging in squamous cell carcinoma of the head and neck. N Engl J Med 1995;332:429–35.

33. Onofre MA, Sposto MR, Navarro CM. Reliability of toluidine blue application in the detection of oral epithelial dysplasia and in situ and invasive squamous cell carcinoma. Oral Surg Oral Med Oral Pathol Oral Radiol Endod 2001;91:535–40.

34. Petruzzi M, Lucchese A, Baldoni E, et al. Use of lugol's iodine in oral cancer diagnosis;an overview. Oral Oncol 2010;46:811–3.

35. Genden EM, Ferlito A, Silver CE, et al. Contemporary management of cancer of the oral cavity. Eur Arch Otorhinolaryngol 2010;267:1001–17.

36. Kowalski LP, Sanabria A. Elective neck dissection in oral carcinoma: a critical review of the evidence. Acta Otorhinolaryngol Ital 2007;27:113–7.

37. Stuckensen T, Kovacs AF, Adams S, et al. Staging of the neck in patients with oral cavity squamous cell carcinomas: a prospective comparison of PET, ultrasound, CT and MRI. J Craniomaxillofac Surg 2000; 28:319–24.

38. Schoder H, Carlson DL, Kraus DH, et al. 18F-FDG PET/CT for detecting nodal metastases in patients with oral cancer staged N0 by clinical examination and CT/MRI. J Nucl Med 2006;47: 755–62.

39. Vandenbrouck C, Sancho-Garnier H, Chassange D, et al. Elective versus therapeutic radical neck dissection in epidermoid carcinoma of the oral

cavity: results of a randomized clinical trial. Cancer 1980;46:386–90.

40. Kligerman J, Lima RA, Soares JR, et al. Supraomohyoid neck dissection in the treatment of T1/T2 squamous cell carcinoma of the oral cavity. Am J Surg 1994;168:391–4.

41. Ebrahimi A, Ashford BG, Clark JR. Improved survival with elective neck dissection in thick early-stage oral squamous cell carcinoma. Head Neck 2011. DOI:10.1002/hed.21809. [Epub ahead of print].

42. Fasunia AJ, Greene BH, Timmesfeld N, et al. A meta-analysis of the randomized controlled trials on elective neck dissection versus therapeutic neck dissection in oral cavity cancers with clinically node-negative neck. Oral Oncol 2011;47:320–4.

43. Civantos FJ, Zitsch RP, Schuller DE, et al. Sentinel lymph node biopsy accurately stages the regional lymph nodes for T1-T2 oral squamous cell carcinomas: results of a prospective multi-institutional trial. J Clin Oncol 2010;28(8):1395–400.

44. Ross GL, Soutar DS, Gordon MacDonald D, et al. Sentinel node biopsy in head and neck cancer: preliminary results of a multicenter trial. Ann Surg Oncol 2004;11(7):690–6.

45. Hurtuk A, Agrawal A, Old M, et al. Outcomes of transoral robotic surgery: a preliminary clinical experience. Otolaryngol Head Neck Surg 2011;145(2):248–53.

46. White HN, Moore EJ, Rosenthal EL, et al. Transoral robotic-assisted surgery for head and neck squamous cell carcinoma: one and 2 year survival analysis. Arch Otolaryngol Head Neck Surg 2010; 136(12):1248–52.

47. Genden EM, Park R, Smith C, et al. The role of reconstruction for transoral robotic pharyngectomy and concomitant neck dissection. Arch Otolaryngol Head Neck Surg 2011;137(2):151–6.

48. Selber JC. Transoral robotic reconstruction of oropharyngeal defects: a case series. Plast Reconstr Surg 2010;126(6):1978–87.

49. Weinstein GS, O'Malley BW Jr, Cohen MP, et al. Transoral robotic surgery for advanced oropharyngeal carcinoma. Arch Otolaryngol Head Neck Surg 2010;136(11):1079–85.

50. Strong MS, Jako J. Laser surgery in the larynx. Early clinical experience with continuous CO_2 laser. Ann Otol Rhinol Laryngol 1972;81:791–8.

51. Strong MS, Vaughan CW, Healy GB, et al. Transoral management of localized carcinoma of the oral cavity using the CO_2 laser. Laryngoscope 1979;89:897–905.

52. Clayman L. Transoral resection of oral cancer. In: Clayman L, Kuo P, editors. Lasers in maxillofacial surgery and dentistry. New York: Thieme; 1997. p. 85–110.

53. Seone J, Caballero TG, Urizar JM, et al. Pseudodysplastic epithelial artefacts associated with oral mucosa CO_2 laser excision: an assessment of margin status. Int J Oral Maxillofac Surg 2010;39:783–7.

54. Fisher SE, Frame JW. The effects of the carbon dioxide surgical laser on oral tissues. Br J Oral Maxillofac Surg 1984;22(6):414–25.

55. Henstrom DK, Moore EJ, Olsen KD, et al. Transoral resection for squamous cell carcinoma of the base of the tongue. Arch Otolaryngol Head Neck Surg 2009;135(12):1231–8.

56. Van der Hem PS, Nauta JM, van der Wal JE, et al. The results of CO2 laser surgery in patients with oral leukoplakia: a 25 year follow up. Oral Oncol 2005;41(1):31–7.

57. Jerjes W, Upile T, Hamdoon Z, et al. Prospective evaluation of outcome after transoral CO(2) laser resection of T1/T2 oral squamous cell carcinoma. Oral Surg Oral Med Oral Pathol Oral Radiol Endod 2011;112(2):180–7.

58. Lubek J, El-Hakim M, Salama AR, et al. Gingival carcinoma: retrospective analysis of 72 patients and indications for elective neck dissection. Br J Oral Maxillofac Surg 2011;49:182–5.

59. Edge SB, Byrd DR, Compton CC, et al, editors. AJCC cancer staging manual. 7th edition. New York: Springer; 2010. p. 21–101.

60. Soo KC, Spiro RH, King W, et al. Squamous carcinoma of the gums. Am J Surg 1988;156:281–5.

61. El-Hafez YG, Chen CC, Ng SH, et al. Comparison of PET/CT and MRI for the detection of bone marrow invasion in patients with squamous cell carcinoma of the oral cavity. Oral Oncol 2011;47:288–95.

62. Shingaki S, Nomura T, Takada M, et al. Squamous cell carcinoma of the mandibular alveolus: analysis of prognostic factors. Oncology 2002;62:17–24.

63. Chen YL, Shih-Wei K, Fang KH, et al. Prognostic impact of marginal mandibulectomy in the presence of superficial bone invasion and the nononcologic outcome. Head Neck 2011;33:708–13.

64. Montes DM, Carlson ER, Fernandes R, et al. Oral maxillary squamous carcinoma: an indication for neck dissection in the clinically negative neck. Head Neck 2011;33:1581–5.

65. Mourouzis C, Pratt C, Brennan PA. Squamous cell carcinoma of the maxillary gingiva, alveolus and hard palate: is there a need for elective neck dissection? Br J Oral Maxillofac Surg 2010;48:345–8.

66. Simental AA Jr, Johnson JT, Myers EN. Cervical metastases from squamous cell carcinoma of the maxillary alveolus and hard palate. Laryngoscope 2006;116:1682–4.

67. Lin CS, Jen YM, Cheng MF, et al. Squamous cell carcinoma of the buccal mucosa: an aggressive cancer requiring multimodality treatment. Head Neck 2006;28:150–7.

68. Jan JC, Hsu WH, Liu SA, et al. Prognostic factors in patients with buccal squamous cell carcinoma: 10-year experience. J Oral Maxillofac Surg 2011;69:396–404.

69. Chiou WY, Lin HY, Hsu FC, et al. Buccal mucosa carcinoma: surgical margin less than 3 mm not 5 mm predicts locoregional control. Radiat Oncol 2010;5:79.

70. Le QT, Fu KK, Kaplan MJ, et al. Lymph node metastasis in maxillary sinus carcinoma. Int J Radiat Oncol Biol Phys 2000;46:541–9.

71. Le QT, Fu KK, Kaplan MJ, et al. Treatment of maxillary sinus carcinoma a comparison of the 1997 and 1977 American Joint Committee on Cancer staging system. Cancer 1999;86:1700–11.

72. Guo GF, Yang AK, Xie RH, et al. Prognostic analysis of 151 patients with maxillary sinus malignant neoplasms. Ai Zheng 2004;23:1546–50 [in Chinese].

73. Paulino AC, Fisher SG, Marks JE. Is prophylacyic neck irradiation indicated in patients with squamous cell carcinoma of the maxillary sinus? Int J Radiat Oncol Biol Phys 1997;39:283–9.

Index

Note: Page numbers of article titles are in **boldface** type.

A

Abscess, parapharyngeal space, 202–203
   peritonsillar and parapharyngeal, 201–202
Acute sinusitis. *See* Sinusitis.
Adjuvant chemoradiotherapy, for squamous cell
   carcinoma of oral cavity and oropharynx, 309–310
Agger nasi cells, anatomic variations in, 177
Allergic rhinitis, **205–217**
   diagnostic strategies, 208–210
      physical examination, 208
      skin testing, 208–210
         in vitro, 210
         intradermal, 209–210
   epidemiology, 205–206
   pathophysiology, 206–208
      Samter triad, 207–208
   treatment strategies, 210–215
      environmental exposure monitoring, 210
         indoor allergens, 210
         outdoor allergens, 210
      immunotherapy, 213–215
         injection, 214
         mechanisms, 214
         sublingual, 214–215
      pharmacotherapy, 210–213
         antihistamines, 210–212
         decongestants, 212
         intranasal corticosteroids, 212
         leukotriene receptor antagonists, 212–213
         mast cell stabilizers, topical anticholinergic,
            and mucolytics, 213
         monoclonal antibody therapy, 213
Alloplastic material, for closure of oroantral
   communication, 245
Ameloblastic fibroma, of the paranasal sinuses, 258
Ameloblastoma, of the paranasal sinuses, 257–258
Anatomy, for endoscopic surgery, 276–277
      nose and lateral nasal wall, 276–277
      paranasal sinuses, 277
   for imaging the paranasal sinuses, 176–177
      anatomic variants, 177
      outflow tracts, 176–177
   in epistaxis, 219
   of nasal obstruction, 229–231
      nasal turbinates, 229–230
      nasal valve, 230–231
   of tonsils and adenoids, 197–198
   relevant for examination of ear, nose, throat, and
      sinus, 167–170

surgical, of major salivary glands, 295–296, 300,
   301–302
   parotid gland, 295–296
   sublingual gland, 301–302
   submandibular gland, 300
surgical, of nasal cavity, **155–166**
   lateral wall, 157–159
   lower lateral nasal cartilages, 156
   nasal septum, 156–157
   upper lateral nasal cartilages, 155–156
surgical, of paranasal sinuses, **155–166**
   ethmoidal sinus, 159–161
   frontal sinus, 164–165
      blood supply, 165
   maxillary sinus, 161–162
      anatomic relationship with teeth, 162–163
      blood supply and innervation, 163–164
      clinical significance of septa, 163
      ostium of, 163
      superior alveolar nerves, 163
      vital structures, 162–164
Angiofibroma, of the paranasal sinuses, 256–257
Anticholinergics, topical, for allergic rhinitis, 213
Antihistamines, for allergic rhinitis, 210–212
Antrostomy, endoscopic middle meatal, 282

B

Benign cysts, of paranasal sinuses, **249–264**
   extrinsic, 250–253
      dentigerous cysts (follicular, primordial),
         250–252
      lateral periodontal cyst (radicular), 252
      neurogenic, 252–253
   fissural, 253–255
      globulomaxillary (lateral bony inclusion
         cyst), 253
      median palatal (palatine) cyst, 254–255
      nasopalatine duct cyst (incisive canal cyst),
         253–254
   intrinsic, 249–250
      cholesteatoma (keratoma,
         epidermoidoma), 250
      mucocele (mucus extravasation
         phenomenon), 250
      mucous retention cyst (salivary duct cyst),
         249
      serous cyst, 250
   odontogenic, 258

Oral Maxillofacial Surg Clin N Am 24 (2012) 317–324
doi:10.1016/S1042-3699(12)00061-1
1042-3699/12/$ – see front matter © 2012 Elsevier Inc. All rights reserved.

Printed and bound by CPI Group (UK) Ltd, Croydon, CR0 4YY

03/10/2024

01040357-0008